P. P. Rickham · R. T. Soper · S0-EKC-858

Synopsis of Pediatric Surgery

with contributions by
P. Dangel · M. Lehner · M. Perko · P. P. Rickham · R. T. Soper
U. G. Stauffer · M. Zachmann

283 Figures, 10 Tables

1975

Year Book Medical Publishers, Inc.

Georg Thieme Publishers

Year Book Medical Publishers, Inc. 1975

ISBN 0-8151-7325-3
Library of Congress Catalog Card Number 75-4094

This book is dedicated to our wives
Elizabeth,
Hélène,
Ellen
without whose help we could not have completed the work

Foreword

Pediatric Surgery is the youngest branch of General Surgery, having enjoyed rapid development only since World War II. Although at least half of all children admitted to hospital suffer from surgical conditions and although one-fourth of all operations are performed on children, there does not exist a textbook for students on this subject either in the German-speaking countries or in North America. Students are therefore forced to learn what they can about surgical conditions in childhood by reading general textbooks of Surgery or Pediatrics, which often deal with this subject inadequately, or to read the large specialist volumes which are far too advanced for their needs.

In trying to write a short, illustrated student's textbook on Pediatric Surgery simultaneously in English and German, we believe we may fill a void which has become apparent to us when giving lectures, tutorials and bedside teaching to undergraduates. Much of Pediatric Surgery is still in the developmental phase and views on the etiology, pathology, clinical history and treatment differ widely. In a book of this kind long discussions of the various theories seem out of place and we have tended to be dogmatic in order to be concise. For the sake of brevity we have also omitted all those important surgical and pediatric considerations which the student can learn by reading the appropriate textbooks on this subject. For the same reason we have also tended to omit some of the rare conditions one meets in pediatric surgical practice and have concentrated on the clinical aspects of the more common diseases. This is not a book for surgeons, and the technique of the various operations is only described in the barest outlines.

Although this book is mainly directed toward medical undergraduates, we hope that it may be of some use also to those in General Practice and even to the busy Pediatrician who finds it time-consuming to read through the large pediatric surgical textbooks and literature. Pediatric Nurses and certain paramedical personnel might also benefit from the book.

The fact that the co-authors were or are still working together with me has, we hope, ensured that although this is a book written by a number of authors, there is a certain uniformity of doctrine.

We gratefully acknowledge the help we have received in preparing this book from the Georg Thieme Verlag Stuttgart and especially from Dr. (h. c.) G. Hauff.

P. P. R.

The Authors

P. P. Rickham, M.D., M.S., F.R.C.S., D.C.H.

Surgeon in Chief, University Children's Hospital, Zürich. Professor of Pediatric Surgery, University of Zürich, Switzerland. Formerly Senior Surgeon, Alder Hey Children's Hospital, Liverpool, and Director of Surgical Studies, University of Liverpool, England.

R. T. Soper, M.D.

Chief of Pediatric Surgical Section and Professor of Surgery, The University of Iowa College of Medicine, Iowa City, Iowa, U.S.A.

U. G. Stauffer, M.D.

Associate Surgeon, University Children's Hospital, Zürich. Lecturer in Pediatric Surgery, University of Zürich, Switzerland.

Contributors

Peter Dangel, M.D.

Chief of Pediatric Anesthesia, University Children's Hospital, Zürich.

Margaret Lehner, M.D.

Chief Assistant in Pediatric Surgery, University Children's Hospital, Zürich.

Milivoj Perko, M.D.

Facio-Maxillary Surgeon, University Children's Hospital, Zürich. Associate Professor of Facio-Maxillary Surgery, University of Zürich.

Peter P. Rickham, M.D., M.S., F.R.C.S., D.C.H.

Surgeon in Chief, University Children's Hospital, Zürich, Professor of Pediatric Surgery, University of Zürich.

Robert T. Soper, M.D.

Chief of Pediatric Surgical Section and Professor of Surgery, The University of Iowa College of Medicine, Iowa City, Iowa.

Urs G. Stauffer, M.D.

Associate Surgeon, University Children's Hospital, Zürich. Lecturer in Pediatric Surgery, University of Zürich.

Milo Zachmann, M.D.

Pediatric Endocrinologist, University Children's Hospital, Zürich. Lecturer in Pediatrics, University of Zürich.

Contents

1 Pediatric Surgery and the Child in Hospital

P. P. RICKHAM

Why do we practice pediatric surgery and why should students learn pediatric surgery as a distinct surgical discipline? Is it a branch of general surgery or is it just the miniaturized surgery of adults? Pediatric surgery has rightly been termed "the whole of surgery applied to a special age group". For essentially the same reasons which justify separation of children with medical problems (Pediatrics) from their adult counterparts, we feel that children with surgical disease require special consideration because of the profound physical and psychological differences which are age-related. The best results in the surgery of childhood are clearly obtained by teams of doctors and nurses specialized in the management of children, preferably working in institutions designed for this purpose. Every medical student should be aware of the fundamental physical and psychological differences in the surgical management of children and adults.

Physical Differences

1. Cell division in the adult occurs largely to repair the wear and tear of the body and also of course for reproductive purposes. In contrast, cell division is greatly increased in children to allow for growth. This is especially noticeable during the first four weeks of life (neonatal period) and to a lesser extent during puberty.

2. This increased rate of cell division explains the tremendous healing power of the infant compared with that of adults, especially the very elderly. It also explains the child's great resistance to physical trauma and the rapidity with which normal body functions are reestablished following a traumatic insult. In general, the younger the child, the more rapid his growth and the greater his resistance to physical trauma. On the other hand, the more active the rate of cell division, the lower is the resistance to roentgen radiation and cytotoxic drugs; neonates are very prone to injury from these agents.

3. Surgery in neonates is further complicated by the fact that the organism after birth is in a transitional state between the parasitic existence in utero (where the infant is maternally dependent not only for his nutrition, oxygenation, etc., but where his body functions are also largely influenced by maternal hormones) and an independent existence after birth. During this transition period the infant's metabolism changes markedly as his own hormones take over the steering of body functions. In addition, some of the newborn infant's organs do not function quite as well as they do later in life; often maximal

efficiency is not achieved until several days, weeks and even months have passed.

4. Another important factor markedly affecting the surgery of childhood is the difference in the defenses against infections in children compared with that of older age groups. In the neonate the defense against infection only builds up slowly. At first he has little resistance apart from the passive immunity derived from the mother via the placenta. Active defenses against infection gradually develop, provoking in older children a violent reaction to infection often accompanied by more complications than we observe in adults. The lymphatic system is the main source of the body's anti-infection activities, and in children this system is extremely well developed.

5. Today adults admitted for surgery suffer mainly from four groups of conditions: Malignant tumors, functional diseases such as cholecystitis and peptic ulcers, degenerative processes and trauma. In children the most important conditions necessitating surgery are congenital malformations, which may be so severe that unless they are immediately corrected will kill the newborn within a few days. Other malformations may be relatively trivial in nature and can be corrected later on in life. Trauma is also frequently encountered in childhood, but the types of trauma and their management differ markedly from those of adult life. Malignant tumors are less common but paradoxically rank second to trauma as a cause of death in children in developed countries. Adult malignancies most commonly arise from epithelial tissue. In contrast, malignancies in children arise mainly from embryonic tissue and are extremely malignant. Fortunately some of these tumors are very sensitive to cytostatic drugs and the prognosis, which until recently was virtually hopeless, has now become quite favorable in certain cases. As previously stated, children frequently contract infections and often react to these infections much more violently than do adults. Surgical infections such as appendicitis, osteomyelitis, etc. are not only common in childhood but their management differs widely from the same disorders occurring in the older age groups.

Psychological Differences

1. Doctor/Patient Relationship

In the surgical treatment of adults there are usually only two people involved, the surgeon and his patient; it is vital to have satisfactory contact between these two. In the very young, personal communication between surgeon and patient is virtually impossible and a clinical history or even a description of his symptoms are often difficult to obtain. Therefore, the surgeon depends on other persons, usually the parents and particularly the mother. Even when the child gets older, the surgeon has to deal with him as well as his mother, and this fact complicates the doctor-patient relationship. Mothers are on the whole very observant and hence good witnesses, but they are naturally anxious and tend involuntarily to exaggerate their children's symptoms. The doctor has to take this into account and avoid asking leading questions. While in adults it is at times difficult to be frank with the patient, it is usually possible to be quite candid about the prognosis of a child during discussions with the parents. The doctor must avoid being too gloomy, even if the outlook is desperate. He needs the parents' cooperation and cannot afford their breaking down at this critical moment. Furthermore, children have such vast recuperative powers that one should hardly ever give up hope even under the most difficult circumstances.

2. The Child in Hospital

Children should be admitted to hospital only if it is absolutely inevitable. Hospitalized children run the risk of contracting infections from other patients. Toddlers and children under five years of age not only suffer the separation from their parents and accustomed surroundings, but it is also difficult to explain to them the reasons for undergoing such unpleasant experiences as injections, intravenous therapy, gastric suction and operations. Much can be achieved by helping parents to intelligently prepare their children before a hospital admission. Conversation with the parents and instructive booklets play important roles in directing this preparation. Frequent visits of the parents are also essential and the special difficulties which this entails in surgical wards must be overcome. There is a great advantage in having the mother living in the hospital with the child, although this is not always possible because of home commitments and distances between home and hospital. Great care is taken to shield the child from unpleasant or upsetting impressions from other patients in the ward. The child's stay in hospital should be as short as possible, the surgeon constantly asking himself whether the treatment could not be equally well given at home. If prolonged hospitalization is required, the child's time must be suitably occupied including instruction by hospital teachers of the older child. Many of the non-emergency operations have to be carried out at a certain specific time in the child's life. (See Chapter 2.) If there is no special urgency, it is always better to postpone the operation until the child is old enough to understand the parent's and doctor's explanation of the need for the various tests and manipulations and operations. Most important, all the hospital personnel who deal with children must not only try to be kind to them but to make contact with them, talk to them and if possible play with them and demonstrate a real personal interest. There is no greater reward in pediatric surgery than a child in the followup clinic who exhibits a willingness to return to hospital again after a lengthy and often uncomfortable period of hospitalization. There is no greater failure than the child with a successful operation but who bears severe psychological scars following his hospital admission.

2 Timetable for Pediatric Surgical Operations

U. G. STAUFFER

General Remarks

In non-urgent cases, the optimum time for pediatric surgical repair depends on a number of different considerations:

1) The risk of the disease or the malformation to the patient.
2) The risk of operation to the patient.
3) Surgical-technical aspects of the operation.
4) Possible spontaneous cure of the condition.
5) Psychological considerations.

The Risk of the Disease to the Patient

This decisively influences the choice of the age for operation. For example, severe hydronephrosis and hydroureter in a child of only a few weeks of age demands early surgical repair. To wait longer could jeopardize the life of the patient (renal insufficiency). On the other hand, corrective repair of a cleft palate, polydactyly, etc., can be postponed until a more suitable time.

The Risk of the Operation to the Patient

Thanks to modern anesthesia, better knowledge of pre- and post-operative care and establishment of well-designed intensive care units in practically all pediatric surgical centers, it is now possible to perform pediatric surgical operations without any special risk at almost any age. At present, the risk of the operation does not materially influence the timing of the operation. An exception is the neonatal period, when operations are generally limited to correction of congenital malformations which otherwise would jeopardize life or the limb of the patient (diaphragmatic hernia, esophageal atresia, intestinal atresia, etc.).

Surgical-Technical Aspects

Complicated operations may be postponed for purely technical reasons, since a waiting period may improve chances for a successful operation. For example in babies with Hirschsprung's disease or high rectal atresia a minor operation to save the child's life (i. e.

colostomy) is carried out during the newborn period, reserving the definitive corrective operation until the child is older.

Possible Spontaneous Cure of the Condition

Awareness of possible improvement or cure of the disease influences the timing of proposed operations. For instance, an umbilical hernia or hydrocele often disappears spontaneously during the first year or two of life, and surgical correction is therefore postponed for this length of time.

Psychological Aspects

These play an especially important part in smaller, non-urgent pediatric surgical operations.

The Significance of Separating the Child from His Parents

After about the sixth month of life a baby becomes aware of strangers. Separation from the mother after this age is a painful experience. Therefore, a baby should be admitted to hospital after the first six months of life only if an operation is really necessary. Hospitalization for children two to four years old is a traumatic experience; children who are removed from home at this time feel deserted in spite of the efforts of sympathetic nurses and doctors. To children over four years of age the purpose of hospitalization can be relatively well explained, and the separation is made easier. Thus, hospitalization between the ages of two and four years should be avoided if possible.

Psychological Effects of the Original Disease

This must not be neglected. Children with visible malformations (bat ears) or with abnormalities of the genitals (hypospadias), especially when combined with incontinence (epispadias) are often teased by other children in school and come to realize that they are different from others. These repairs should therefore be accomplished before the children have reached kindergarten or school age.

Cooperation of the Child during the Postoperative Phase

Cooperation of certain patients is very important for pre- and post-operative treatment, e. g. for physiotherapy after operations for funnel chest, which may have an effect on the cosmetic result.

The Psychological State of the Parents

Parental fears frequently affect the timing of operation. For instance, a hernia repair may properly be performed in a young infant if the parent's constant fear of incarceration jeopardizes the whole family's life style.

Optimal Time for Non-Urgent Operations

Table 2.1 summarizes the optimal time for non-urgent pediatric surgical operations. This timetable is important for the family physician, who is usually the first to be consulted. For this reason the average ages at operation are added. A discussion of the optimum time for the more important conditions follows.

Inguinal Hernia

(Chapter 16)

An inguinal hernia practically never heals spontaneously. Further, there is a 5—15 % risk of incarceration. Therefore, repair is best performed one to two weeks after diagnosis. In premature infants and small neonates hernia repair may be postponed until the third month of life.

Umbilical Hernia

(Chapter 19)

Many newborn infants develop umbilical hernia. Most umbilical hernias spontaneously disappear during the first one to three years of life. They rarely disturb the patient. Umbilical hernias should therefore not be operated before the third year of life.

Phimosis

(Chapter 17)

In the first year of life phimosis is almost a physiological condition; most spontaneously disappear before the second birthday. A corrective operation should therefore not be attempted before the third year of life. However, phimoses with complications (balanitis, urinary infections, paraphimosis) are exceptions to this rule.

Table 2.1.   **Timetable for Non-Urgent Surgical Repairs**

	Operation Time	Average Length of Hospitalization
Craniostenosis	from 2nd month	10 days
Meningocele	3rd–6th month	10 days
Harelip	3rd–9th month	5 days
Cleft Palate	18th–36th month	14 days
Bat Ears	4th–5th year	2 days
Branchial Fistulae and Cysts	4th–5th year	3 days
Torticollis	2nd–5th year	2 days
Inguinal Hernia	from 3rd month	1 day
Umbilical Hernia	4th–5th year	1 day
Incompletely Descended Testis	from 2nd year	5 days
Phimosis	3rd–5th year	2 days
Hypospadias	3rd–5th year	5–14 days
Exstrophy of the Bladder —Turn in	1st–3rd month	3–4 weeks
— Continence operation	4–5 years	7–10 days
Hydrocele	from 3rd year	1 day
Kidney, Ureter, Bladder Operations (pelvi-ureteric stricture, vesico-uretal reflux)	from 3rd month	2–4 weeks
Hirschsprung's Disease def. Correction	3rd–6th month	2 weeks
Anal and Rectal Atresia def. Correction	6th–12th month	2 weeks
Polydactyly	3rd–6th month	7 days
Syndactyly	2nd–4th year	1 week
Funnel Chest	4th–5th year	2 weeks
Exostoses	10th–12th year	7 days
Bone Cysts	from 5th year	1–2 weeks
Hemangioma	5th–10th year	2–5 days

Incompletely Descended Testis

(Chapter 16)

According to recent data, degenerative changes may develop in an incompletely descended testis during the first two years of life. Therefore, orchidopexy is performed during the second year of life in some centers. Orchidopexy is technically difficult in these small children, and the possibility of testicular injury is considerable in our view.

We therefore withhold repair until the third year of life. Formerly, the waiting period was often longer.

Hypospadias
(Chapter 17)

Repair should be completed before the child begins school. If two operations are necessary (meatotomy and straightening of the penis), the first stage is performed during the third year of life. If the meatal stenosis is severe, the meatotomy may be carried out still earlier.

Ectopia Vesica
(Chapter 17)

The time of operation depends on the operative method. Reconstruction of the bladder is carried out in the first few months of life, or even in the neonatal period. Correction of continence and repair of the penis may be postponed until the child is four to five years of age.

Craniosynostosis
(Chapter 8)

Since premature ossification of all the cranial sutures may influence development of the brain, its surgical correction must be performed as soon as the diagnosis is established. However, if only one suture is involved, correction is carried out mainly for cosmetic reasons. The earlier the repair, the better the cosmetic result. Therefore, we operate on craniosynostosis as early as the second month of life.

Fistulae and Cysts of the Neck
(Chapter 11)

For psychological reasons, excision may generally be postponed until the child goes to school (4 to 5 years of age) if no infection is present. However, if the sinus becomes infected it is difficult to remove in toto and may recur after operation. This risk must be explained to the parents.

Polydactyly

This should be corrected early so that the hand or foot can develop normally. Pedunculated skin appendages can be tied off in the neonatal period. Excision of fully developed extra digits is postponed until the third to fourth months of life. Correction should be carried out on both hands and feet for both cosmetic and functional reasons.

Syndactyly

In general only the hands are surgically corrected. Operation should be postponed until the age of two to four years because before this age separation of the fingers is technically difficult. The best functional improvement occurs when the patient can cooperate in performing exercises postoperatively. Progressive contracture of one of the fingers may necessitate earlier operation.

Exostoses

(Chapter 23)

These are removed only if they cause pain or functional disturbances. When possible, excision is postponed until after the tenth or twelfth year of life. If the patient is operated upon before this age, recurrence is common.

Hemangioma

(Chapter 20)

Flat capillary hemangiomas and small cavernous hemangiomas frequently regress after an initial growth spurt during the first two years of life. Spontaneous regression may occur until at least the fifth year of life. Exceptions to this rule are hemangiomas in unfavorable areas (face or genitals) or ones with complications (bleeding, erosion and infection). These may require earlier treatment.

Torticollis

(Chapter 11)

In most cases, physiotherapy corrects torticollis during the first 12 months of life. If not, surgical correction is carried out during the second year of life.

Hydrocele

(Chapter 16)

Hydroceles are very common in infants and young children. Many disappear spontaneously within one to two years, and therefore operation is delayed until the third year of life. Early correction of a communicating hydrocele is indicated since it practically never disappears spontaneously.

3 Pre- and Postoperative Management

P. DANGEL

Introduction

The aim of pediatric surgery is not only to reduce the mortality of surgical disease, but also to assure that the surviving children are as normal as possible psychologically and physiologically. This is possible only if measures are immediately taken which prevent or minimize damage secondary to complications of the disease. These measures restore and preserve normal respiration, circulation, body temperature, energy and electrolyte balance and acid-base equilibrium. The same principles apply when the patient is under anesthesia in the operating room as well as during the postoperative phase.

In addition to good general treatment, the ill child should receive the best possible psychological care; the doctors must retain close contact with the parents to prevent the psychological disturbances to which any hospitalized child is prone. Only when all these measures are carried out satisfactorily will the child be discharged physically and psychologically normal.

There are few surgical conditions where immediate surgery is mandatory: airway obstruction, massive hemorrhage, etc. As a rule there is enough time to take a good clinical history, perform a thorough clinical examination, undertake appropriate radiographic and laboratory investigations and to discuss the patient's state of health with the parents.

Psychological Management

Every hospitalization disturbs the relationship between the child and his family. Most affected are young children in hospital for prolonged periods, or who have to be operated and anesthetized more than once. The child's attitude towards hospitalization and his natural fear of unpleasant experiences (examinations, injections, anesthesia, pain, operation and especially the uncertainty of what will actually happen to him) can be markedly influenced by psychologically preparing him for admission to hospital while he is still at home. This necessitates conveying to the parents adequate information about these facts. There are a number of brochures and picture books available for small children which help to prepare them for hospitalization. These brochures should be made available to the parents.

On the day of admission the surgeon, the anesthetist and the nurse should prepare the patient for the upcoming experiences in language appropriate to his age. The child is truthfully informed about the coming operation, injections, change of dressings, intravenous infusions, etc. in simple language but without dwelling on the more unpleasant details. The patient has a right to know whether he will be given an injection into his arm or an inhalation anesthesia, the location and length of the incision and postoperative pain. In emergency cases there is unfortunately much less time to prepare the patient in this way, but even here is it possible to speak with the child for a few minutes explaining to him what is going to happen.

If the child must remain in hospital after operation it is preferable to admit him on the day before operation. This allows him to become accustomed to the new surroundings and acquainted with the doctors and nurses.

The parents should visit the child as often as possible, touch him and talk to him. The mother's confidence is enhanced by allowing her to carry out simple nursing procedures such as feeding the child, changing diapers, washing and bathing him. Parents must be encouraged not to lose contact with a child who is hospitalized for prolonged periods. This is especially true in neonates who are directly transferred to the pediatric surgical area from the maternity department. If parents are taught to take the same hygienic measures as doctors and nurses, one can allow them to handle the infant lying in an incubator. The highly technical machinery used in a modern intensive care department must be explained to the parents in simple terms when they first visit their child. Daily discussions are held between doctor and parent as long as the child is dangerously ill. The doctor should listen to the parents' fears and problems, rather than burden them with his own worries about the patient's medical condition. The nurse in charge should attend these discussions whenever possible.

Transport of Pediatric Surgical Emergencies

Major pediatric surgery, especially of newborns, can only be carried out in special centers because of the need for specially trained doctors and nurses as well as special apparatus and instruments. It is often necessary to transport the patient over considerable distances to such centers. Since prognosis relates directly to the patient's general condition on arrival, it is important that he be transported without additional risks. However urgent the condition of the baby, it is senseless to transport him to a neonatal center if he were to die or deteriorate during transport. Patients with disturbances of respiration and circulation (shock) are transported only when all functions necessary to life have been restored to normal, with maintenance support administered during transport.

To obviate the disaster of aspirating gastric content, all emergency cases and especially all neonates should have a stomach tube passed and aspirated at frequent intervals. Patients who may vomit and all unconscious patients are transported on their side or in the prone position. Patients with severe respiratory difficulties are intubated and artificial respiration instituted before transport. Hemo- or pneumothorax should be recognized and drained before transport. Patients with an oxygen deficit need adequate oxygen therapy during transport, especially if the child is to be transported by air. Since atmospheric pressure diminishes with increasing altitude, any air collection in the body increases rapidly in volume as altitude is gained. Partial oxygen pressure decreases with higher altitudes, with the danger of hypoxia developing during air transport.

Hypovolemic shock is treated before and during transport. Intravenous infusions in neonates who must be transported long distances are best given with the aid of an electric infusion pump.

Mechanical respirators cannot be sufficiently controlled during transport. If assisted ventilation is needed, it is best administered by positive pressure respiration by hand. The strictest cleanliness and asepsis are necessary during transport, especially of neonates.

Severely sick or injured children can also be transported without danger if they have been adequately prepared and if there is good supervision during transport by qualified assistants. Infants must be guarded against excessive loss of temperature, preferably by transporting them in a portable incubator.

Preoperative Management

The clinical examination of each patient must include documenting his length, body weight, temperature, head circumference and calculating his surface area. Routine laboratory tests include hemoglobin, hematocrit and urine analysis. The temperature must be taken. Special notice is taken of the state of respiration, circulation, fluid and electrolyte and acid-base balance.

Respiration

Signs of disturbed respiration include flaring of the ala nasi, tachypnea (for normal values see Table 3.1), suprasternal retraction, grunting respiration, forced expiration and cyanosis.

Cyanosis becomes detectable only after the pO_2 of arterial blood has been considerably lowered. Evaluating respiratory status in neonates

Table 3.1. **Normal Values for Different Ages**

Age	Weight	Pulse at rest/ min	Respiration at rest/ min	Blood pressure mm Hg	Hb gm%	Blood volume ml
Premature	1000–2000 g 2000–3000 g 3000 g	140	50	50/26 60/32 70/45	16–20	85–100 ml/kg
Fullterm	3.4 kg	125	30–50	70/50	16–20	275 ml
3 months	6 kg	120	30	80–90/50	12	450 ml
1 year	10.3 kg	110	25–30	90–100/60	10–12	750 ml
5 years	20 kg	100	20–25	90–100/60	10–12	1500 ml
10 years	32 kg	90	20	100/65	12–14	2400 ml

with an oxygen dissociation curve shifted to the left is even more difficult than in older children, because the hemoglobin is adequately saturated even with low pO_2 values, and hypoxia and cyanosis occur relatively late. The other clinical signs of neonatal hypoxia (increased ventilation rate, tachypnea, restlessness, tachycardia, raised blood pressure) are also not marked. Thus, whenever a suspicion of respiratory dysfunction arises, a blood gas analysis (including arterial pO_2 is necessary.

The air passages are kept patent by frequent pharyngeal or tracheobronchial suction. Dyspneic neonates and young infants often breathe better when nursed in the prone position. Neonates with esophageal atresia should undergo tracheal intubation immediately after admission, usually before any radiological investigations are carried out. Tracheal intubation and assisted ventilation is also indicated in any neonate who tires because of respiratory difficulties, especially newborns with congenital diaphragmatic hernia. The question of whether a patient should be intubated hinges on the blood gas analysis. Intubation is mandatory if the pH is below 7.2, the pCO_2 above 70 and the pO_2 under 40 to 50 mmHg when taken with an oxygen concentration in the inspired air of between 70 and 80 %. Dyspneic children with a distended abdomen need constant suction of the stomach (negative pressure of between 25 to 50 cm of water) supplemented by repeated unblocking and hand aspiration of the catheter. Dyspnea always demands a chest radiograph.

Circulation

The circulation is restored to normal before operation. The skin of the extremities should be pink and warm, the pulse and blood pressure should be within normal limits and urine excretion should be at least 1 ml per kg per hour.

Hypovolemic shock occurs after hemorrhage, extensive injuries, burns, prolonged vomiting or after severe respiratory difficulties, especially in the respiratory distress syndrome of newborn infants.

Signs and symptoms of *hypovolemic shock* are:

Pale, cool skin (peripheral vasoconstriction).

Apprehension, restlessness, apathy, tachycardia (difficult to evaluate in the newborn).

Decreased arterial pressure (may initially be normal because of peripheral vasoconstriction).

Acidosis (inadequate perfusion of tissue leads to oxygen deficiency and anaerobic metabolism).

Increased difference between arterial and venous oxygen concentration.

Tachypnea, possibly dyspnea, falling central venous pressure. Oliguria.

Possible signs of coagulation defect resulting from disseminated intravascular thrombosis.

Edema does not exclude the possibility of hypovolemia!

Management of Shock

In children the principles governing the treatment of shock are the same as in adults. The sequence of the various treatment modalities is of importance.

1) **Adequate respiration** is mandatory, if necessary by artificial respiration. The oxygen concentration in the inspired air should approximate 40 to 50 %.

2) The patient should be nursed flat with elevation of the legs.

3) **External hemorrhage** must be controled, if necessary by direct pressure.

4) **A central venous catheter** is placed to measure central venous pressure. With experience, a central venous catheter can be passed percutaneously via the brachial, external jugular, subclavian or femoral vein. Central pressure is accurate only when the tip of

the catheter lies in the superior or inferior vena cava or in the right atrium. With peritonitis or gross abdominal distension, pressure in the inferior vena cava may be higher than in the right atrium.

5) **Intravenous therapy** aims toward restoring normal blood volume as quickly as possible. Ringer's lactate solution is a suitable infusion fluid for shock. Blood loss is replaced by whole blood, hypoproteinemia is corrected by albumin solution. All infusions are controlled by observing the patient's general condition at short intervals. The arterial blood pressure can be determined accurately even in neonates by the ultrasonic technique. Frequent evaluation of the central venous pressure protects against overtransfusion. It is impossible to calculate in advance the amount of fluid required to restore the circulation to normal; one must infuse or transfuse until the circulation parameters have returned to normal.

6) **Acidosis** occurs regularly with severe shock and must be quantitated and then corrected by intravenous sodium bicarbonate. Before treating acidotic neonates and young infants, the 8.4 % molar solution of sodium bicarbonate is best diluted with the same volume of 5 % glucose water.

Hypotonic fluids contain too few electrolytes; it is not advisable to use them in treating shock as they produce water intoxication if too quickly administered.

If the central venous pressure rises over 20 cm of water one must consider the possibility of heart failure versus overinfusion. If pulmonary edema develops the child is intubated and positive end expiratory pressure respiration is started. Cardiac glycosides are necessary only with signs of cardiac decompensation (cardiac enlargement, hepatic enlargement, tachycardia).

Disturbances in the Fluid, Electrolyte and Acid-Base Equilibrium

Vomiting, diarrhea and "third space" fluid losses disturb the fluid, electrolyte and acid-base balance, and must be corrected before operation. When starting infusion therapy, the following points should be considered:

1) Treat shock, if present.

2) Administer the normal 24 hours' requirement.

3) Replace existing deficits.

4) Replace ongoing pathological losses of fluid.

Treatment of Shock

Hypovolemic shock is treated as described above.

Normal Fluid and Electrolyte Requirements

The normal requirements per day are seen in Table 3.2. The fluid may be given as a mixture of one part 0.9 % NaCl and 4 parts 10 % glucose solution. The resulting solution contains about 31 mEq of sodium per liter. The amount of glucose does not cover the daily calorie requirements, but it prevents hypoglycemia. The potassium requirement is met by adding 3 mEq KCl per kg per day. Serum electrolytes are estimated preoperatively and on the day after operation.

Table 3.2. **Normal 24-Hour Requirements of Fluid and Electrolytes**

Fluids:	Newborns		85 ml/kg
	Infants under 3 months		120 ml/kg
	Children over 3 months		1800—2000 ml/m^2
Electrolytes:	Na$^+$ 35—50 mEq/m^2	or 3—4 mEq/kg	
	K$^+$ 30—40 mEq/m^2	or 2—3 mEq/kg	
	Cl$^-$ 30—40 mEq/m^2	or 2—3 mEq/kg	
Calories:	Newborn, first day of life		50—60 Cal/kg
	Newborn after first week of life		120—150 Cal/kg
	Children		1700 Cal/m^2
Quantity of Urine	1000—1500 ml/m^2		
	Minimal excretion 1 ml/kg/hour		

Extra Fluid Requirements

Preexisting dehydration or elevation of body temperature demand fluids in addition to maintenance needs. Table 3.3 shows the fluid deficit with different degrees for dehydration expressed as a percentage of body weight. This extra amount for dehydration is added to the normal fluid requirements. In addition, normal daily fluid requirements are increased by 10 % for each degree C rise in body temperature.

Replacement of Pathological Losses from the Gastrointestinal Tract

To simplify matters, we replace all abnormal losses from different parts of the alimentary tract by the same infusion mixture containing

Table 3.3. **Intravenous Therapy for a Preexisting Deficit**

Degree of Dehydration Weight Loss in %	Clinical Signs	Fluid requirements necessary for correction (in addition to normal daily requirement and if patient not in shock)
mild 5 %	Irritability, dry mucosa. skin warm and pink. Slightly decreased skin turgor. Oliguria, possibly thirst.	25—50 ml/kg
medium 5—10 %	Anxious expression, restlessness, sunken eyes, decreased intraocular pressure, skin pale. Markedly decreased skin turgor. Fever, tachycardia, oliguria, high pitched cry, sunken fontanelle.	50—75 ml/kg
severe 10—15 %	Patient looks very ill. Apathy or semiconscious, hypotonia, sunken eyes with marked decreased intraocular pressure. Skin pale or cyanotic, cold, no turgor. Hyperpyrexia, possibly convulsions. Pulse weak, blood pressure low. Fontanelle markedly depressed.	75—120 ml/kg

1 part 0.9 % of NaCl solution and 1 part 10 % glucose solution to which is added 10 mEq KCl/Liter. This solution must be given slowly as it may produce high blood sugar levels and an osmotic diuresis.

If the fluid replacement is accurate and if there is adequate diuresis, hyperkalemia practically never occurs. On the contrary, patients who are dehydrated or in shock after massive operation, or who suffer respiratory and metabolic acidosis or salt loss secondary to renal insufficiency often develop hypokalemia. Thus, the potassium deficit should be replaced only when diuresis has started or when hypokalemia has been proved by serum analysis.

Fluid Replacement During Operation

If an infusion is necessary during operation, Ringer's lactate solution with added 5 % glucose is given in quantities of 10 ml per kg of body weight per hour. If the preoperative hemoglobin is normal, operative blood losses of 10 %/o of the patient's total blood volume can be replaced by Ringer's lactate solution. Only when blood loss exceeds 10 %/o of the total blood volume must it be replaced by blood transfusions.

Postoperative Fluid Therapy

Here the same rules apply that were discussed under preoperative fluid therapy. Antishock measures, normal daily fluid requirements, preexisting deficits and pathological fluid losses must be calculated and replaced. Potassium is given when diuresis has started or for proven hypokalemia. Whenever all the fluid requirements must be given by infusion, serum electrolytes should be determined daily. A constant infusion speed is very important in newborns and young infants, best achieved by infusion machines (roller pumps, electrical syringes, etc., Fig. 3.1 and 3.2). Daily recording of body weight (Fig. 3.3) and urine output help monitor the fluid and electrolyte status while infusions are given.

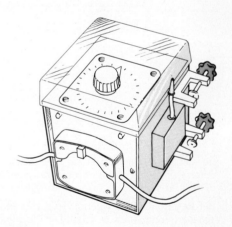

Fig. 3.1. Roller pump

Anemia and Blood Transfusions

The normal hemoglobin concentration of different age groups is shown in Table 3.1. There are no absolute minimal hemoglobin concentrations below which blood transfusions are mandatory. Children with normal respiration and circulation tolerate a hemoglobin concentration of 8 to 10 g%/o without difficulty. However, patients with dyspnea or circulatory disturbances require a higher hemoglobin concentration than is normal for the age group. Patients with cyano-

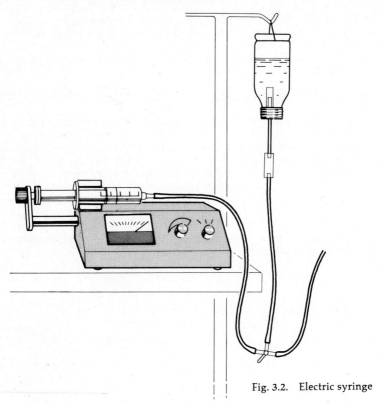

Fig. 3.2.   Electric syringe

tic congenital heart lesions, pneumonia and all neonates with the respiratory distress syndrome demand a hemoglobin concentration of at least 16 g⁰/o.

Before one decides whether to give a blood transfusion the patient's special circumstances should be evaluated. The danger of serum hepatitis must be balanced against the advantages of a higher hemoglobin concentration. As a rule, transfusions of 20 ml of blood per kg of body weight are well tolerated, even in patients with border-line cardiac reserve.

Special Problems of the Newborn

After aspirating the newborn infant's pharynx, he should be dried and examined. Special notice is taken of respiratory and circulatory

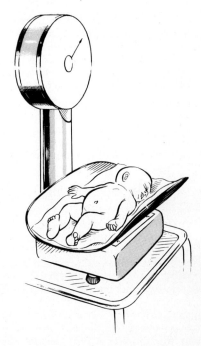

Fig. 3.3. Infant weighing machine

function and visible malformations. In high risk newborn, blood pH, hemoglobin concentration, hematocrit and blood sugar should be determined immediately. In addition, immature or high risk newborns should be kept warm and an adequate respiratory status assured, if necessary by administering oxygen and parenteral glucose. These measures help the low weight-high risk newborn establish normal adaptation to extrauterine life.

Adaptation Disturbances of Respiration

Immature newborns often develop the so-called "idiopathic respiratory distress syndrome" (hyaline membrane disease), especially in association with asphyxia, acidosis, hypothermia or hypovolemia. These newborns develop diffuse pulmonary atelectases with a characteristic radiographic picture, a condition brought about by deficiency of surface tension factors in the alveoli. In addition, hypoxia and acidosis encourage continuation of the fetal circulation in which blood bypasses the lungs via the foramen ovale and the ductus arteriosus. This results in a vicious circle with progressive hypoxia and acidosis, associated with frequent mortality. Clinically, one observes tachypnea, mild cyanosis in spite of nursing the infant in an oxygen-rich atmosphere, inspiratory retraction of the pliable thoracic cage and expiratory grunting. Chest radiography reveals diffuse atelectasis, poor aeration and air bronchograms. Early treatment has reduced the mortality to about 20 %:

maintaining normothermia by nursing the baby in an incubator, adjusting the oxygen content of the inspired air to maintain normal arterial pO_2, correcting acidosis and giving an intravenous infusion of 10 % glucose solution. Severe cases require mechanical respiration with positive endexpiratory pressure.

Adaptation Disturbances of Circulation

As we have seen, hypoxia and acidosis increase resistance in the pulmonary vessels, triggering a rise of pressure in the right atrium to reopen the foramen ovale and prevent closure of the ductus arteriosus. A right to left shunt develops, excluding the pulmonary circulation. Symptoms resemble the respiratory distress syndrome: tachypnea, cyanosis in spite of added oxygen, shock and mild respiratory and metabolic acidosis. Treatment consists of improving respiration by tracheobronchial suction, administration of oxygen and possibly by mechanical respiration. The baby is warmed, acidosis, hypovolemia and anemia are corrected and calories are administered in the form of 10 % glucose solution. The differential diagnosis between this condition and a congenital cardiac malformation is often not easy. If the arterial pO_2 remains below 100 mmHg in spite of pure oxygen being given by face masks for 5 to 10 minutes, a cardiac malformation with right to left shunt can be excluded.

Adaptation Disturbances in Temperature Regulation

A newborn exposed to a cold environment cannot maintain normal body temperature by increasing his metabolism via muscle contractions, shivering and visible goose pimples, but rather increases metabolism by burning the still-present brown fatty tissue of the body. Concomitantly, heat loss is minimized by marked peripheral vasoconstriction. Since any increase in metabolism requires more oxygen and glucose, newborns with inadequate energy reserves or deficient energy supplies tolerate hypothermia poorly. Especially at risk are premature and low-weight infants, as well as newborns who are hypoxic, shocked, hypoglycemic and infected as well as those who cannot be fed early. If the increased oxygen requirements of hypothermia cannot be met because of respiratory difficulties, hypoxia with all its dangers will result.

Prevention of hypothermia is all-important: the newborn is quickly dried and wrapped in aluminium foil prior to nursing him in an incubator with air temperature of 36°C. During operation the newborn's temperature must be kept normal by such measures as raising the room temperature (26° to 28°), placing the child on a heated water mattress, humidifying the respiratory gases, warming infused fluids, etc. When warming hypothermic infants (i. e. rectal temperature of below 36°) one must not be too drastic. The rectal temperature should not rise faster than 1°C per hour, and if this produces vasodilatation and hypovolemia it must be compensated for by intravenous infusion. Examination, observation and treatment of the high-risk neonate should be carried out in the incubator at a temperature set at 32° to 34°C for full-term and 34° to 36° for low-weight infants. The temperature in the incubator as well as the patient's skin and rectal temperature are monitored frequently.

Adaptation Disturbances of Metabolism

Even normal full-term infants possess energy reserves which suffice for only 24 to 36 hours. Low weight and premature newborns have even smaller energy reserves, especially in the face of increased metabolic demands from respiratory difficulties. Hypoglycemia can occur during the first few hours after birth, manifested by seizures, cyanosis, apathy, decreased muscle tone and unstable body temperature. Even subclinical hypoglycemia may produce central nervous system damage. A full-term newborn can be said to have hypoglycemia if the blood sugar drops below 30 mg%; in premature and low weight infants values below 20 mg% are pathological. Newborns especially prone to hypoglycemia are premature, low-weight and overweight infants, babies of diabetic mothers, infants with asphyxia or low body temperature as well as those with Rh incompatibility. Prevention consists of feeding the infant within the first 4 hours after birth or administering 10% glucose solution by infusion. All newborns at risk should have periodic blood sugar investigations.

Hyperbilirubinemia

Part of the unconjugated (indirect) bilirubin exists as free bilirubin and is toxic for the central nervous system, producing kernicterus. The indirect bilirubin should not excede 15 mg% in premature infants or 20 mg% in full-term infants. Especially prone to kernicterus are newborns with asphyxia, acidosis, hypothermia, hypoproteinemia (under 4% total plasma proteins) and when certain drugs are administered: sulphonamides, caffeine, furosemide, digoxin, gentamycin, etc. These drugs increase the risk of kernicterus as they displace bilirubin from its combination with albumin, or lower the blood/cerebrospinal fluid barrier. In these special patients hyperbilirubinemia must be treated earlier than normal, i. e. in premature infants with a serum bilirubin of 12 mg⁰/o and in full-term infants with a bilirubin of 15 mg⁰/o. The serum bilirubin must be measured repeatedly in all jaundiced newborns. The plasma proteins should be kept above 4.5 g⁰/o. When a dangerous bilirubin level is reached, exchange transfusion is indicated. Phototherapy with ultraviolet light does not replace exchange transfusions; however, if used early it can cause excretion of part of the non-conjugated bilirubin and discourage further rise in the bilirubin level.

Calcium Metabolism

Hypocalcemia is heralded by tremors and convulsions, and occurs during the first 48 hours of life in premature infants, in babies of diabetic mothers, after asphyxia and after correction of metabolic acidosis. Under these circumstances the serum calcium must be measured and, if necessary, calcium infusions given.

General Preparations

Newborn and Young Infants

These patients should be left no longer than 4 hours without feeds or glucose administration. If operation is delayed beyond this time, a glucose infusion should be started preoperatively. The last feed should consist of 5⁰/o glucose solution. If an operation becomes urgent shortly after a feeding has been given, the stomach is emptied by nasogastric tube aspiration.

Older Children

Older children receive their last normal meal the evening before operation and are allowed to drink clear liquids until 6 hours before operation. The colon does not need to be emptied preoperatively, but the child should be encouraged to empty his bladder.

Premedication

For elective operations under general anesthesia, children are given a sedative, an analgesic and drugs which depress vagal activity. This is done to keep the patient quiet, allay fears and depress excessive secretions and dangerous vagal reflexes. Since children resent injections, these drugs may be administered per os or per rectum. Any necessary local preparations as well as laboratory and radiographic investigations are carried out before giving the premedication. Before emergency operations at least a vagal depressive drug should be given.

A child who has been properly prepared psychologically should sleep well without medicines on the night before operation. Very excitable and anxious patients may need a sedative: Valium (Diazepam) in dosages of 6 to 10 mg per square meter of body surface is given intramuscularly or intravenously. Children with severe pain may require an analgesic before operation.

Postoperative Treatment

After general anesthesia the child is observed continuously until he has awakened completely. The state of consciousness is observed as well as the respiration, skin color and pulse rate. After extensive operations and if there is danger of further hemorrhage, arterial blood pressure and central venous pressure are taken at intervals.

Newborn and young infants require constant monitoring of body temperature. They are best nursed naked in an incubator. Pediatric electrocardiogram and body temperature monitors have been developed, but monitoring respiration is still problematic. Continuous monitoring of arterial pO_2 and pCO_2 is not yet feasible.

Maintenance of Normal Respiratory Functions

The same principles hold good as discussed under preoperative management. Airway obstruction and pulmonary atelectasis are obviated by repeatedly aspirating the pharynx and frequently changing the position of the patient. This is especially important after big operations and in unconscious patients. Expectoration of sticky mucus is facilitated by humidifying the inspired air. Regrettably, humidifiers do increase the danger of infection. In certain cases additional measures (percussion of the thorax in various positions) are necessary, facilitated by trained physiotherapists. If the patient cannot raise secretions by coughing, tracheobronchial suction is carried out and the sputum is cultured. In most cases the bronchoscope is not necessary to perform tracheobronchial toilet in young infants and children.

If there are profuse secretions or if mechanical respiration is necessary, it is wise to aspirate secretions periodically via a nasotracheal tube, especially in infants and toddlers (Fig. 3.4). Oxygen therapy is

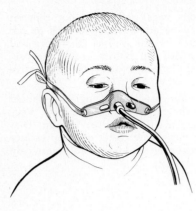

Fig. 3.4.   Oxygen therapy through nasal catheter

especially needed in immature infants. However, arterial oxygen values above 100 to 120 mmHg can cause blindness secondary to retrolental hyperplasia in newborns. This danger is minimized by frequently measuring arterial pO_2 and keeping the oxygen content of inspired air at or below 40 %.

The air-oxygen mixture is humidified to 80 to 100 % and warmed to body temperature. Administration of oxygen is a problem in children who are not intubated. 1 liter of oxygen per minute introduced via

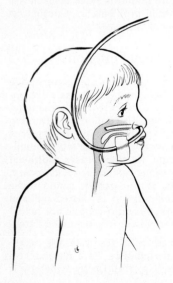

Fig. 3.5.   Nasopharyngeal tube

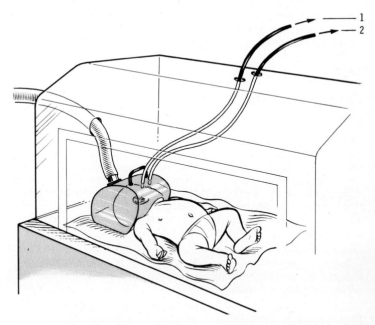

Fig. 3.6. Oxygen therapy in incubator

a small catheter placed into one nostril (for a distance corresponding to that from nostril to ear lobe) raises the oxygen contents of inspired air in a newborn to between 50 % and 60 % (Fig. 3.5). Older children need a flow of between 2 and 4 liters of oxygen per minute. Oxygen tents only minimally increase oxygen concentration of inspired air, even when relatively large amounts of oxygen are administered; the same holds true for incubators. Infants who need an oxygen concentration higher than 40 % should be nursed in a plastic hood (Fig. 3.6) which delivers a constant oxygen concentration to the baby. If this type of oxygen therapy is used, the inspired air should be warmed.

Maintenance of Circulation

This has already been described; the same rules hold for postoperative therapy. The extra respiratory efforts displayed in newborns with heart failure constitute grave additional stress; intubation and mechanical respiration may be indicated. In emergency situations, babies with brachycardia and falling blood pressure in spite of adequate circulatory volume require adrenergic drugs. The speed of infusion of drugs is varied according to the results obtained while monitoring pulse rate, arterial blood pressure and central venous pressure.

Postoperative Fluid-Electrolyte and Acid-Base Metabolism

Similarly to the practice discussed under preoperative treatment, volumes are calculated on the basis of normal daily requirements plus preexisting deficit plus further pathological losses. Blood gases are measured after every major operation as well as in patients with respiratory trouble, hypoxia, shock, renal failure or continuing losses from the gastrointestinal tract. Blood pH below 7.3 is corrected by administering sodium bicarbonate as described under preoperative management.

One must remember that patients with acidosis have a higher serum potassium concentration than when blood pH is normal. Thus, hyperkalemia in an acidotic patient does not necessarily contraindicate potassium administration.

Postoperative Feeding

After *smaller operations* without complicatons, older children can receive clear liquids at the latest 4 hours after operation, provided they are completely awake and do not vomit. If tolerated, the feedings are increased and enlarged. In premature and newborn infants (with danger of aspiration) the stomach is aspirated by tube before each feed. For the composition of normal feedings for neonates and infants the reader should consult a pediatric textbook.

After *major operations* the nasogastric catheter is put on suction with a negative pressure of between 25 and 50 cm of water. The catheter is irrigated with saline from time to time to prevent blockage. It usually takes 24 to 48 hours until the patient can be fed, depending on the severity and type of operation. The patient is given clear liquids to drink as soon as peristalsis returns and when only small amounts of gastric contents are aspirated.

In premature and small neonates with a gastrostomy tube in place and where the danger of regurgitation and aspiration exists, feedings are initiated via the gastrostomy catheter. Feedings are poured into the outer sheath of a plastic syringe suspended 10 to 15 cm above the child (Fig. 3.7); this enables the gastric contents to be pushed up into the syringe when the child strains, only to return to the

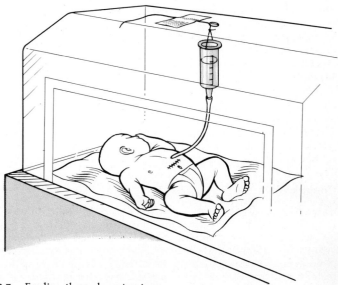

Fig. 3.7. Feeding through gastrostomy

stomach afterwards. Measures to start intestinal function (enemas and anticholinesterase injections) should not be routinely employed.
Whenever the gastrointestinal tract cannot be used for feeding purposes for lengthy periods of time, some sort of parenteral nutrition support must be given. By proper parenteral support, even infants can be given all the nutritional elements necessary for normal growth and development. Commercially prepared solutions of suitable mixtures of amino acids, electrolytes, vitamins, trace elements and concentrated glucose solutions are available in the United States; they are hypertonic and must be delivered into a central vein via a silastic catheter, infusion pump and millepore filter. Otherwise, they must be prepared by hand under strict aseptic conditions and a laminar air flow hood; this is expensive, tedious and risky from the standpont of infection. In either event, strict asepsis and frequent monitoring of the patient make total parenteral nutrition difficult at best. Further, we do not yet know all the possible harmful effects on the young, growing organism of administering synthetic or natural amino acid mixtures on the development of the central nervous system. It is difficult to keep a central venous catheter infusion going for 4 to 6 weeks without encountering complications such as phlebitis, thrombosis, emboli or septicemia. Constant careful observation of the patient is necessary.

The Management of Complications

Postoperative *hyperthermia* is encountered with dehydration, infection or respiratory distress. Dehyration fever can be easily prevented. Hyperpyrexia in conjunction with cerebral edema should raise the suspicion of water intoxication (excessive administration of water) or respiratory insufficiency.

High body temperature increases oxygen consumption and is especially dangerous in children with respiratory distress or heart failure. Treatment consists of adequate fluid therapy, antishock measures, returning electrolyte balance to normal, antipyretics and if necessary, cooling of the skin by tepid sponging and ventilator fanning.

Convulsions

Convulsions must be carefully observed. A unilateral fit is important diagnostically. The convulsion must be stopped as quickly as possible by administering appropriate drugs. We favor *Diazepam* intravenously in dosages of 10 mg per m² of body surface. *Barbiturates* in dosages of 100 to 300 mg per m² of body surface or *chloralhydrate* rectally in dosages of 2 to 3 g per m² may also be used. Neonatal convulsions must raise the suspicion of hypoglycemia or hypocalcemia and demand appropriate investigation and treatment.

Infection and Antibiotic Therapy

When severely ill patients, some with defective antibacterial defense mechanisms, are nursed together without proper isolation precautions, pathologic bacteria may spread quickly from one to the other in an epidemic manner. In a humid atmosphere gram-negative bacilli are commonly encountered. Humidifiers, respirators, incubators, oxygen tubes, gastric and infusion tubes as well as endotracheal catheters are all well-known fomites. Careless doctors and nurses greatly enhance the danger of infection epidemics.

Before entering an intensive therapy unit gowns must be donned and rings and watches removed. Hands and forearms are scrubbed and disinfected before examining each patient. All instruments used for diagnosis or treatment are effectively sterilized or disinfected. All this is time-consuming and demands sufficient nursing personnel. The greatest care must be exercised when mixing intravenous infusions.

These hygienic measures cannot be supplanted by administering antibiotics. Routine prophylactic use of antibiotics should be condemned; it does not reduce infection and does favor growth of resistant organisms. On the other hand, antibiotics are still a powerful weapon against infection when the causative organism and its bacterial resistance are known.

All newborns, and especially premature infants, are prime candidates for septicemia when exposed to pathogenic organisms. Neonatal sepsis is often difficult to diagnose, heralded by such non-specific findings as unstable body temperature, hypothermia, poor peripheral circulation, anemia, jaundice, shock, hypotonia, vomiting, attacks of hypoglycemia, thrombopenia and leukopenia. If several of these symptoms occur together, one must consider giving antibiotics even if the causative organism is as yet obscure. The same holds true if it is known that the mother harbored an infection during labor.

Special Conditions

Aspiration of Foreign Bodies

Acute attacks of suffocation, coughing, stridor, dyspnea or cyanosis in a small child often signify that he has aspirated a foreign body. As a rule the respiratory sounds are diminished on the affected side of the thorax (usually the right side); percussion hyperresonance and radiographic overinflation support the diagnosis. Initially a valvular mechanism exists which allows inspiration but inhibits expiration. It usually takes several days or weeks before the bronchus becomes completely blocked to produce atelectasis.

Hanging the child head down and percussing his back are not usually successful in dislodging a foreign body from the hypopharynx or larynx; since there is imminent danger of suffocation an attempt should be made to remove the foreign body with the finger. The extremely dyspneic child should be given positive pressure respiration through a mask or mouth-to-mouth breathing until an endoscope can be passed to remove the foreign body. This allows sufficient ventilation even if spontaneous respiration has ceased. Endoscopic removal of the foreign body should be carried out as soon as possible, but is rarely emergent.

Pneumothorax

This condition may develop after thoracic trauma (Chapters 4 and 22), major upper abdominal operations or during assisted ventilation through an endotracheal tube. An extensive pneumothorax can be diagnosed clinically: hypertympany, decreased breath sounds and contralateral shift of the trachea and heart. Tension pneumothorax is especially dangerous, requiring immediate treatment perhaps even before radiographic confirmation of diagnosis. A pneumothorax can also develop while a patient with deficient compliance of the lungs is on a respirator.

Posttrauma pneumothorax is treated by inserting a chest tube connected to underwater seal drainage. A tension pneumothorax may be punctured immediately with a thick bore needle, through which a thin catheter is passed for drainage. Only in a quite small pneumothorax is a single aspiration with needle and syringe justified.

The combination of pneumothorax, pneumomediastinum and pneumopericardium is not uncommon in small children. In newborn infants pneumopericardium can be treated by percutaneous introduction of a tube. Most cases of severe mediastinal air and subcutaneous emphysema are cured by tube draining the pneumothorax and giving the patient 100 % oxygen to breathe; this must not be done in newborn infants because of the danger of retrolental fibroplasia.

Drainage of a pneumothorax is more efficient and expansion of the lungs occurs more quickly if suction is employed rather than the simpler underwater drainage. The strength of the suction depends on the patient's size and condition. As a rule a negative suction of between 30 and 40 cm of water is sufficient. The tube is removed when no further accumulation of air or fluid occurs after the tube has been clamped for several hours.

4 Respiratory Distress Syndrome

U. G. STAUFFER

Anatomy

The respiratory tract of infants is anatomically different from that of adults. Serious respiratory disturbances occur quickly and may have grave consequences:

1) The respiratory tract is relatively narrow in diameter and inflammatory processes, foreign bodies or tumors very quickly obstruct it.

2) Newborns' ribs lie horizontally, the intercostal muscles are relatively underdeveloped and respiratory exchange is achieved by the respiratory diaphragm. The ability to compensate for respiratory distress by respiratory muscles, therefore, is small.

3) The thorax of newborns is narrow and relatively malleable, and excessive respiratory force may cause its deformation (retraction).

4) In small infants the abdomen is relatively large. Additional enlargement by increased intraabdominal pressure (mechanical and paralytic ileus, ascites, hepatomegaly, etc.) may quickly inhibit diaphragmatic descent and thereby directly impair respiratory exchange.

5) The oxygen requirements of infants and children are up to 50 % greater than that of adults.

Clinical Symptoms

The respiratory distress syndrome of the newborn presents clinically with tachypnea, dyspnea and in serious cases with cyanosis.

Tachypnea

By definition tachypnea refers to an abnormally rapid respiratory rate. The newborn infant normally breathes about 30 times per minute and the adult 10 to 15 times per minute.

Cyanosis

Severe respiratory distress results in cyanosis. Cyanosis indicates that more than 5 g % of hemoglobin are not combined with oxygen. Therefore, patients with severe breathing difficulties who have a low hemoglobin level may not exhibit cyanosis which would be severe if the same patient had a very high hemoglobin concentration.

Gasping, Gurgling, Stridor

If the respiratory obstruction is situated at the level of the nasal passages (posterior choanal atresia or stenosis) a gasping type respiratory pattern is seen. If the obstruction lies in the pharynx (large tongue, underdeveloped lower jaw) a gurgling noise is common. If the respiratory obstruction is found in the area of the larynx and upper trachea, an inspiratory stridor occurs. If both inspiratory and expiratory stridor are present, the obstruction involves the trachea.

Dyspnea

In newborns and older infants laborious and difficult breathing manifests itself by retraction of the thoracic wall and of the supraclavicular fossae during inspiration. Children with a moderate dyspnea often appear anxious and restless. In serious cases an increasing apathy is present ("CO_2 anesthesia").

Causes of Dyspnea

Most dyspneic newborns have problems which are mainly of medical interest (asphyxia neonatorum, aspiration, hyaline membrane disease, etc.). Similarly, medical problems cause most cases of dyspnea in older babies and small children (infections of the upper respiratory tract, laryngismus stridulus, bronchitis, pneumonia, aspiration of foreign bodies, etc.). Only a few cases are of surgical import.

Emergency Treatment

In serious or dangerous cases of dyspnea no time should be lost over etiological considerations. If respiration is unsatisfactory, mechanical respiration must be started. Mouth-to-mouth or mouth-to-nose insufflation by trained helpers is helpful in emergencies which occur outside hospital. Every medical student must be proficient in this technique. The length of the first asphyxial phase is often decisive for the quality of survival. In hospital, emergency intubation and artificial respiration may save a life. Emergency tracheotomy can practically always be dispensed with later.

Surgical Causes for Respiratory Disturbances in Newborn Children and Small Infants

A small percentage of newborns and small babies harbor respiratory disturbance which is amenable to surgery. These are mostly congenital malformations at sites somewhere between the nose or mouth and the diaphragm. The most important ones are discussed below.

Posterior Choanal Atresia

In choanal atresia the normal connection of the posterior nasal passageway with the nasopharynx is blocked. The blocking septum usually consists of bone or cartilage, but in 10 to 20 % of cases is composed only of a mucous membrane. The atresia may be either unilateral or bilateral.

Bilateral Choanal Atresia

Clinical Symptoms. The newborn instinctively breathes through the nose. Only later does he learn to breathe through the mouth. A baby with bilateral choanal atresia may therefore die of asphyxia. Immediately after birth these infants make enormous efforts to breathe, showing intercostal and supraclavicular retractions, becoming blue and sucking the lower lip inwards.

Treatment. An oral tube or a nipple with the end cut off immediately relieves this emergency and the babies start to breathe normally. To confirm the diagnosis a fine rubber tube is then inserted through both nostrils; if it does not reach the pharynx, the nasal passage is filled with contrast medium to confirm diagnosis radiologically (Fig. 4.1). Operative correction is generally performed transpalatally; postoperatively, the choanae are splinted for several weeks with inlying plastic tubes (Fig. 4.2).

Unilateral Choanal Atresia

Unilateral choanal atresia is a little more common than the bilateral variety. The clinical symptoms are less typical and less impressive. Difficulties occur with breastfeeding when the patent nostril is compressed. Later, there is a constant discharge from the appropriate nostril and a tendency to sinusitis. Unilateral choanal atresia is operated on in the same way as bilateral choanal atresia. The condition is usually recognized in older children.

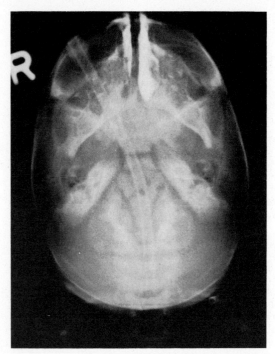

Fig. 4.1.   Bilateral choanal atresia outlined by contrast medium which does not flow from the nose into the pharynx

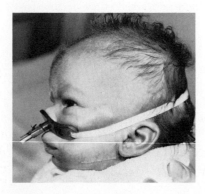

Fig. 4.2.   Splinting with tubes after operation for choanal atresia

Pierre Robin Syndrome

This syndrome combines a hypoplastic lower jaw with cleft palate. The small mandible and its attached tongue are relatively unfixed, airway obstruction ensuing when the tongue prolapses back into the thorax when the baby lies supine.

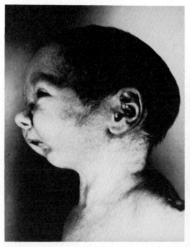

a

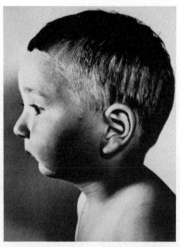

b

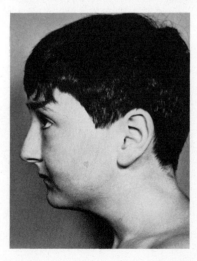

c

Fig. 4.3. Pierre Robin Syndrome:
a) in the newborn,
b) same child when 2 years old,
c) same child when 12 years old. The mandible has grown considerably

Clinical Signs

Children with a Pierre Robin syndrome may show dangerous respiratory disturbances in the neonatal period. The posterior position of the tongue causes severe breathing difficulties with gurgling, stridor, tachypnea, dyspnea and cyanosis. In severe cases difficulties in feeding occur characterized by attacks of choking and asphyxia.

Treatment

Placing the newborn child in the prone position prevents or relieves the acute airway obstruction. The babies are difficult to nurse and supervision by trained staff in an appropriately equipped center is essential. Seriously ill children have to be fed through a nasogastric tube for several weeks. A small dental plate prevents the tongue from gliding upwards through the cleft into the nasopharyngeal space, and often after several weeks normal peroral feeding becomes possible. Mild cases of Pierre Robin syndrome have only drinking difficulties, which are easily prevented with the aid of a dental plate. The babies should be fed in the prone position. In time, the lower jaw recovers from its retardation of growth (Fig. 4.3). At the age of 2 to 3 years the cleft palate is repaired in the usual way.

Pleuroperitoneal Diaphragmatic Hernia

The incidence of diaphragmatic hernia is about 1 in 1000 stillbirths and 1 in 3000 live births. This is the most urgent emergency in the whole spectrum of neonatal surgery. An arrest in diaphragmatic development during the 8th to 10th week of pregnancy causes in-

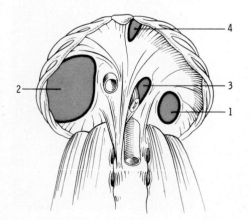

Fig. 4.4. Congenital defects in the diaphragm.
1) posterolateral defect (Bochdalek),
2) right-sided defect,
3) hiatal defect,
4) sternocostal defect (Morgagni)

complete separation of the pleural from the abdominal cavity by the diaphragm. There is a hole in the diaphragm usually in its left posterolateral aspect (Fig. 4.4). During inuterine life the abdominal viscera migrate upwards through this hole, filling the pleural cavity with the whole of the small intestine, portions of colon, the spleen and sometimes even the left lobe of the liver (Fig. 4.5). After birth the intestines start to fill with swallowed air. The lung on the affected side collapses, and heart and mediastinum are displaced towards the opposite side. Additional compression atelectasis of the lung on the opposite side thus ensues often causing death of the patient within a few minutes or hours after birth. Nearly half the afflicted babies die before reaching a pediatric surgical center. The causes of death given are usually neonatal asphyxia, aspiration, prematurity, etc., but post mortem documents the true cause. These very grave cases exhibit extensive diaphragmatic defects. The complete hemidiaphragm is sometimes not developed at all. The lung is often hypoplastic, commonly on the affected side, but also sometimes on the opposite side.

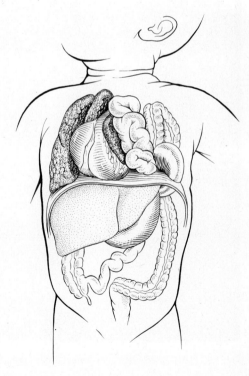

Fig. 4.5.
Left-sided pleuroperitoneal diaphragmatic hernia. The spleen and most of the small and large intestine are in the left hemithorax. The mediastinal structures are shifted to the right side

Clinical Features

Shortly after birth babies with a pleuroperitoneal hernia usually exhibit quickly worsening dyspnea and cyanosis. Breath sounds are absent on the affected side and intermittent intestinal gurgling is often heard. Diagnosis is confirmed by radiography (Fig. 4.6).

Treatment

In distinction to most major surgical anomalies in newborns, babies with diaphragmatic hernia often travel badly. At the start of the

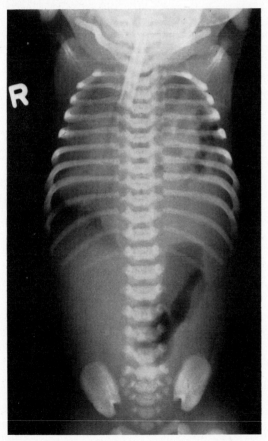

a) Roentgenogram 3 hours after birth with intestinal shadows in the left hemithorax, shifting of the mediastinum towards the right and compression of right lung. There is little air in the abdomen

Fig. 4.6.   Left-sided pleuroperitoneal diaphragmatic hernia.

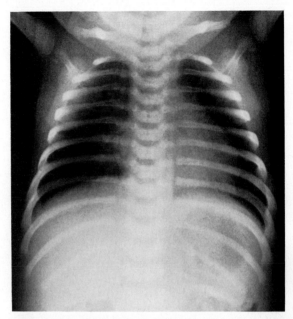

Fig. 4.6.   b) Same patient 14 days after succesful operation

journey the baby may be pink and only slightly tachypneic; within minutes his condition can drastically deteriorate so that upon arrival at a treatment center the baby may be moribund or already dead. Therefore, the measures taken immediately after establishing diagnosis and during transport are of the utmost importance.

1. A catheter is introduced through the nose into the stomach. Every 5 minutes this catheter is aspirated with a syringe. The suction prevents distention of the stomach and intestines with swallowed air.

2. Intubation and artificial respiration must be started. Artificial respiration with a mask must be avoided, since some air always enters the stomach and the child's condition may deteriorate even further. The respiratory pressure is often so high that a pneumothorax may develop as an additional complication. This possibility must be taken into consideration if the condition of the child deteriorates during transport. Puncture of the pleural cavity with a needle to let the air out may save the patient's life. During transport the child should be nursed on the affected side, which facilitates artificial respiration of the normal lung.

In serious cases, operation must be started immediately on arrival at hospital. Most surgeons operate through an abdominal incision.

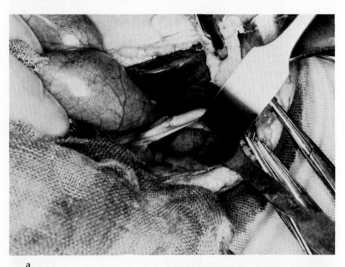

a

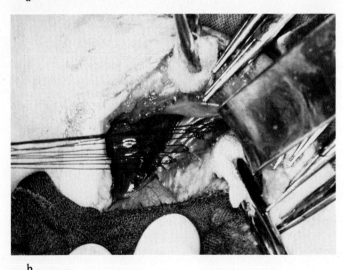

b

Fig. 4.7.   Same patient as in Fig. 4.6. a) Abdominal view during operation: intestine still partly in thorax. b) The defect has been closed

After the herniated viscera are returned to the abdominal cavity, the dangerous respiratory status immediately improves. In most cases the diaphragmatic defect is closed easily by suturing together its edges (Fig. 4.7). If this is not possible, a prothesis of plastic material is inserted, or a muscle flap may be used to bridge the hole in the diaphragm.

Prognosis

In large series the chances of survival are about 50 %. This high mortality rate is occasioned by additional associated malformations, cardiac defects, hypoplasia of the lung, premature and small-for-date babies. Delayed diagnosis and incorrect emergency treatment may cause death of the patient.

Diaphragmatic Eventration

Congenital eventration of the diaphragm is generally defined as an abnormal elevation of part or all of a hemidiaphragm in a newborn. The cause is either failure of the diaphragm to muscularize properly,

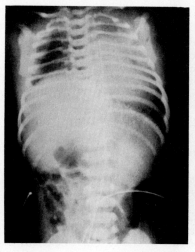 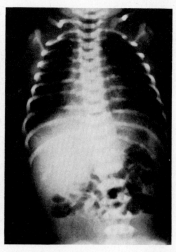

a) Massive eventration right; shifting of mediastinum to left: Paradoxical movements of diaphragm on screening

b) result of operation 6 months later.

Fig. 4.8.   Right-sided diaphragmatic eventration following birth trauma: there was a phrenic nerve palsy

or a traumatic phrenic nerve paralysis produced during delivery. The latter usually occurs with a brachial plexus paresis (Erb-Duchenne). In very severe cases the clinical course of a baby with diaphragmatic eventration may be as dramatic as that of the pleuroperitoneal diaphragmatic hernia. The paradoxic respiration of the affected diaphragm is largely responsible for the dangerous respiratory disturbances. Mild cases exhibit only tachypnea and feeding difficulties. Radiography of the thorax establishes diagnosis (Fig. 4.8).

These children are subject to recurrent infections of the upper respiratory disturbances. Older children tolerate a unilaterally elevated diaphragm relatively well.

Treatment

Operative plication of the diaphragm may be lifesaving in seriously afflicted newborns. In babies who are only mildly symptomatic, it may be extremely difficult to decide if a diaphragmatic eventration should be treated conservatively or operatively.

Esophageal Atresia

This is a relatively common malformation (1 in 3000 births). It is caused by a developmental defect of the tracheo-esophageal septum which forms during the 4th to 6th week of pregnancy. In 90 % of cases the proximal esophageal pouch ends blindly and there is a distal tracheo-esophageal fistula (type 3a and 3b) (Fig. 4.9). As the fetus is unable to swallow and thus to absorb amniotic fluid in utero, the mothers usually suffer from hydramnios.

Babies with esophageal atresia are unable to swallow their saliva and commonly develop laryngotracheal aspiration. This is dangerous, especially in premature infants with underdeveloped swallow and cough reflexes. However, a more serious problem is the tracheo-esophageal fistula. With each cry there is a forced expiration against the closed glottis; this increases intratracheal pressure so that air is forced through the fistula to dilate the stomach. If the intragastric pressure is high and the baby does not cry, stomach contents reflux into the lungs. Relative incompetence of the stomach, especially in the premature child, facilitates regurgitation.

Clinical Features

Soon after birth infants with esophageal atresia exhibit excess salivation, dyspnea, cough and at times cyanosis. Attempts to feed aggra-

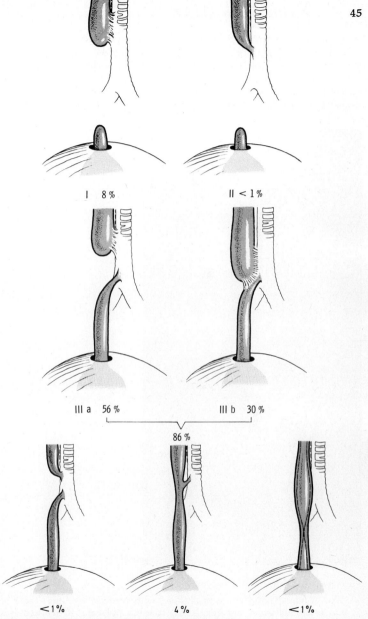

I 8 %   II < 1 %

III a 56 %   III b 30 %

86 %

<1%   4 %   <1%

Fig. 4.9. The various types of esophageal atresia

vate these symptoms and the feeding is regurgitated through mouth and nose. Aspiration occurs quite frequently. If diagnosis is not promptly made, prognosis is worsened due to additional lung complications. Some neonatologists routinely pass a catheter into the stomach of each newborn; the diagnosis of esophageal atresia is made in babies only a few minutes of age if this attempt fails.

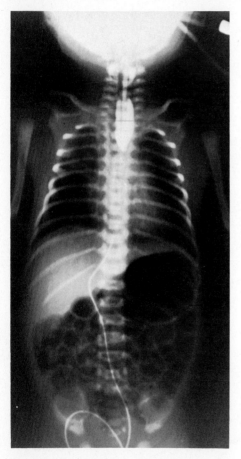

Fig. 4.10.   Esophageal atresia type 3 b:

a) The proximal blind pouch is outlined with contrast medium; there is air in the abdomen and therefore a tracheoesophageal fistula must be present

Treatment

The first measures that are taken in the maternity hospital often decide the fate of babies with esophageal atresia. The following measures are recommended:

1) A fine catheter is passed through the nose into the blind upper pouch. Every 10 minutes the secretions are aspirated via this catheter. This prevents laryngotracheal aspiration.

2) The baby is placed in the prone position with the head lower than the rest of the body, in order to avoid aspiration.

3) Radiographic confirmation of diagnosis is not necessary.

4) The baby is transported as an emergency to the nearest pediatric surgical center.

Treatment in the Pediatric Surgical Center

The diagnosis is confirmed by passing a stiff nasopharyngeal tube which will arrest about 10 cm from the tip of the nose. In most

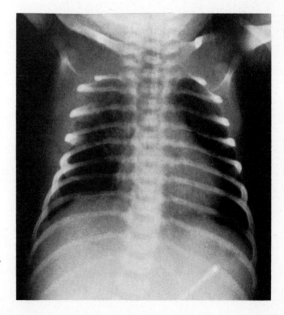

b) The proximal blind pouch is outlined by air blown into it through a catheter

centers no confirmation of diagnosis by contrast media is carried out; if so, the patient is first intubated (Fig. 4.10). The blind pouch is usually outlined just as well by air injected through the nasopharyngeal tube, or by using a simple radiopaque catheter. A roentgenogram shows the level of the proximal blind pouch (Fig. 4.10). Air in the stomach indicates the presence of a tracheo-esophageal fistula.

Term infants in good condition are treated by surgical ligation of the tracheo-esophageal fistula and primary end-to-end anastomosis of the two esophageal segments (Fig. 4.11). Premature infants or

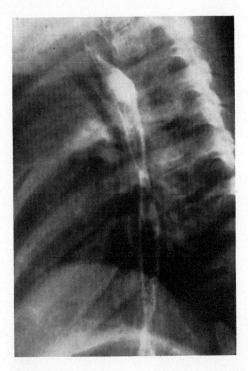

Fig. 4.11. Esophageal atresia type 3 b: primary end-to-end anastomosis; barium swallow radiograph taken 10 days postoperatively. The anastomosis is still somewhat narrow. The child drinks normally

those with anatomically difficult problems or associated anomalies are treated only by fistula ligation and gastrostomy. The definitive corrective operation is performed at a later date. If the distance between the upper and lower esophageal pouches is too large, a segment of colon or stomach may have to be interposed later (Fig. 4.12).

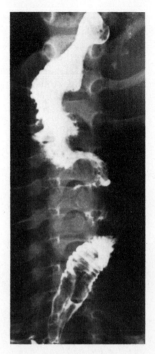

Fig. 4.12. Esophageal atresia type 1. The wide distance between the two segments has been bridged by a piece of colon. Barium swallow radiograph 6 months after operation. The child has no complaints

Prognosis

This depends on the individual case. A term baby harboring the most common type of esophageal atresia (Fig. 4.8) without additional malformations or preoperative aspiration pneumonia enjoys a 90 % chance of survival. Unfortunately, about half of the babies with esophageal atresia also possess other malformations. These associated malformations are so serious that in a quarter of the babies they endanger life and influence the prognosis extensively. One fourth of the babies with esophageal atresia have birth weights less than 2500 gram. These patients suffer the additional complications caused by the low birth weight (respiratory distress syndrome, intracranial hemorrhage).

Congenital Lobar Emphysema

This is relatively rare. It produces a quickly-increasing distention of one or (rarely) several lobes of the lungs. A rapidly worsening respiratory distress syndrome with dyspnea and cyanosis develops shortly after birth in seriously afflicted babies. Diminished breath sounds and hyperresonance to percussion herald the disease clinically. Radiography reveals massive distention of the affected lung (Fig. 4.13). Careful examination prevents confusing a tension pneumothorax with lobar emphysema. In lobar emphysema the lungs extend to the thoracic wall; the left upper lobe is most frequently affected, less often the right middle lobe and least often the right upper lobe (Fig. 4.13). Involvement of both lower lobes is very rare.

Etiology of the condition is obscure in over half the cases. Pathological examination shows disturbances in the anatomy of the bronchial wall with dysplasia of the cartilages, folds in the mucous membrane, etc. in about 50 % of cases. Extrinsic obstruction of the bronchus leading to the involved lobe is occasionally produced by an abnormal vessel.

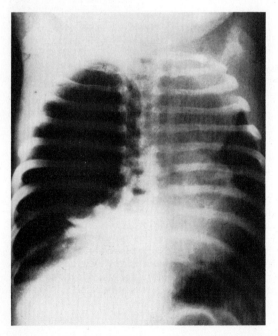

Fig. 4.13.   Congenital lobar emphysema of the right upper and middle lobes:
a) Preoperatively: the right lower lobe is atelectatic. The mediastinum is shifted to the left

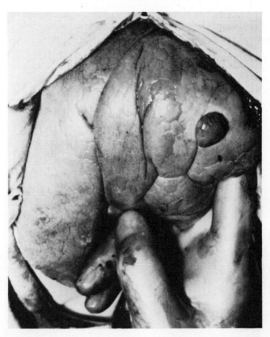

b) Operative findings in the same patient as a. Massive distention of upper and middle lobes

Emergency lobectomy of the affected lobe of the lung is the treatment of choice.

The Respiratory Distress Syndrome in the Small Child

Aspiration of a Foreign Body

Sudden occurrence of dyspnea in an older infant or young child often indicates aspiration of a foreign body. Aspiration of parts of a nut, especially peanuts, are relatively common. The foreign body may lodge in one of the larger bronchi, usually in the right lung. The children show increasing dyspnea, diminished respiratory exchange in the involved part of the lung and sometimes expiratory stridor and a hyperresonant percussion note on the affected side. Radiography of the thorax initially reveals distention of the affected lobe (Fig.

4.14); on inspiration air still flows into the lobe, but on expiration it does not flow out, the foreign body acting in a valve-like manner. If obstruction becomes complete due to inflammatory reaction, atelectasis and pneumonia develop. If diagnosis is delayed a lobectomy may have to be performed at a later date.

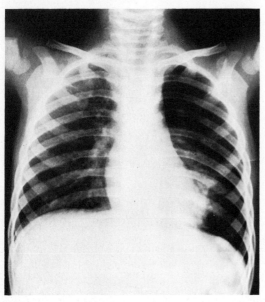

Fig. 4.14. Aspiration of a peanut. Overexpansion of the left upper lobe. Partial atelectasis of left lower lobe. Shift of the mediastinum toward the right

Empyema

During or following an episode of pneumonia a pleural empyema may develop. Most frequently this complicates the dreaded staphylococcal pneumonia of infants. If a pleural empyema cannot be effectively drained within a period of 3 weeks, operative decortication may be necessary; the pyogenous membranes and adhesions of the lung to the thoracic cage have to be completely removed. If neglected, a thick fibrous coat envelops the lung to inhibit its respiratory excursion and may subsequently lead to scoliosis (for further information see textbooks on pediatrics).

The Respiratory Distress Syndrome in Older Children and Adolescents

Respiratory distress syndrome is relatively rare in older children and adolescents. Most common is a spontaneous pneumothorax (Fig. 4.15), which is heralded by sudden, acute pleuritic in the involved chest, with dyspnea. Frequently, spontaneous rupture of small congenital pulmonary cysts produce spontaneous pneumothorax. These are usually located in the upper lobes, suddenly bursting to cause a leak of air into the pleural cavity. Within minutes a dangerous ten-

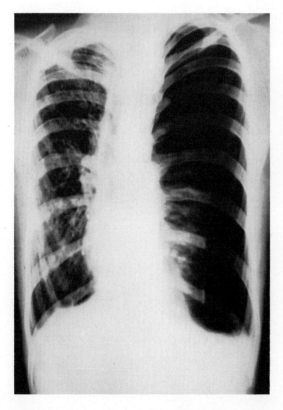

Fig. 4.15.   Spontaneous pneumothorax left (12-year-old boy). Shift of the mediastinum toward the right

sion pneumothorax results. Emergency puncture of the pleural cavity with a needle is lifesaving. In hospital spontaneous pneumothorax is treated by a chest tube connected to under water suction drainage. Recurrent pneumothorax may require obliteration of the pleural space by injection of an irritating fluid, i. e. 10 % glucose solution.

5 Vomiting

R. T. SOPER

Introduction

General

Vomiting is one of the most common manifestations of disease throughout infancy and childhood. Vomiting occurs from such diverse causes as dietary indiscretions, teething, systemic infections and appendicitis. The act itself, therefore, cannot be ascribed exclusively to gastrointestinal disease. However, vomiting that persists or recurs generally implies gastrointestinal disease.

There are many important characteristics in the vomiting pattern which suggest diagnosis and aid in planning treatment:

Color of Vomitus

Clear vomitus. Cloudy, grayish vomitus of a very low pH is invariably of gastric origin. Partially altered food in the vomitus elevates its pH. Persistent vomiting in this pure pattern implies obstruction proximal to the ampulla of Vater.

Bilious vomiting. Bile in vomitus generally has a near-neutral pH and implies a free regurgitation of intestinal contents across the pylorus. Bilious vomiting is associated with intestinal obstruction anywhere downstream from the ampulla of Vater or with paralytic ileus.

Bloody vomitus. Blood in the vomitus implies mucosal ulceration at some point proximal to the ligament of Treitz. Bright red vomitus indicates active, arterial bleeding and is associated with a higher incidence of hypovolemia and shock than when the blood is of venous origin and maroon in color. Regardless of origin, if the blood remains in the stomach for more than a few minutes before being vomited it is broken down by gastric acid and enzymes to form the classic "coffeegrounds" appearance of altered blood. Effortless regurgitation of bright red blood usually implies esophageal origin, as from bleeding esophageal varices.

Feculant vomitus. Vomitus which has the appearance and odor of feces simply implies lengthy stagnation, generally within small bowel loops, wherein bacterial action ferments the succus entericus. It must be clearly distinguished from actual fecal vomiting, which only occurs in the rare gastrocolic fistula.

Volume and pH of the Vomitus

The volume and pH of the vomitus dictate the systemic effects from loss of body fluids, and guide replacement therapy. Dehydration and electrolyte imbalances arise within a matter of hours, and are quantitatively more severe the younger the patient. Pure gastric outlet obstruction produces the classical hypochloremic, hypokalemic alkalotic dehydration occasioned by a pure loss of hydrogen, potassium and chloride ions and water; a saline solution containing potassium is used in treatment. Bilious vomiting produces a more balanced electrolyte and pH loss repaired with a more balanced electrolyte solution, such as lactated Ringer's solution. Bloody vomitus demands replacement with whole blood.

The Act of Vomiting

Vomitus that trails out of the corner of the mouth effortlessly, especially when the patient is supine, suggests simple gastroesophageal reflux (chalasia or hiatus hernia). At the other extreme is the projectile vomiting so characteristic of all forms of gastric outlet obstruction, of which hypertrophic pyloric stenosis is the classic example. In this condition the vomitus is forcefully projected out of the mouth, often arching over the side of the crib to baptize the floor or interested parties standing nearby. In between these extremes is vomiting of ordinary force.

Abdominal Contour

Abdominal contour often suggests the location and nature of the disease producing the vomiting. A sunken, scaphoid abdomen suggests a very high obstruction in the gastrointestinal tract, with collapsed distal bowel. At the other extreme, a grossly distended abdomen with shiny skin and visible subcutaneous veins implies either a mechanical obstruction well distal in the bowel (terminal ileum or colon) or a paralytic ileus stagnating gas and fluid throughout the gastrointestinal tract. A distended epigastrium suggests obstruction in the proximal small intestine, whereas lower abdominal distention implies an obstructed colon with a competent ileocecal valve that allows no regurgitation back into the small intestine. A generally distended abdomen dull to percussion suggests fluid either within bowel loops or the peritoneal cavity, whereas a tympanitic percussion note occurs with gas within bowel or peritoneum.

Bowel Function

Not surprisingly, bowel function relates inversely to the volume and duration of vomiting. With complete bowel obstruction, once the distal bowel is completely evacuated, no further gas or stool is passed per rectum. Partial bowel obstruction produces less severe vomiting, with an occasional small stool passed per rectum. Severe paralytic ileus generally is associated with complete obstipation.

Neonatal Vomiting

First Two Weeks of Life

General

Persistent neonatal vomiting has a different and often more serious significance than vomiting at any later period in life. First, the newborn suffers more from vomiting than older children because of low body fluid, electrolyte and nutritional reserves. Further, the newborn tends to aspirate vomitus to trigger cardiopulmonary arrest, a disaster best prevented by effective gastric decompression. Nearly one-third of vomiting newborns are premature, further complicating the problem. These factors combine to interject a sense of urgency for prompt diagnosis and management of the vomiting newborn.

Workup

The vomiting neonate needs to have his stomach evacuated to obviate aspiration of vomitus. This is best achieved by passing a #14 French catheter through the mouth and into the stomach for hand-aspirating the stomach to retrieve the curds and particles that obstruct tubes of finer caliber. Then, a fine nasogastric tube can be taped into place for intermittent or continuous aspiration.

Next, blood is drawn for appropriate laboratory studies and a dependable route for administering intravenous fluids is established. Appropriate fluids and electrolytes are then infused, tailored to body needs as judged by clinical and laboratory evaluation.

The history should query the family members for inheritable causes of vomiting: Hirschsprung's disease, mongolism with its propensity for congenital duodenal atresia, cystic fibrosis and its association with meconium ileus. Also, the history should evaluate the first trimester of pregnancy for exposure of the mother and fetus to teratogenic drugs, irradiation, viral infections, etc., as well as questions regarding oligodramnios and polyhydramnios. Anything that upsets the cyclic flow of amniotic fluid in utero (swallowed by the fetus, absorbed in the proximal half of the fetal small bowel, circulated as tissue fluid, plasma and cerebrospinal fluid, and finally manufactured into urine by the kidneys and excreted back into the amniotic sac) alters this delicate balance, producing abnormalities of amniotic fluid volume.

History of the color, volume and duration of vomiting and the passage of meconium provide additional clues as to the cause of the vomiting, as indicated above. Pigmented meconium implies staining by bile, which begins to enter the fetal intestine at the end of the first trimester of pregnancy. Pale, grayish meconium therefore implies an obstruction which originated somewhere distal to the ampulla of Vater during the first trimester of gestation. Evaluating dehydration, abdominal contour, palpation and auscultation of the abdomen and a carefully performed rectal digital exam (using the little finger) are the key features of the physical examination. A complete blood count, urinalysis, serum electrolyte studies and plain upright radiographs of the chest and abdomen complete the workup of the obstructed newborn, pinpointing the problem accurately enough to launch definitive therapy. Non-intestinal causes for the vomiting are unearthed, and mechanical intestinal obstruction sites are bracketed accurately enough to allow laparotomy, where more precise diagnosis and appropriate surgical care is carried out. Rarely are radiocontrast studies of the gastrointestinal tract necessary.

Salvage

Table 5.1 estimates the salvage rate of newborns with congenital gastrointestinal obstruction. The salvage rate is very good when the baby is term and harbors no other major anomalies. When the baby is both premature and suffers from other congenital anomalies, the salvage rate is very poor. The influence of opening the bowel is clear from this table, as is the inability of the newborn to fight bacterial peritonitis secondary to gastrointestinal obstruction. The overall salvage rate of 75 % is twice what it was 15 years ago.

Table 5.1. **Survival Rates of Neonates with Congenital Malformations of the Gastrointestinal Tract.**

Full term, no additional malformations	95 %
Premature, dysmature, additional severe malformations	10 %
Intestine opened during operation	60 %
Intestine not opened during operation	90 %
Peritonitis	50 %
Total survival rate	75 %

At present, delay in diagnosis is the only one of these variables that physicians can influence. Expediency of diagnosis cannot be over-emphasized. The most common cause of death in an obstructed new-born is aspiration of vomitus into the lungs, triggering acute cardio-pulmonary arrest. This disaster is avoided by effective decompression of the stomach. Perforation of an obstructed intestine occurs with delay in diagnosis (Fig. 5.1) resulting in death of half the newborns with this dread complication.

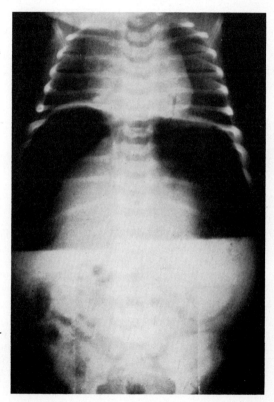

Fig. 5.1.
Upright plain radio-graph revealing a huge air fluid level in a newborn with massive perforation of bowel

Specific Entities

Non-Surgical

Some of the more common non-surgical causes for neonatal vomiting are listed below (Table 5.2):

Table 5.2.   **Continuous Vomiting in the Neonatal Period: Medical Causes.**

Feeding problems:
>   too much, too little

Infection:
>   intestinal, extraintestinal

Intracranial pressure:
>   intracranial hemorrhage, cerebral edema, hydrocephalus

Urinary tract malformations

Endocrine and metabolic disturbances:
>   adrenogenital syndrome
>   hypoglycemia, galactosemia, glycogenesis etc.
>   tetany

Gastrointestinal allergy

Miscellaneous:
>   chalasia, pylorospasm

Feeding Problems

Newborns who are overfed or not burped properly after feeding tend to spit up small amounts of non-digested milk. Underfed babies swallow considerable air with crying and may reflect this by spitting up, as well as exhibiting a distended abdominal contour. Commercial formulas that are mixed improperly (generally less water being added than necessary, producing a hypertonic feeding) often have vomiting as one manifestation of the resultant serum osmolar abnormalities.

Septicemia

Systemic infection, whatever the source or organism, is associated with vomiting and abdominal distention, due probably to paralytic ileus. A low white blood cell count, jaundice and blood cultures help in diagnosis.

Increased Cerebrospinal Pressure

Elevated intracerebral pressure from whatever the cause (birth trauma with cerebral edema and bleeding, hydrocephalus) generally produces vomiting as part of its clinical manifestation. Careful examination of the fontanelle and neurologic system help in diagnosis.

Obstructive Uropathy

Congenital anomalies interfering with the flow of urine produce rapidly progressive uremia postnatally, with vomiting as one expression of the uremic state. Blood urea nitrogen, urinalysis and intravenous pyelography help sort out this cause of neonatal vomiting.

Maternal Drug Dependency

Babies born of mothers who are hard drug addicts often develop withdrawal symptoms of abdominal distention and vomiting, jittery episodes and convulsions during the first few days of life.

Endocrine and Metabolic Factors

The adrenogenital syndrome, hypoglycemia and neonatal tetany can produce vomiting, often with abdominal distention. Evaluation of serum electrolytes, glucose and calcium help in diagnosis.

Cardiac Malformations

Often present in the newborn with vomiting and failure to thrive.

Surgical Causes of Neonatal GI Obstruction

A glance at Table 5.3 indicates that atresias are responsible for the majority of congenital neonatal gastrointestinal obstructions. The word "atresia" implies a complete congenital obstruction, either with a separation of the two ends of bowel or with a mucosal diaphragm (external continuity of the bowel preserved). Incomplete mucosal membranes produce only partial obstruction. It is clear that the extreme ends of the gastrointestinal tract (esophagus and ano-

Table 5.3.   **Neonatal Intestinal Obstruction.**

Atresia		80 %
Esophagus	30 %	
Anorectal	30 %	
Small intestine	20 %	
Hirschsprung's disease		10 %
Malrotation		6 %
Meconium ileus		2 %
Others		2 %

rectum) are more commonly involved than the intervening bowel. Atresia of the duodenum is likely a retention of the "solid stage" of embryonic intestinal development (the "solid stage" is present only in the duodenum of the human embryo) coupled with the complex splitting away of the pancreaticobiliary tree from the duodenum. Vascular insufficiency to the developing fetal intestine is the clear and reproducible cause of the atresia of the jejunum, ileum and colon.

Hirschsprung's disease is the most common non-mechanical cause of neonatal gastrointestinal obstruction. Midgut rotational problems and obstruction to the ileum of inspissated, undigested meconium (meconium ileus secondary to cystic fibrosis of the pancreas) round out the more common causes of neonatal gastrointestinal obstruction.

Esophageal Obstruction

Esophageal atresia is the only common cause (see Chapter 4).

Obstructions of the stomach and pylorus

Truly neonatal obstructions of the stomach and pylorus by membranes are extremely rare. Persistent clear vomiting is the clinical hallmark and plain or contrast radiographs confirm diagnosis. Surgical resection or bypass suffices for therapy.

Duodenal Obstructions

For its relatively short length, the neonatal duodenum is more commonly obstructed by a greater diversity of mechanisms than any similar length of bowel between the esophagus and anorectum.

Atresia and Stenosis. Atresia (and stenosis) is the most common cause of congenital duodenal obstruction. Regrettably, about 25 % of the cases occur in mongoloid babies. The majority of atresias are juxtaposed to the ampulla of Vater. If the obstruction lies below the ampulla, the vomitus is consistently bile-stained but it is clear in the smaller fraction of cases where the obstruction is proximal to the ampulla. Mild epigastric distention characterizes all forms of congenital duodenal obstruction. Upright plain radiographs of the abdomen and chest reveal the classic "double bubble" sign: air-fluid levels within stomach and duodenum, respectively (Fig. 5.2). Absence of downstream gas indicates that the obstruction is complete (atresia), whereas small driblets of gas downstream imply an incomplete obstruction (stenosis). Small amounts of pigmented meconium may be passed per rectum even in the face of complete duodenal obstruction from atresia, indicating that the obstruction occurred in utero after bile had passed into the distal bowel.

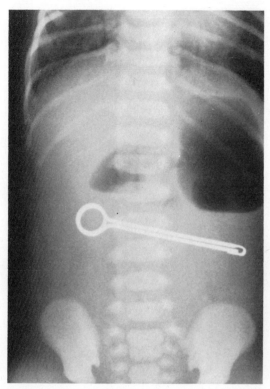

Fig. 5.2.
Upright plain radiograph in a newborn with bilious vomiting; the two air fluid levels (in stomach and duodenum only) characterize complete congenital duodenal obstruction

The diagnosis is verified at laparotomy (Fig. 5.3), and surgical treatment is directed toward bypassing the obstruction by anastomosing the duodenum just upstream from the atresia to the duodenum just downstream. Duodenojejunostomy is also acceptable.

Midgut Malrotation

Rotational problems of the midgut constitute the second most common cause of congenital duodenal obstruction. Since the obstruction is occasioned by an extrinsic band, it is often incomplete. The vomitus is bile-stained; vomiting is intermittent if the obstruction is only partial. In high grade obstruction plain radiographs show the same "double bubble" picture as duodenal atresia; this study only documents the *site* and *completeness* of the obstruction, not its cause. Radiocontrast studies of the colon provide additional clues suggesting

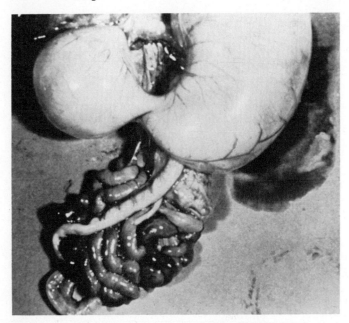

Fig. 5.3.   Duodenal atresia with loss of duodenal continuity

the duodenal obstructions which are due to malrotation rather than atresia. Since there is real urgency in the surgical correction of malrotation, this additional information often expedites treatment.

To understand midgut malrotation, one must first understand normal midgut rotation. During the first three weeks of gestational life, the gastrointestinal tract is a midline, straight tube suspended by both dorsal and ventral mesenteries (Fig. 5.4). The ventral mesentery disappears except for the definitive gastrohepatic ligament. During the fourth gestational week, the stomach and duodenum (the foregut) rotate 90 degrees in a counterclockwise direction (as one views the developing fetus from the front), bringing the left vagus nerve and wall of the stomach anterior and the right vagus nerve and stomach wall posterior; the original ventral wall of the stomach becomes its lesser curvature and the dorsal-wall its greater curvature. The duodenum lies to the right of the midline in its accustomed position (Fig. 5.5). This completes rotation of the stomach and duodenum.

The midgut, nourished by the superior mesenteric artery, participates in this initial 90 degree clockwise thrust so that the duodenojejunum occupies the right hemiabdomen (Fig. 5.5). During the fifth and sixth

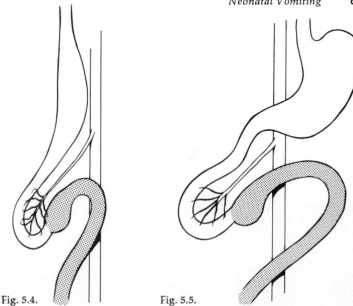

Fig. 5.4. *Lateral* view of gastrointestinal tract early in fourth gestational week. Stomach is just beginning to sacculate; colon is stippled, vessel arising from the aorta is the superior mesenteric artery which nourishes the midgut (Figs. 5.4 to 5.7 from: R. D. Liechty and R. T. Soper: Synopsis of Surgery. Mosby, St. Louis, Mo., 1972)

Fig. 5.5. *Anterior* view of gastrointestinal tract late in fourth gestational week; stomach and duodenum have rotated 90 ° clockwise

gestational weeks an enormous linear growth of midgut occurs, such that the bulk of the midgut is forced out through the umbilical ring into the extracelomic pouch. During the eighth and ninth weeks the midgut begins returning to the abdominal cavity in an orderly manner from proximal to distal. Coincident with this return the midgut undergoes an additional 180 degrees clockwise rotation, bringing the duodenojejunum behind (underneath) the superior mesenteric artery, where it is anchored by the ligament of Treitz with the proximal jejunum filling the left hemiabdomen (Fig. 5.6).

The ileocolon, comprising the distal half of the midgut, returns to the abdominal cavity last and also rotates 270 degrees counterclockwise, bringing the transverse colon across above (in front of) the superior mesenteric artery with the cecum residing in the right upper abdominal quadrant (Fig. 5.7). This is the situation that pertains during the 10th to 12th weeks of gestational life; the only change

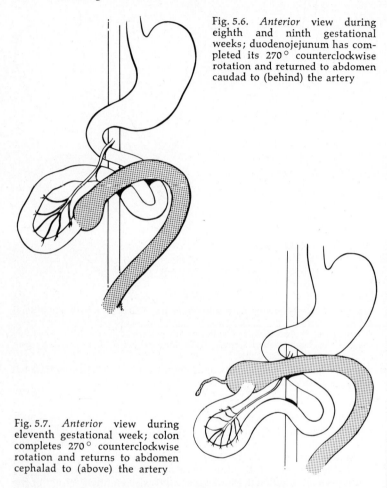

Fig. 5.6. *Anterior* view during eighth and ninth gestational weeks; duodenojejunum has completed its 270° counterclockwise rotation and returned to abdomen caudad to (behind) the artery

Fig. 5.7. *Anterior* view during eleventh gestational week; colon completes 270° counterclockwise rotation and returns to abdomen cephalad to (above) the artery

which occurs during the latter two trimesters of gestation is a gradual descent of the cecum toward the right lower quadrant and its ultimate fixation (generally postnatally) in that characteristic location.

Almost all of the abnormalities referred to as "midgut malrotation" involve an *arrest* of rotation after the initial 90 degrees of counterclockwise rotation. The duodenojejunum remains in the right upper quadrant, the small bowel resides in the right hemiabdomen and the colon occupies the left hemiabdomen upon its return to the abdominal cavity (Fig. 5.5). Sometimes the intestine sits in this malrotated position throughout life producing no or relatively few symptoms. However, two potential complications produce symptoms in the majority of cases.

The most common misadventure produces congenital duodenal obstruction. This is occasioned by a band that traverses the interval from the right posterior abdominal parietes to the cecum and ascending colon (which are in the left epigastrium), in transit crossing the duodenum. This so-called "Ladd's" band indents, extrinsically compresses and obstructs the duodenum distal to the ampulla of Vater; the vomitus is therefore bile-stained.

When the obstruction is complete, plain radiographs reveal a "double bubble" indistinguishable from duodenal atresia. Radiocontrast swallows clarify diagnosis if the obstruction is incomplete. Radiocontrast enemas suggest malrotation if the majority of the colon occupies the

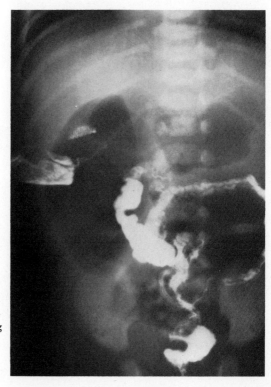

Fig. 5.8.
Barium enema in newborn with obstructed duodenum (gas shadow on the left) showing the unused "microcolon" to reside entirely in the left hemiabdomen

left hemiabdomen (Fig. 5.8) with the cecum in some ectopic upper abdominal position. Surgical division of "Ladd's" band relieves the duodenal obstruction, allowing the cecum to swing freely into the left hemiabdomen.

The second complication of malrotation is *volvulus of the midgut*. In malrotation the upper midgut (duodenojejunum) and the lower midgut (ascending colon) lie juxtaposed to one another (Fig. 5.5), forming a very narrow axis around the superior mesenteric artery and vein, with all of the small bowel (about 200 cm in length) sus-

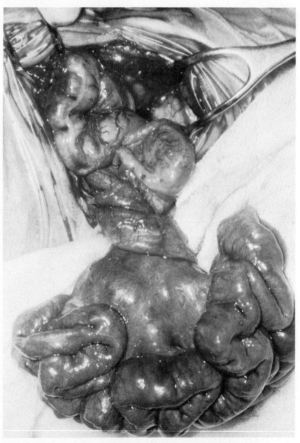

Fig. 5.9.   Midgut volvulus (270° twist); midgut plethoric and edematous but still viable

pended below the two. Midgut volvulus occurs when the voluminous apron of midgut twists around the narrowed axis of the proximal superior mesenteric vessels (Fig. 5.9). This occurs in about one-half of the symptomatic patients with midgut malrotation, the volvulus or twist always occurring in a clockwise direction as one views the patient from the front. This immediately puts the entire midgut in jeopardy because of obstruction first to the lymphatic and venous outflow from the gut (as in Fig. 5.9) and finally shutting down the arterial inflow to the midgut as the volvulus progressively twists the vascular axis. Midgut strangulation ensues with first hemorrhagic and later ischemic necrosis. Further, a closed loop mechanical obstruction of the midgut is produced.

Volvulus of a malrotated midgut is heralded by a sudden, acute worsening in the general condition of a newborn or young infant with vomiting characteristic of partial or complete duodenal obstruction. The abdomen becomes distended and tender, and the patient's general condition deteriorates rapidly. Plain radiographs show either a "gasless" abdomen or many dilated, air-filled loops of bowel. Radiocontrast studies of the colon confirm its malposition, suggesting that volvulus is the likely cause of the patient's rapid deterioration. In this situation, the patient needs aggressive supportive care (nasogastric suction, rapid rehydration, systemic antibiotics) and immediate laparotomy.

Ischemic midgut is salvaged by surgical derotation of the volvulized midgut to bring the relationships back to their original malrotated state. Ladd's band is surgically divided. Clearly necrotic bowel needs to be resected, with continuity restored by end-to-end anastomosis.

Another extrinsic congenital duodenal obstruction arises at the normally rotated duodenojejunal junction by an unusually *thick and narrow ligament of Treitz*. In this situation the normally gentle duodenojejunal curve is replaced by acute angulation producing complete or partial obstruction at this point (Fig. 5.10). It may be suspected preoperatively by air or radiocontrast material traveling across to the midline in the fourth portion of the duodenum with failure to progress normally downstream from this point. Surgical treatment consists of excising the ligament of Treitz.

Annular Pancreas

This condition consists of encirclement of the second part of the duodenum by pancreatic tissue which restricts or completely shuts off the lumen at this point. Vomiting is almost always bile-stained in nature. It is distinguished from duodenal atresia or from malrotation at the operating table. Annular pancreas results from a failure of the ventral pancreatic bud to rotate around the duodenum. Treatment

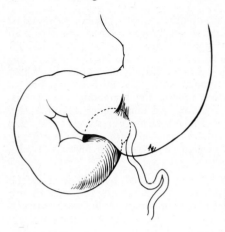

Fig. 5.10.   Diagram of obstruction at duodenojejunal junction by extrinsic bands (ligament of Treitz)

consists of bypass, best achieved by side-to-side anastomosis of the duodenum just proximal to the annular pancreas to that just distal to the obstruction. Duodenojejunostomy also suffices.

Congenital Obstructions of the Jejuno-Ileum

Congenital obstructions of the jejuno-ileum occur fairly frequently, the majority due to either *atresia* or *stenosis*. Bilious vomiting, passage of only small amounts of sometimes grayish meconium and abdominal distention of varying degrees characterize the condition clinically. The number of the air-fluid levels on an upright radiograph help estimate whether the obstruction is relatively proximal or relatively distal (Fig. 5.11 and 5.12) in the bowel. Laparotomy shows: 1) a dilated upstream bowel which narrows significantly at a point of an incomplete internal membrane (stenosis) 2) bowel which retains its external continuity but sharply diminishes in diameter at the point where an internal membrane completely obstructs the lumen, or 3) loss of continuity of bowel (Fig. 5.13). In the latter case the upstream bowel is very dilated from obstruction whereas the tiny downstream bowel is closed off at its proximal end with often a V-shaped defect in the mesentery between the bowel ends. Occasionally significant lengths of small bowel are missing between the two blind ends of atretic bowel (Fig. 5.14). In 15 % of cases the atresias are multiple (Fig. 5.15).

Atresias of the jejunum, ileum and colon occur from ischemic infarction of fetal bowel rather than from other embryonic misadventures. The above-described three forms of atresia can be reproduced in the

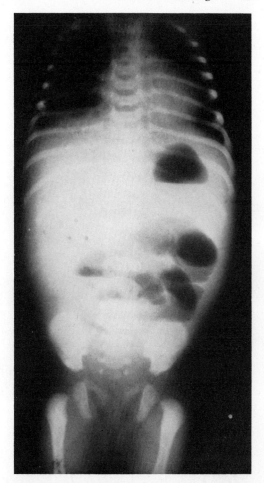

Fig. 5.11.
Upright radiograph
showing a modest
number of air fluid
levels indicating mid
jejunal obstruction.

fetal puppy by devascularizing different lengths of intestine. Because the content of the developing fetal intestine is sterile, only a modest chemical peritonitis ensues rather than the lethal peritonitis of bacterial origin which is occasioned by postnatal bowel devascularization.

Surgical correction of atresias and stenoses of jejunum and ileum require resecting dilated, atonic proximal bowel with restoration of luminal continuity by end-to-end anastomosis (Fig. 5.16). In the

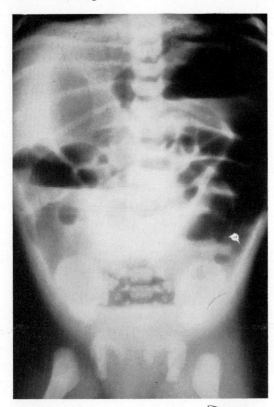

Fig. 5.12.
Upright radiograph
showing innumer-
able air fluid levels
indicating obstruc-
tion of lower colon

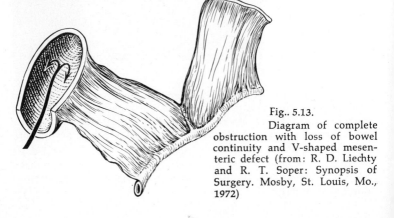

Fig.. 5.13.
Diagram of complete
obstruction with loss of bowel
continuity and V-shaped mesenteric defect (from: R. D. Liechty
and R. T. Soper: Synopsis of
Surgery. Mosby, St. Louis, Mo.,
1972)

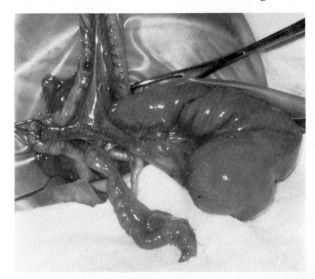

Fig. 5.14. Jejunal atresia (right), mesenteric defect and tiny terminal ileum (below) in newborn who had lost all the intervening small bowel in utero (estimated 180 cm)

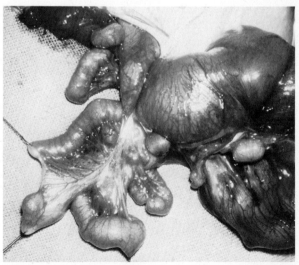

Fig. 5.15. Thirteen areas of atresia studded the small bowel of this newborn

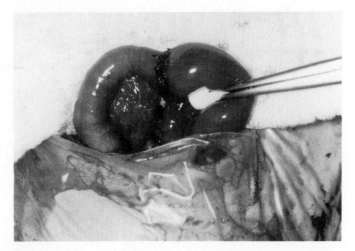

Fig. 5.16.   End-to-end anastomosis after resection of atretic bowel

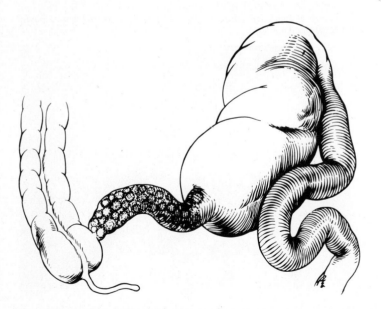

Fig. 5.17. Diagram of meconium ileus

unusual baby with loss of extensive segments of small bowel, major fluid and electrolyte imbalance, diarrhea and malnutrition occur post-operatively. Lengthy total intravenous nutrition is a helpful adjunct in the long term care of these patients, allowing time for compensatory enlargement of the remaining bowel to occur before oral alimentation is instituted.

Meconium Ileus

Here the distal ileum is plugged by inspissated, undigested and often non-pigmented meconium (Fig. 5.17). Since it is always associated with cystic fibrosis of the pancreas, the meconium inspissation is clearly secondary to lack of digestion. Why it occurs in only 5—10 % of patients with cystic fibrosis is unknown. The pellet-like masses of sticky meconium mechanically occlude the lumen of the distal ileum with a dilated and obstructed proximal bowel. Bilious vomiting and abdominal distention from birth characterize the condition clinically. Occasionally small bits of calcium are visible on plain abdominal radiographs (Fig. 5.18), attesting to antenatal rupture of the obstructed bowel with the production of a chemical peritonitis

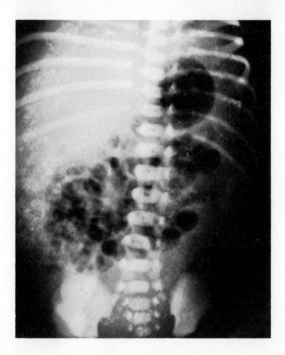

Fig. 5.18.
Intra-abdominal calcification of meconium peritonitis

(so-called *"meconium peritonitis"*). The condition is suspected pre-operatively from a history of cystic fibrosis in the family. It is also suggested by obstructed bowel loops of different sizes and peculiar absence of air-fluid levels (due to the sticky, inspissated and thick meconium) on upright radiographs of the abdomen (Fig. 5.19). Bubbles of air within meconium is the final radiographic sign of meconium ileus. Occasionally one can palpate the pellet-like masses of inspissated meconium.

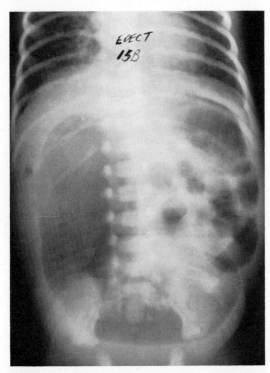

Fig. 5.19. Upright plain radiograph on newborn with meconium ileus; note bowel loops of different sizes, absence of air fluid levels

If one suspects the diagnosis clinically and if there are no complications already present (like perforation) then the obstructing plugs of meconium may be flushed out by water-soluble contrast material administered as an enema under fluoroscopic control. If this fails, or if it is thought that a complication exists, laparotomy is indicated. At surgery, the intestine is temporarily exteriorized just upstream from the point of obstruction, through which saline, enzymes or

N-acetylcysteine (Mucomist) is injected downstream to flush out the inspissated meconium (Fig. 5.20). The obstruction is resolved in this manner within three or four days, allowing surgical reconstitution of bowel continuity. Serious postoperative morbidity from pulmonary complications of the disease makes nonoperative treatment of meconium ileus very attractive.

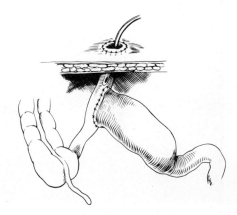

Fig. 5.20.   Diagram of surgical correction of meconium ileus.

Obstruction of the anorectum

Meconium Plug Syndrome

This may be associated with cystic fibrosis of the pancreas or Hirschsprung's disease, or may occur in an otherwise normal baby. A sticky plug of meconium lodges in the rectum and rectosigmoid producing a temporary mechanical obstruction (Fig. 5.21) representing a portion of those 5 % of newborns who fail to pass meconium during the first 24 hours of life. Clinically, it is heralded by a progressively enlarging abdomen in a newborn who may vomit and refuse feeds. The offending plug of inspissated meconium is later expelled either spontaneously, after a rectal digital examination or administration of cleansing or radiocontrast enemas used in treatment and diagnosis. Many of the babies with the meconium plug syndrome are thereafter perfectly normal, but a proportion of them turn out to have Hirschsprung's disease or cystic fibrosis. For this reason they need close followup and re-evaluation.

Anorectal atresia (Chapter 6) and *Hirschsprung's disease* (Chapter 9) can produce neonatal vomiting, but will not be discussed here.

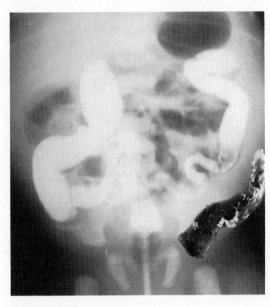

Fig. 5.21.
Meconium plug superimposed on barium enema study performed on newborn with the meconium plug syndrome

Vomiting in Infancy

1 month to 18 months of age

General

Infants 1 month to 18 months of age vomit more commonly than newborns. They vomit for a great variety of reasons, many of them non-specific such as hyperthermia, while teething, during upper respiratory tract infections, etc. Further, they are host to a significant number of gastrointestinal tract infections, both bacterial and viral, which generally include vomiting in their course.

Workup

The initial workup is carried out coincident with necessary resuscitative and supportive measures; nasogastric suction, blood drawn for the same electrolyte and laboratory determinations as the newborn, administration of electrolyte and laboratory determinations as the newborn, administration of electrolyte-containing parenteral fluids to correct dehydration and electrolyte and pH abnormalities. If the youngster is acutely ill, blood should be crossmatched and urine output monitored.

Physical examination includes evaluating for signs of dehydration: sunken fontanelle, sunken and soft eyeballs, dry mucous membranes and loss of skin elasticity (skin which remains in an upright position when pinched by the fingers). Abdominal tenderness, contour and masses are noted. The evaluation of bowel sounds is more meaningful than in a newborn. The physician should bring up a chair and sit comfortably at cribside while listening for five to ten minutes over different portions of the abdomen with a stethoscope. Percussion note and its response to changes of position carry the same significance as they do in the newborn. Rectal digital examination evaluates stool color and appearance; a careful bimanual examination allows palpation of the lower one-third of the abdominal cavity for masses or bulging loops of bowel.

Plain Radiographs of the Chest and Abdomen

On the upright or decubitus film one looks for free air or fluid within the abdominal cavity or for air-fluid levels within distended loops of intestine. Air-fluid levels which are at the same level in a single loop of dilated bowel, with gas present from the stomach to the rectum, are the radiographic hallmarks of paralytic ileus. Air-fluid levels at different levels within each loop, with absence of gas in the rectum, signify a mechanical obstruction. In general, the greater the number of these air-fluid levels in mechanical obstruction, the lower down the bowel is the obstruction located. A ground-glass appearance to the x-ray signifies fluid, either free within the abdominal cavity or entrapped within bowel. In both mechanical and paralytic ileus, the size of the bowel loops and the thickness of the intervening walls relate to the duration of obstruction. Radiopaque foreign bodies (aspirated foreign objects, fecaliths, etc.) are looked for.

If mechanical intestinal obstruction is likely, contrast studies of the colon are often helpful even if they show only a normal colon, and are diagnostic, of course, if the obstruction lies within the colon. Contrast material given by mouth is rarely indicated in mechanical intestinal obstruction.

Specific Entities

Free Gastroesophageal Reflux

Both **hiatus hernia** and its non-surgical first cousin **chalasia** will be discussed together, since the most significant problem (vomiting) of both these entities is produced by free gastroesophageal reflux. Chalasia is defined as simply an absence of a competent and functioning mechanism to prevent gastroesophageal reflux. Since most babies spit up some feedings, the term "chalasia" should probably be reserved for young infants with persistent or excessive vomiting of feedings. This situation can be satisfactorily handled empirically by sitting up the infant 24 hours each day, or at least for a period of time after each feeding, allowing gravity to help discourage the gastroesophageal reflux. Placing the baby into a prone, rather than a supine, position also discourages gastroesophageal reflux. No more sophisticated workup or treatment is generally needed.

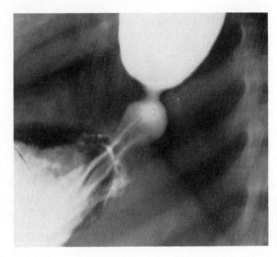

Fig. 5.22.
Small hiatus hernia
shown on barium
swallow

Hiatus hernia occurs when a portion of the fundus of the stomach herniates through the diaphragmatic esophageal hiatus. It probably happens in young infants much more commonly than hitherto realized, at least intermittently. In the incipient stages, congenital hiatus hernia often is intermittent and unless the contrast swallow is obtained at just the right time with careful fluoroscopic inspection (Fig. 5.22), it may be missed. In its florid form, with the fundus of the stomach more or less permanently resident within the lower thorax, an upper GI contrast swallow is always diagnostic (Fig. 5.23). The major danger of a hiatus hernia is bathing of the esophagus with irritating, low pH gastric material which inevitably induces esophagitis. If neglected, esophagitis leads to ulceration with hemorrhage and fibrous stricture (Fig. 5.23) after many weeks of esophageal spasm, inflammation and irritation.

Clinically, hiatus hernia is heralded by a baby who persistently vomits after feedings, and later in-between feedings, accentuated when

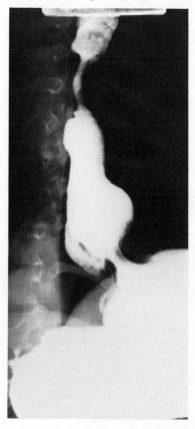

Fig. 5.23. Large hiatus hernia shown on barium swallow. The middle esophagus is narrowed by a stricture

he is supine. The "vomiting" is generally an effortless regurgitation of gastric content out of the corner of the mouth. Hematemesis secondary to esophagitis is common. The neglected patient with esophageal stricture ultimately develops dysphagia with prompt regurgitation during feedings. Recurrent aspiration pneumonia and failure to thrive supervene.

Treatment of a baby with established congenital hiatus hernia begins by upright positioning in an infant seat 24 hours day and night, feeding him alkali and thickened feeds frequently in small amounts. In early or mild cases the stomach fundus gradually descends below the diaphragm to resume its normal intra-abdominal position with a return of gastroesophageal competency. If the hiatus hernia and/or gastroesophageal reflux persist after two or three months of this intensive medical treatment, then surgical correction is necessary to preclude the chronic complications of hiatus hernia related above. Surgical treatment includes snugging up the crura around the esophagus, suturing the reduced stomach to the abdominal wall or creating an anti-reflux valve at the gastroesophageal junction.

In about 10 % of infants, hiatus hernia is secondary to some form of gastric outlet obstruction (a membranous web in the antrum of the stomach or the pyloric channel, hypertrophic pyloric stenosis). In these babies, treatment is directed at relieving the gastric obstruction.

Hypertrophic Pyloric Stenosis

Hypertrophic pyloric stenosis is the most common surgically correctable cause of vomiting in young infants. It occurs about once in every 200—400 male infants and once in every 400—800 female infants. About 15 % have a family history of hypertrophic pyloric stenosis in previous generations of the same family, or in older siblings. The firstborn male of a family seems more predisposed than later siblings. The majority of infants with hypertrophic pyloric stenosis enjoy a one to three week vomiting-free interval immediately after birth. Non-bile-stained vomiting then begins sporadically after feedings, gradually increasing in frequency and force. Constipation gradually ensues as less food is delivered into the small bowel.

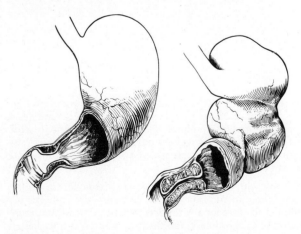

Fig. 5.24.   Diagram of normal pyloric muscle (left) contrasted with hypertrophic pyloric stenosis (right)

The condition results from a progressive diminution in size of the pyloric channel at the gastric outlet, occasioned by a hypertrophic thickening (not hyperplasia) of the circular muscles of the pyloric sphincter (Fig. 5.24). The thickened muscle tissue encroaches upon the pyloric channel lumen because the tough serosa prevents an outward protrusion. The cause for hypertrophy of the pyloric muscle is unknown. The condition spontaneously remits in most cases, but this process may take several months.

Because the obstruction is proximal to the ampulla of Vater, the vomitus is never bile-stained, although with prolonged and forceful vomiting it occasionally becomes tinged with altered blood. As the gastric outlet obstruction gradually increases in severity, the stomach dilates and its walls thicken as excessive demands are placed upon gastric peristalsis to force food through an everdiminishing pyloric channel. This results in the classical gastric hyperperistaltic waves which travel from left to right across the upper abdomen after feeding (Fig. 5.25); their reversal produces forceful (so-called "projectile") vomiting which characterizes the condition.

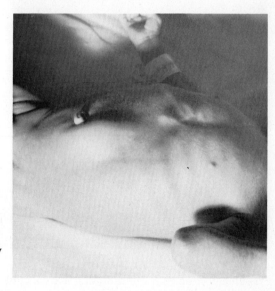

Fig. 5.25.
Visible gastric hyperstaltic waves traveling from left to right side of epigastrium in baby with hypertrophic pyloric stenosis

It is understandable that some degree of dehydration ultimately ensues. The steady loss of potassium and chloride ions in the vomitus produces the hypochloremic, hypokalemic alkalosis epitomizing the metabolic alterations of the condition.

Diagnosis rests upon a typical history of non-bilious postprandial vomiting which begins during the second or third week of life. Gastric hyperperistaltic waves are visible after feeding, and a firm, mobile, "olive-shaped" mass is palpated just above and to the right of the umbilicus (the hypertrophied pyloric muscle). A typical history and physical findings require no additional diagnostic workup. If the history is atypical or the pylorus not palpable, then a diagnostic plain radiograph (Fig. 5.26) or upper gastrointestinal contrast study (Fig. 5.27) is indicated. A narrow, elongated pyloric channel is the confirmatory radiographic sign of hypertrophic pyloric stenosis.

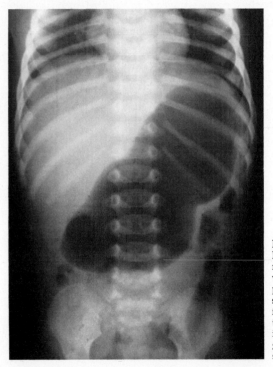

Fig. 5.26.
Plain abdominal radiograph in baby with hypertrophic pyloric stenosis showing dilated air-filled stomach with thick walls and indentations of gastric hyperperistaltic waves

Treatment commences with passing a large tube (14 to 16 French) through the mouth and into the stomach for aspirating all the curdled feeding within the stomach, then lavaging the stomach with saline. The gastric lavage should be done with the baby on his side in the head-down position to obviate aspiration. This large tube is then removed and a finer soft catheter passed through the nose and into

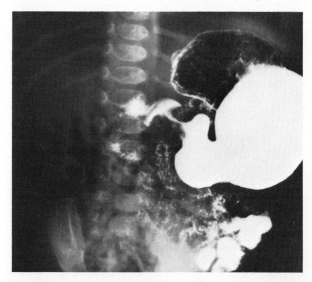

Fig. 5.27. Upper GI barium study showing narrow, elongated pyloric channel characteristic of hypertrophic pyloric stenosis

the stomach to maintain gastric decompression. Serum electrolytes and blood gases document the metabolic upset and guide parenteral fluid replacement. Surgical treatment of pyloric stenosis is never an emergency, and should be delayed until all of the fluid, electrolyte and pH abnormalities are totally corrected.

Pyloromyotomy (Ramstedt's operation) is the best treatment for hypertrophic pyloric stenosis. The operation is simple, enjoying the lowest morbidity-mortality rate and the highest expectation of cure of any surgical procedure commonly performed. It involves a longitudinal splitting of the serosa and muscle of the pylorus, spreading the split muscle edges apart to allow the entrapped (but intact) mucosa to bulge through the breach in the muscle (Fig. 5.28). Glucose feedings by mouth are often resumed within four hours of operation with the child placed in the right lateral position (to improve gastric emptying by gravity) after each feeding. The feedings are increased to dilute and then full strength formula such that by 48 hours after operation the average infant is ready for discharge.

The medical treatment of hypertrophic pyloric stenosis (nasogastric suction, antispasmodics, parenteral fluids, periodic trials of feeding) is only successful in about two-thirds of patients. It generally requires several weeks in hospital for spontaneous resolution of the

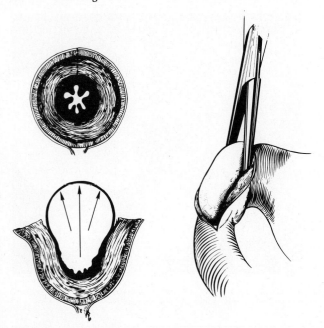

Fig. 5.28.   Upper left: line of seromuscular incision used in pyloromyotomy. Lower left: intact pyloric mucosa bulges through when cut muscle edges are spread apart. Right: completed pyloromyotomy

pyloric hypertrophy to occur, and if it fails operation is required anyway. For these reasons, prompt surgical correction is the best treatment.

Duplications of Intestine

These rare enteric anomalies produce a variety of symptoms, of which vomiting is but one. Intestinal duplications may occur from the esophagus to the anus, but the majority involve duodenum and ileum. Duplications generally lie within the bowel mesentery, assuming either a spherical or tubular form depending upon whether they communicate with the lumen of the normal gastrointestinal tract.

The more common spherical duplications have no communication and often share blood supply and muscularis with the parent bowel. Symptoms occur when secretions within the cyst increase in volume

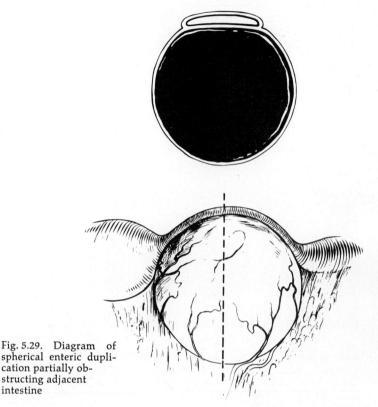

Fig. 5.29. Diagram of spherical enteric duplication partially obstructing adjacent intestine

and pressure enough to encroach upon adjacent structures, including the lumen of parent bowel (Fig. 5.29). In contrast, tubular duplications retain a connection with the gastrointestinal tract lumen, often at one end of the duplication (Fig. 5.30 and 5.31). In addition to the mucosa normal to that segment of bowel which is replicated, duplications often contain ectopic gastric mucosa, thus adding inflammation, peptic ulceration, bleeding and perforation to the clinical picture of intestinal obstruction.

Most duplications come to diagnosis in the latter part of the first year of life or during the first few years of childhood. Spherical duplications gradually encroach upon adjacent bowel, producing signs and symptoms of mechanical intestinal obstruction which, when coupled with a relatively non-tender abdominal mass, heighten the diagnostic likelihood. Gastrointestinal hemorrhage prompts laparo-

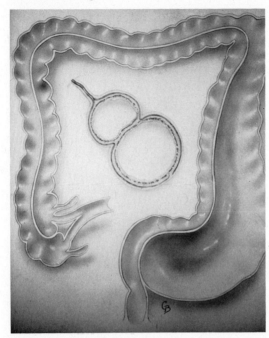

Fig. 5.30.
Diagram of tubular
duplication of
terminal ileum and
colon (from R. T.
Soper: Surgery 63:
998—1004, 1968)

tomy in those containing both ectopic gastric mucosa and a connection with the parent gastrointestinal tract, and perforation in those lacking luminal connection to bowel. Intrathoracic duplications produce respiratory symptoms and show up as masses on chest x-ray.

The cystic duplication is resected with the adjacent normal bowel which shares a common wall and blood supply. Tubular duplications not intimately connected with the parent bowel are safely resected. Tubular duplications that share a wall and blood supply with the parent bowel are resected only if the length of residual bowel is not compromised; those lacking ectopic gastric mucosa need only to be anastomosed to the parent lumen. Lengthy tubular duplications with gastric mucosa and a common wall and blood supply require only mucosal stripping of the duplication.

Omphalomesenteric Remnant

The embryologic connection of the bowel to yolk sac, normally existing only during the first few weeks of gestational life, is retained into postnatal life in about 2 % of individuals. By far the

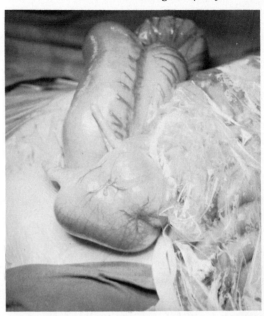

Fig. 5.31.
Operative photo-
graph of duplicated
appendix and right
colon in patient in
Fig. 5.30

most common remnant is the **Meckel's diverticulum** (Chapter 13);
the rare counterparts include a patent connection between distal
ileum and umbilicus draining meconium through the fistula, a band
from the distal ileum to the underside of the umbilicus around which
bowel can become obstructed and varying combinations of bands
and cysts. Surgical treatment consists of excising the bands, cysts,
fistulas or diverticulum. Asymptomatic ones are discovered incidentally at laparotomy or postmortem.

Intussusception

Idiopathic intussusception generally occurs in youngsters somewhere
between three and 18 months of age, in males more often than
females in 3:2 ratio. It generally involves the terminal ileum tele-
scoping or intussuscepting into itself and then into the cecum and
on around the colon (Fig. 5.32). Intussusception is characterized clinically by abrupt episodes of periodic abdominal colic during which
the youngster turns pale, screams and draws up his knees for a
minute or two, followed by a symptom-free interval of 5 to 15
minutes before another attack occurs. After several hours of these
classical episodes, dark-red blood is passed per rectum which resem-

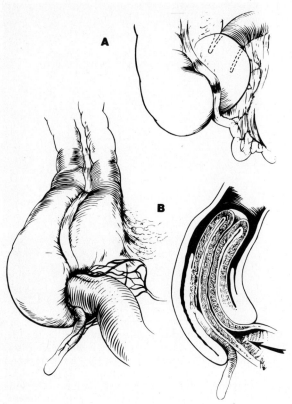

Fig. 5.32.   Diagram tracing the evolution of an ileocolic intussusception (early)

bles red currant jelly. If neglected, abdominal distention, bilious vomiting and signs of mechanical intestinal obstruction supervene.

Diagnosis is suspected from the history of intermittent abdominal colic in a previously well youngster 3 to 18 months of age. If examined during the symptom-free interval, he is often pale but has a flaccid abdominal wall. This is the ideal time to palpate the tubular mass usually transversely oriented in the right upper abdominal quadrant which is separate from liver, movable and only mildly tender. Abdominal wall spasm is triggered by the pain episodes and crying, prohibiting palpation of the mass during the episodes. High-pitched borborygmi of intestinal obstruction may be heard in the late case. Rectal examination may detect the currant jelly stool described above; occasionally one can palpate the lead point of the intussusception as a cervix-like mass if it has progressed this far distally.

Radiocontrast barium study of the colon confirms diagnosis by the "coil spring" filling defect seen at the leading point of the intussusception (Fig. 5.33). Hydrostatic reduction under fluoroscopic control with the barium bag not more than 100 cm above the table may

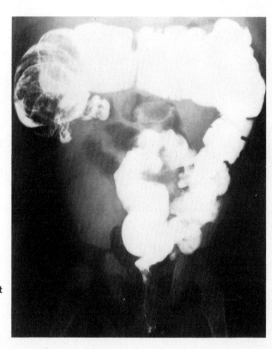

Fig. 5.33.
Barium enema
showing the "coil
spring" filling defect
in the ascending
colon characteristic
of ileocolic intussusception

be attempted if the history is less than 24 hours' duration and if the patient has no signs of peritoneal irritation or frank intestinal obstruction. In about 70 % of cases, intussusception is completely reduced by this hydrostatic technique, confirmed when the barium retrogradely flows freely into the terminal small bowel. About 10 % of intussusceptions reduced hydrostatically recur, generally during the first few days. In the 30 % not completely reduced hydrostatically, or in those suspected of having necrosis, perforation or mechanical intestinal obstruction, surgical reduction is required (Fig. 5.34). Surgical reduction is impossible with necrotic bowel, requiring resec-

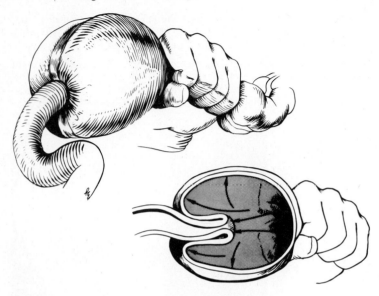

Fig. 5.34. Diagram showing "milking" technique for operative reduction of intussusception

tion and end-to-end anastomosis. Resection is required in only about 5 % of patients with intussusception.

Only 5 % of infants harbor a mechanical cause for the intussusception, such as an intestinal polyp or an inverted Meckel's diverticulum. In these cases, resection of the polyp or diverticulum is a necessary adjunct to surgical reduction. The older the child who develops intussusception, the more commonly does he harbor such a mechanical or anatomic cause. However, the majority of intussusceptions occurs in the 3 to 18 month age group.

Cases of intussusception tend to occur periodically or seasonally, commonly preceded by upper respiratory tract infections, and the intussusception constantly originates in the terminal ileum. Recent studies suggest that an adenovirus infection might be the offending causal agent, inducing lymphoid hyperplasia within the Peyer's patches so plentiful in the submucosa of the infant's terminal ileum. The hyperplastic lymphoid tissue then protrudes into the lumen much as a polyp, to serve as the leading point allowing intestinal peristalsis to trigger the intussusception. This theory of origin is still speculative, but attractive because it satisfies many otherwise in-explicable features of the common idiopathic ileocolic intussusception.

Incarcerated Inguinal Hernia

About 15 % of indirect inguinal hernias in infants and children are complicated by incarceration of intestine and vomiting. This is discussed in detail in Chapter 16.

Vomiting in Childhood

2 Years to 15 Years of Age

In general, the older the child the less frequently he vomits. This is certainly true in terms of surgical causes for vomiting, which diminish greatly after the first two years of life. Considerably greater reserves of body fluids, electrolytes, nutrition and pH-conserving mechanisms allow the surgeon time to launch fairly sophisticated studies, if necessary.

Specific Entities

Non-Surgical

Gastrointestinal infections, bacterial or viral in origin, are common causes for vomiting in childhood. The more serious ones are usually associated with bilious vomiting, abdominal colic, mild generalized distention of the abdomen, hyperactive but not obstructive bowel sounds and diarrheal stools. Dietary indiscretions are a fairly common cause of childhood vomiting: overeating, ingesting food tainted by Staphylococcus, eating too many green apples, etc.

Paralytic Ileus

Paralytic ileus is more common in the older child than the newborn or young infant. Most children with paralytic ileus have some intra-abdominal inflammatory disease producing abdominal pain, discussed in Chapter 12.

Intussusception

Intussusception occurs much less frequently in older children, with an ever-increasing statistical likelihood that it is caused by some mechanical or anatomic abnormality such as a small bowel tumor, polyp or an inverted Meckel's diverticulum.

Incarcerated Hernias

Incarcerated indirect inguinal hernias (see Chapter 16) occur less frequently in childhood than infancy.

Rarely, an **internal hernia** incarcerates. By internal we mean a herniation of bowel through an aperture located intraabdominally rather than one involving the abdominal wall. Characteristically, these apertures are juxtaposed to the duodenum at the ligament of Treitz, or adjacent to the ileocecal angle. Internal abdominal hernias are very rare, are manifested clinically as mechanical intestinal obstruction but with the specific cause identified only at laparotomy. The intestine is withdrawn from the internal hernia sac and the aperture through which it herniated is surgically closed.

Adhesive Intestinal Obstruction

It is likely that any patient with a surgical scar on his abdominal wall who later develops persistent, bile-stained vomiting has intestinal obstruction from adhesions. Adhesions represent scar tissue formed at points of injury to visceral or parietal peritoneum. The incidence of postoperative adhesive obstruction is therefore diminished by gentle handling of bowel at operation, shielding peritoneum from trauma, dessication and cautery injury.

With time, adhesions thicken and foreshorten to obstruct bowel either by angulating the intestine or by providing a band around which intestine drapes itself. Abdominal distention, persistent bile-stained vomiting and abdominal colic herald the mechanical obstruction clinically. Physical examination confirms the abdominal distention, and auscultation discloses the characteristic high-pitched peristaltic rushes. Plain radiographs of the abdomen in the supine and upright position confirm diagnosis. Treatment begins with nasogastric suction and parenteral repair of fluid, electrolyte and pH disturbances. Prompt laparotomy to divide or excise the offending adhesions is proper treatment.

Recurrent bouts of postoperative adhesive obstruction occasionally are relieved by passing a long tube weighted with mercury at its tip through the nose and into the stomach, where peristalsis carries it downstream into small intestine. Suction on the tube siphons out the gas and fluid from the bowel upstream to the obstruction, and occasionally unkinks the bowel to relieve the obstruction without operation. In patients operated upon for recurrent adhesive small bowel obstruction, a tube may be directly placed into the small intestine to serve as a splint for 10—14 days postoperatively; often the adhesions that then reform tend to encase the bowel in gentle loops and curves dictated by the tube to diminish the likelihood of subsequent adhesive obstruction. Suction applied to these internal splint tubes facilitates intestinal decompression during the first few postoperative days.

Bezoars

Older children who are mentally retarded or emotionally disturbed occasionally eat undigestible material (hair, persimmon seeds) which collects into a ball in the stomach to induce partial gastric obstruction. Trichobezoars (hair) or phytobezoars (vegetable matter) or combina-

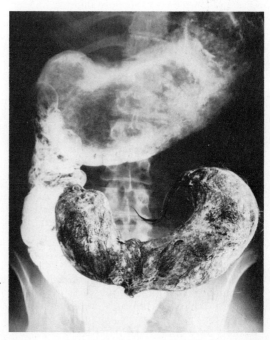

Fig. 5.35.
Trichobezoar super-
imposed upon upper
GI contrast study
showing gastric
filling defect it
created

tions of the two are the most common examples. Vague abdominal discomfort and tenderness, intolerance to solid foods and clear vomitus characterize the clinical picture. Examination reveals a movable epigastric mass in a disturbed child who generally has alopecia. Upper gastrointestinal contrast studies reveal a characteristic filling defect in the stomach (Fig. 5.35). Surgical removal is occasionally necessary.

6 Deformity and Disease of the Anorectum

R. T. SOPER

General

There is a strange reluctance to include the anorectum in the physical examination of the newborn and child, but it is just as important as auscultating the heart or palpating the abdomen. These examinations are never omitted from a physical examination, but somehow anorectal examination is commonly slighted.

In the newborn, inspection and digital examination of the anus is vital, since anorectal abnormalities constitute one of the more common congenital anomalies of the gastrointestinal tract. It is embarrassing, to say the least, to discover such an abnormality when evaluating a newborn several days of age with abdominal distention and vomiting. A soft catheter should be passed into the anus as a routine part of every physical examination of a normal newborn. In addition, a gently performed digital examination with the well-lubricated little finger of the examiner is safe in all but the smallest newborns, yielding much relevant information as to the nature of the meconium, the internal anatomy of the pelvis and masses in the lower portion of the abdominal cavity.

In the older infant and child, rectal digital examination should be one of the last maneuvers of the physical examination, since its discomfort provokes crying and may rob the examiner of whatever favorable rapport he has established with the patient.

Normal Bowel Control

Normal fecal control depends on effective function of the puborectalis muscle. This sling-like muscle is the anteriormost portion of the levator ani muscle; both ends are tethered to the pubic bone. In the male, only the urethra and rectum lie within the puborectalis sling, to which the vagina is added in the female.

When the patient is ready to have a bowel movement, he voluntarily relaxes the puborectalis muscle, unpinching the lower rectum coincident with an autonomic relaxation of the smooth muscle internal anal sphincter to allow expulsion of gas and/or stool from the rectal ampulla. The ampulla then returns to its normal, non-distended size. The striated external anal sphincter muscles add a delicate nuance to bowel control, particularly during the passage of flatus to prevent liquid material from being discharged, but its contribution to fecal continence is minor compared to the puborectalis muscle.

Anorectal Atresia

General

The term *anorectal atresia* encompasses the majority of congenital malformations of the anorectal area. *Congenital anal stenosis* is the most minor abnormality. It involves simply a narrowing of the anal canal, often associated with a delay in the passage of meconium in the immediate neonatal period of life, which is detected by sounding the anal canal with dilators. Congenital anal stenosis should be dilated daily with well-lubricated dilators until one's little finger can be inserted. Digital dilatation of the anus can then be carried out at home by the mother for two to three weeks as the only treatment for this very minor abnormality.

Another anorectal abnormality involves an otherwise perfectly normal anus which simply lies anterior to where it should. The so-called *anterior ectopic anus* (Fig. 6.1) has descended and exteriorized itself in a perfectly normal fashion, except for missing the external anal sphincter fibers in its passage to the perineum. Since the rectum lies

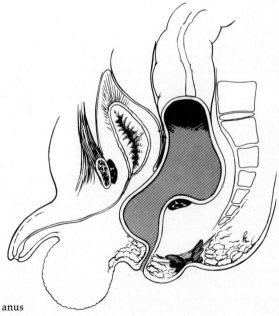

Fig. 6.1.
Anterior ectopic anus

within the puborectalis sling and bowel control is perfectly normal in this situation, one is most reluctant to surgically treat a simple anterior ectopic anus.

The more serious forms of anorectal atresia occur approximately once in every 5,000 live births. Males outnumber female babies in about a 3:2 ratio. Because of its importance to bowel control, the single most important point to determine in babies with major anorectal atresia is the relationship which the terminal atretic rectum bears to the levator ani muscle. In so-called *"high"* anorectal atresia, the rectum terminates at or above the levator sling muscle. In the *"low"* anorectal atresias, the rectum descends in a normal fashion through the puborectalis portion of the levator sling before terminating.

Overall, about 60 % of anorectal atresias are of the "low" variety, and about 40 % "high". Fifty percent of involved male infants have a high atresia contrasted with only 20 % of females. About 75 % of babies with anorectal atresia have congenital fistulas connecting the rectum to some adjacent structure; about 70 % of males and 90 % of females have such a congenital rectal fistula.

Etiology

It is clear that the different types of anorectal atresia result from imperfections in the normal embryologic separation of the hindgut from the anteriorly-located genitourinary apparatus and/or the mechanism by which these separated structures penetrate through to the perineum. In the "high" or supralevator anomalies, the urorectal septum descends imperfectly, or is arrested at some waystation in its descent. In the "low" or infralevator anorectal anomalies, descent of the urorectal septum is complete; the problem centers around establishing connections of the hindgut to the perineum, as well as maldevelopment of the urogenital folds and other perineal tissue primordia.

The birth weight of babies with anorectal atresia is less than 2,000 grams in only about 6% of patients. Another 6% have esophageal atresia associated, the only common remote anomaly. However, significant urologic malformations occur in about a quarter of the patients with anorectal atresias, and are more common in the high anorectal atresia (45%) compared to the low atresias (20%). Some patients with high anorectal atresias harbor associated sacral bony malformations, signaling the likely presence of major urologic abnormalities. If the first three sacral vertebrae are present, the neuromuscular anatomy of the pelvis is generally normal, but with more major or higher sacral malformations, many of the patients have imperfect levator muscles and/or innervation. These latter patients often have no intergluteal cleft. They are understandably poor treatment candidates, because of poor bowel control even with perfect surgical relocation of the rectum.

Low Anorectal Atresias

Low anorectal atresia is suspected when there is no anal outlet visible (Fig. 6.2), if the anus is ectopically located or if a fistula to the perineum (Fig. 6.3) is discovered. Rectoperineal fistulae are generally located near the midline anterior to where the anus normally would lie, but occasionally are present in an occult form by a bluish (meconium-stained) tract extending up the scrotal raphe and sometimes onto the ventral side of the penis in male babies. In the female, the fistula commonly opens onto the perineal body, or onto the vulva just posterior to the vagina. The fistulas are probed (Fig. 6.3) to

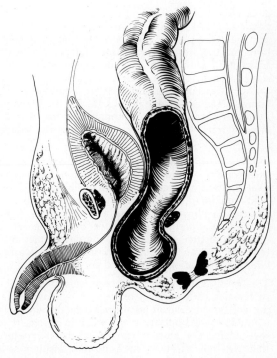

Fig. 6.2. Low anorectal atresia without fistula; rectum has descended through the puborectalis muscle

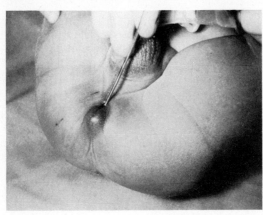

Fig. 6.3.
Low anorectal
atresia with
rectoperineal fistula
("covered anus").
Probe introduced
into fistula

determine more precisely the extent of the rectal descent. Radio-paque material injected through the fistula also helps to objectively document the precise anatomy. The coccyx is determined by palpation, and the presence of an intergluteal cleft by inspection. Perineal stimulation with a pin will document sensation, often eliciting a contraction of the external sphincter muscles to pinpoint their location. X-rays of the sacral vertebral bodies in an anteroposterior and lateral plane are essential, looking for bony anomalies. Intravenous pyelograms and voiding cystourethrograms record the status of the urinary tract. Occasionally, cystoscopy and injecting cystourethrography are justified.

If there is no perineal fistula, a low anorectal atresia (Fig. 6.2) is suggested by a midline perineal bulging when the baby cries. The dilated terminal rectum is seen as a gas-filled shadow on lateral plain radiographs taken after the baby has been inverted for 2–3 minutes to allow gas to displace meconium. A radiopaque marker placed on the perineal skin allows one to measure the distance from terminal rectum to skin. An alternative method is to needle the terminal rectum and inject water-soluble contrast material, after which lateral radiographs are taken.

Treatment is tailored to the precise anatomy of the abnormality. In females with perineal or vaginal fistulas, dilatation often allows normal bowel evacuation through the fistula; formal perineal anoplasty is carried out at several months of age. If probing the fistula reveals that the anus is simply covered by perineal skin (Fig. 6.3) that has not ruptured in a normal fashion, a simple "cutback" anoplasty (Fig. 6.4) may be performed. In this operation, the perineal skin that covers the anus is simply incised posteriorly in the

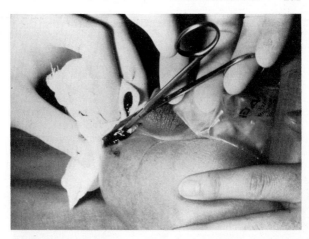

Fig. 6.4 a).   Cutback anoplasty

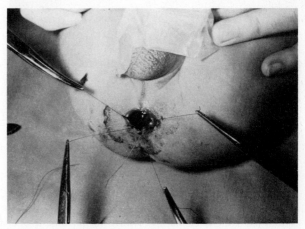

Fig. 6.4 b).   Completion of cutback anoplasty

midline, perineal skin being sutured to rectal mucosa to maintain the opening (Fig. 6.4 b). If a fistula cannot be dilated adequately to allow defecation, a formal transposition of the anus is carried out via the perineal approach, a faradic nerve stimulator precisely locating the external anal sphincter muscles through the center of which the ectopic anus is drawn and sutured to the perineal skin. By these simple measures, the "low" anorectal atresias are satisfactorily treated with expectation of good fecal control.

High Anorectal atresias

One of the varieties of high anorectal atresias should be suspected in a newborn with no anal opening and no rectoperineal or rectovulvar fistula. In the female, passage of meconium per vagina heralds a congenital rectovaginal fistula (Fig. 6.5); dilatation of the fistula usually suffices for early treatment. However, one must clearly determine where the urethral meatus lies: if it is visible, there will be

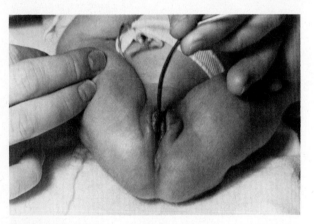

Fig 6.5.   Female with no anus who passes meconium from the vagina. Probe inserted into rectovaginal fistula

no admixture of urine and feces in the vagina and hence no threat of lower urinary tract infection. However, occasionally the urethra cannot be seen from below, which means that it opens ectopically into the anterior vagina; this anatomic condition is referred to as a "urogenital sinus", and when an atretic rectum discharges feces into the vagina (cloaca) through a rectovaginal fistula (rectocloacal fistula) then ascending urinary tract infection is expected, and the fecal stream should be diverted by colostomy.

The male with a "high" rectal atresia has no visible fistula. Indirect evidence of a rectourinary fistula is confirmed by pneumaturia or the passage of meconium in the urine.

Workup includes palpation of the coccyx, inspection of the intergluteal cleft and pinprick evaluation of perineal sensation and contraction of the external anal sphincter muscle group. Often the external anal sphincter muscle group is present only in a rudimentary
and disarrayed form. Lateral radiographs of the pelvis of the inverted
baby may help document where the rectum terminates (Fig. 6.6).
X-rays of the lumbosacral vertebrae, pyelograms and cystourethrograms are essential.

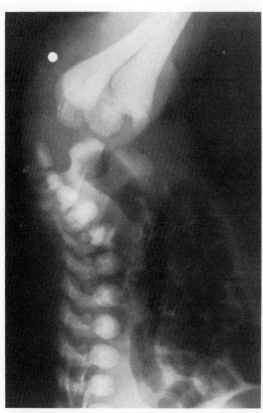

Fig. 6.6.
Lateral radiograph
of inverted newborn
with high rectal
atresia; note the
distance between the
gas in the terminal
rectum and the
radiopaque bead on
the perineal skin
(from: R. D. Liechty
and R. T. Soper:
Synopsis of Surgery.
Mosby, St. Louis,
Mo., 1972)

Treatment

Most surgeons agree that the safest initial treatment of a patient
with a high anorectal atresia is colostomy, to decompress the intestinal obstruction. If performed in the transverse colon, there is

enough bowel distally so that a corrective "pull-through" can later be carried out without disturbing the colostomy. As soon as the colostomy is established and functioning, the bowel distal to the colostomy is flushed out with saline injected via a catheter. The distal bowel is then filled with water-soluble radiocontrast material (Fig. 6.7) to pinpoint the level of atresia and document the presence and location of fistulas.

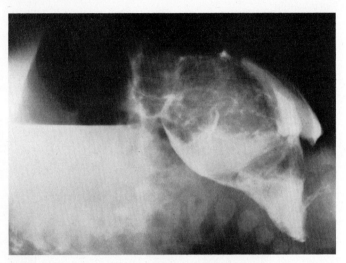

Fig. 6.7. Lateral radiograph after radiopaque dye is injected into the rectum via colostomy in a male baby with high rectal atresia; dye travels through rectourethral fistula and fills the urinary bladder

Definitive surgical correction of high anorectal atresia is generally carried out when the patient is a few months of age, or older. The most important feature of the operation is placing the rectum inside (anterior to) the puborectalis muscle en route to the perineum. Fecal continence, the best final test of the surgical procedure, hinges on this precise anatomic relocation of the rectum.

Anal Fissures

Anal fissure is a longitudinally-oriented superficial tear in the anal mucosa, located most commonly in the anterior or posterior midline. Most fissures result from the trauma of passing firm, bulky stools but, paradoxically, occasionally are seen with diarrhea. Anal fissures are especially common during the first year of life, when they constitute the most common cause of rectal bleeding.

The typical history of anal fissure is an infant or young child who screams while passing a bulky, firm stool which has a few drops of bright red blood clinging to its surface. Occasionally the blood follows the bowel movement, staining the diapers. If diarrhea is associated with the anal fissure, there is often severe perineal skin excoriation.

Blood loss is never severe, as evidenced by lack of pallor and a normal hemoglobin and hematocrit. The blood is on the outside of the firm stool, and not admixed. The fissure is visualized by spreading the buttocks apart and inspecting the now-everted anal mucosa.

Treatment should be directed toward restoring stool consistency to normal. Stool softening agents plus glycerine suppositories placed in the anal canal to lubricate its mucosa are adequate treatment for the majority of anal fissures associated with constipation (See Chapter 9). For those resulting from diarrhea, medical treatment of the diarrhea produces prompt healing of the anal fissure.

Fistulas and Perianal Abscesses

Perianal fistulas and abscesses are seen occasionally in infants but are uncommon in children, except as an external manifestation of Crohn's disease (transmural granulomatous enterocolitis) (see Capter 13). Thus, persistent or recurrent perianal fissures, fistulas or abscesses in older children should prompt sigmoidoscopy and contrast study of the entire gastrointestinal tract to rule out this serious intestinal inflammatory disease as a cause of the perianal problem.

In the simple perianal fistulas and abscesses in small infants the likely pathophysiology is: infection originating in anal glands or crypts which then dissects submucosally superficial to or through the external anal sphincter muscles to involve the subcutaneous fatty tissue in the perianal area. Conservative local treatment should first be tried with warm Sitz baths and local drainage of abscesses. If this does not suffice, surgical opening of the fistula or abscess through the offending anal crypt or gland is required for definitive control. These operations require general anesthesia because of the acute sensitivity of the area.

Hemorrhoids

Hemorrhoids are varicosities of anorectal veins. External hemorrhoids are covered by skin and are visible external to the anus, generally manifesting themselves as exquisitely tender, purplish local swellings in adolescents secondary to thrombi developing in the external hemorrhoidal veins. Warm Sitz baths and avoiding pressure on the area often help, but if these fail, thrombectomy is carried out under local anesthesia.

Internal hemorrhoids are varices of the hemorrhoidal veins above the anus, located within the lower rectum. They are extremely uncommon at any pediatric age except in patients with portal hypertension. In view of their rarity, workup on a pediatric patient with internal hemorrhoids should include evaluation for portal hypertension. Hardly ever is surgical treatment of the internal hemorrhoids necessary in childhood.

Rectal Prolapse

Prolapse of rectal mucosa or full thickness rectal wall (procidentia) (Fig. 6.8) through the anus is fairly common during the first two years of life, and extremely uncommon thereafter. This peculiar age relationship is explained by the relative mobility and lack of fixation of the rectum in the very young, the loose attachment of the rectal

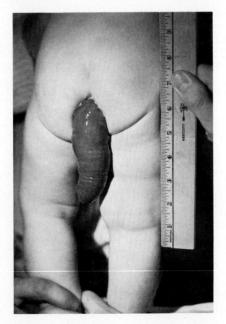

Fig. 6.8.
Complete rectal prolapse

mucosa to the muscularis and the fact that the sacrum is relatively straight in infancy, assuming a greater curvature during later years of childhood. Particularly predisposed to rectal prolapse are children with major neuromuscular disorders in and around the pelvis, i. e. exstrophy of the bladder or myelomeningocele with flaccid paraplegia and absence of rectal sphincters. To a lesser degree, children with constipation and especially those who by habit sit for lengthy periods on the toilet also suffer this alarming complaint. Rarely, polyps lead what amounts to an intussusception of the rectal wall out the anus.

Diagnosis is made at a glance, the radial mucosal folds of a purely superficial mucosal prolapse being easily distinguished from the circumferentially-oriented folds of a full thickness rectal wall prolapse. The prolapse may involve just a centimeter or two of bowel (mostly mucosal), to the extreme varieties where the rectal wall prolapses down to the knees with straining.

Workup includes a careful search for etiologic factors: major neuromuscular disorders, constipation, malnutrition, the bad habit of sitting for lengthy periods on the toilet, etc. Pernicious bowel habits are corrected by parental suggestion, and the constipation by appropriate stool softeners. The rectal prolapse is promptly reduced each time it occurs, taping the buttocks together to hold it reduced.

These simple treatment measures generally suffice in the ordinary case. Rectal prolapse that persists requires admitting the patient to hospital and depositing small amounts of hypertonic saline (30 % solution) just outside of the reduced rectum via a needle inserted just in front of the coccyx. The injection is made while the operator's finger is inside the rectum to assure the saline is deposited into the immediate perirectal tissue. Inflammation and reaction to the hypertonic saline serves to fix the rectum in its reduced position and discourage further rectal prolapse. In the extreme case, generally associated with major neuromuscular disorders, a wire or nylon suture is placed subcutaneously around the anus and tied down snugly while the operator's finger is in the anal canal.

Sacrococcygeal Teratoma

Although not originating in or from the anorectum, sacrococcygeal teratoma will be included in this chapter. It generally produces a rather conspicuous mass adjacent to the anus and rectum (Fig. 6.9) which may displace and compress the lower bowel and urinary tract, producing symptoms which justify its discussion here.

By definition, teratomas consist of tissue derived from all three germinal layers: ectoderm, mesoderm and endoderm. They are gener-

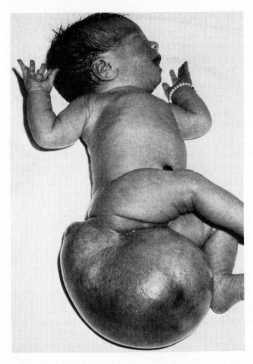

Fig. 6.9.
Huge sacrococcygeal
teratoma

ally located near the midline, often in the vertebral gutter. The sacrococcygeal region is the most common site for teratomas that become clinically evident during the first year of life; retroperitoneal, cervical and intracranial teratomas less often produce enough symptoms to bring the patient to diagnosis during infancy. In contrast, the average age at diagnosis of teratomas arising in the ovary, mediastinum, and testicle is late adolescence or early young adulthood.

The incidence of sacrococcygeal teratoma is in the neighborhood of 1:40,000 births with females outnumbering males by a 3:1 ratio. These teratomas are generally multiloculated cysts with varying amounts of solid tissue in the lobular septa, and are usually rounded and well encapsulated. They vary in size from 1 cm to enormous swellings as large as the baby's head (Fig. 6.9). They either have a stalk which connects the teratoma to the coccyx, or they may extend in front of the sacrum into the retroperitoneal region. Occasionally, appendages or grossly recognizable organs are observed.

About 10 % of sacrococcygeal tumors are malignant. Malignancy is related to age, being extremely uncommon in teratomas excised before the age of three months and increasing progressively in those discovered later in life.

Sacrococcygeal teratoma is generally obvious in the newborn as a roundish cystic or solid mass of the buttocks which displaces anus and rectum anteriorly. The mass usually is midline although extending to one side or the other to some degree. The teratomas are covered with apparently normal skin, with rare exceptions. The larger teratomas may obstruct labor and occasionally rupture during vaginal delivery. Careful rectal digital examination is mandatory to assess the amount of the tumor which lies between the sacrum and rectum. Understandably, teratomas that have large presacral extensions displace rectum and bladder anteriorly and produce obstructive symptoms of constipation and hydronephrosis and occasionally edema of the lower extremities. This is the exception to the rule, however, that usually the genitourinary and bowel functions are normal.

Plain anteroposterior and lateral radiographs reveal calcification within the teratoma in about 40 % of cases. The calcification may be diffuse or may show definitive structures such as partially formed bones or teeth. Teratomas with intrapelvic and retroperitoneal extensions produce dilated loops of bowel with anterior displacement of colon and rarely hydronephrosis.

To be ruled out in the differential diagnosis of sacrococcygeal teratoma is a posterior sacral myelomeningocele which produces a presacral mass only. An especially careful neurologic examination should be carried out. Plain radiographs of the sacrum are crucial, looking for evidence of spina bifida (posterior sacral myelomeningocele) and bony defects in the anterior wall of the sacrum (anterior sacral myelomeningocele). Rarely, combinations of both sacrococcygeal teratoma and myelomeningocele occur, and an accurate diagnosis is possible only at operation. Pressure on the sacral myelomeningocele should cause the open anterior fontanelle to bulge, as an aid in differential diagnosis; when the infant strains or cries the sacral myelomeningocele becomes more tense, whereas the sacrococcygeal teratoma does not.

Surgical excision of sacrococcygeal teratoma is carried out as soon as feasible. There is no benefit in delaying surgery, and there is some danger because of malignant degeneration.

Operation is safely undertaken under general anesthesia, the patient in the jackknife position with the buttocks elevated. The coccyx is always removed with the tumor. When the tumor has been removed, dead space is obliterated by suture and the wound is drained temporarily.

Prognosis is very good if the sacrococcygeal tumor is benign, and if complete excision is achieved. Tissue that is left behind will produce recurrent tumors requiring secondary excision, remarkably increasing the chance for malignancy to develop. Malignant sacrococcygeal teratomas are difficult to safely remove completely because they invade adjacent muscle, rectum, and other tissues. Most babies with malignant sacrococcygeal tumor die from metastases within one year of operation.

7 Malformations of the Spine

U. G. Stauffer

Spina Bifida

Spina bifida is by far the most important malformation of the spine. Under this term we include various serious deformities of the spine, which represent a developmental gap in one or several vertebrae. If the malformation is confined to the spine, it is called a spina bifida occulta; if the overlying tissues (the meninges and the spinal cord) are also affected, it is called a spina bifida cystica. In one only the meninges are affected (meningocele), and in the other the spinal cord is also involved (myelomeningocele).

The different types of spina bifida are easily explained embryologically (Fig. 7.1). In the 14-day-old embryo a strip of dorsal ectoderm thickens to form the *neural plate* (Fig. 7.1 a), which then forms a linear depression known as the *neural groove* (Fig. 7.1 b). Later, the

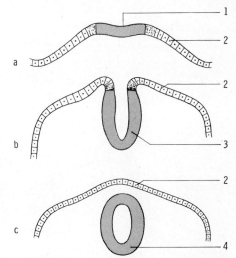

Fig. 7.1. Schematic representation of the developing neural tube from ectoderm:
a) Differentiation of neural plate (1) from ectoderm (2);
b) Formation of neural groove (3);
c) Formation of neural tube (4)

lips of the groove fuse together, forming the *neural tube* (Fig. 7.1 c). This fusion starts in the middle and extends craniad and caudad. Fusion is complete by the end of the third week of pregnancy.

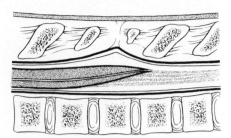

Fig. 7.2.   a) Spina bifida occulta;

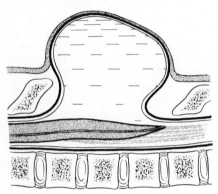
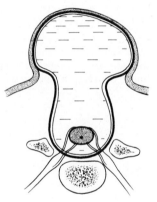

b) Meningocele;

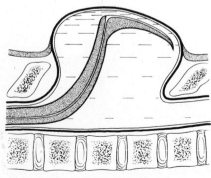
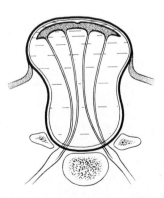

c) Covered myelomeningocele;

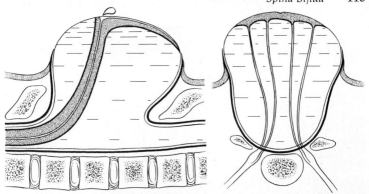

d) Open myelomeningocele; the neural plate is exposed and cerebrospinal fluid drops out of the spinal canal

Simultaneously, the ectoderm fuses dorsally to the neural tube, leaving it buried beneath. Mesoderm invades the space between the neural tube and the body ectoderm, forming the spinal membranes and the vertebral arches. Inhibition of this embryonic process during some phase causes the different types of spina bifida. A disturbance in the differentiation of the mesoderm causes spina bifida occulta (Fig. 7.2 a) or meningocele (Fig. 7.2 b); an earlier disturbance while the neural tube is developing creates a myelomeningocele (Fig. 7.2 c and d).

Spina Bifida Occulta

The defect affects only vertebral arch or arches. The meninges and the spinal cord are intact. Occult spina bifida is frequently discovered accidentally by radiography. Only one or two vertebral arches are usually affected, most frequently the 5th lumbar and the 1st sacral vertebrae (Fig. 7.3). This anomaly is of no significance, occurring in about 10 % of the population. Pigmented nevi, a small patch of hair, a hemangioma, lipoma or a small dimple over the sacrolumbar region are often external clues of the underlying defect (Fig. 7.4).

Spina Bifida Cystica

The precise etiology of spina bifida cystica is still unknown. Frequent occurrence in the same family speaks for a genetic component but definite hereditary factors have not been found. Marked fluctuations

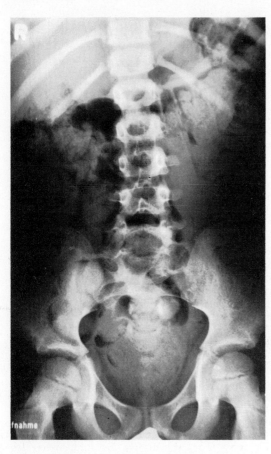

Fig. 7.3.
6-year-old boy;
spina bifida occulta
L_5 to S_1: no neuro-
logical deficits

in its incidence make additional enviromental factors a possibility.
The frequency of spina bifida cystica varies considerably from country to country. It occurs relatively rarely in Switzerland and Japan
(1 in 3000 births), whereas in the U.S.A. its incidence approaches
1 in 1000 births and in England 3 in 1000 births. If one child in a
family is born with spina bifida cystica, the chance of a second child
being similarly afflicted is 1 in 250 births in Switzerland and 1 in
30 births in England. Approximately 10 %/o consist of pure meningoceles, and in the remainder myelomeningoceles are found. Both types
occur most frequently in the lumbosacral region, less often in the
cervical region and least commonly in the thoracic vertebrae.

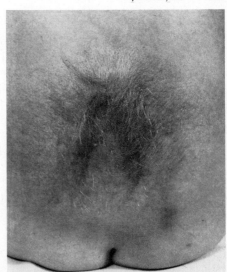

Fig. 7.4. Same patient as in 7.3.: a tuft of hair indicates an underlying spina bifida occulta

Meningoceles

The protruding meninges form a softish or tense sac of variable size. The underlying spinal cord is normal and there is no neurological

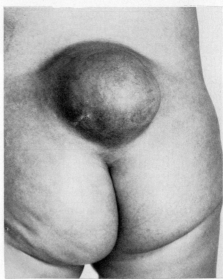

Fig. 7.5. Lumbosacral meningocele: the overlying skin is normal but there is a pale portwine stain

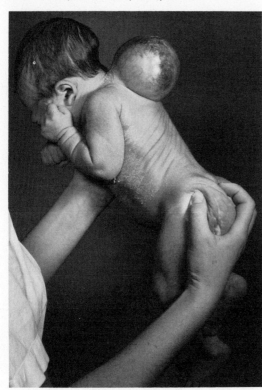

Fig. 7.6.
Large occipital
meningocele: the
skin is thin and in
planes translucent
and bulges on
screaming

deficit. The sac is often covered by normal skin which becomes more tense when the child cries. Occasionally, the skin covering the sac is replaced by a hemangioma (Fig. 7.5). Sometimes the sac is extremely thin, consisting only of a translucent membrane (Fig. 7.6). These thin sacs rupture easily; if rupture is imminent, the meningocele must be excised as an emergency. In all the other cases the meningocele is electively excised when the baby is three to six months of age.

Myelomeningocele

This is one of the most serious and complicated malformations which a pediatric surgeon encounters. In the most serious cases the nerve tissue lies exposed on the body surface without any cover. The denuded neural plate usually appears as an oval, dark red area (medulla vasculosa); the upper and lower ends of the neural plate drain cerebrospinal fluid constantly. A thin, delicate membrane surrounds the actual nerve tissue which corresponds to the pia mater (zona epithelioserosa), which in turn is surrounded by normal skin. The neural plate often lies in the wall of a membranous sac which is filled with cerebrospinal fluid (Fig. 7.7); rarely, it is situated deeply within the sac.

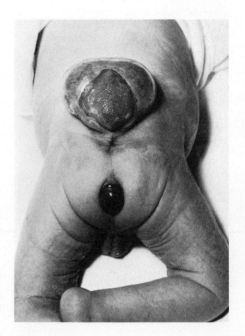

Fig. 7.7. Open lumbosacral myelomeningocele; prolapsed rectum secondary to paralysis of the pelvic muscles

Hardly any other congenital malformation is associated with so many distressing anomalies as myelomeningocele. Some consist of motor and sensory nerve defects, but often there are additional malformations involving other systems of the body.

Effects of Motor and Sensory Loss

Motor Loss of Limb Movements

Depending on the level of the neurological lesion, there is partial or total paralysis of the muscles of the abdomen, the back and the lower extremities. The paralysis is usually of the flaccid type. Sometimes the exact level of the neurological loss is difficult to pinpoint. The voluntary movements of a newborn with a meningomyelocele must be observed and recorded for a long time to document for certain the defect. Often the level of the neurological lesion and the level of the spinal defect do not correspond. This is partly explained by dysplasia of the spinal cord above the site of the myelomeningocele.

Over 50 % of myelomeningoceles are situated in the lower lumbar and upper sacral region. Typically the flexor and abductor muscles of the hips are still intact, wheras the adductor and extensor muscles are paralyzed; the quadriceps muscle and the dorsiflexors of the foot are often not affected. Fig. 7.8 shows this most common type of paralysis in a newborn. The legs are extended at the knee joint, flexed and abducted at the hip. The unopposed muscle pull frequently subluxates or dislocates the hip joint and produces clubfeet.

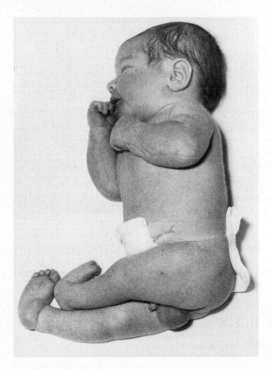

Fig. 7.8. Newborn infant with high lumbo-sacral myelomeningocele (L_2 to S_3). Typical position with hips bent at right angle, knees extended, legs adducted, club feet and paralysis of pelvic muscles

Paralysis of the Pelvic Floor

If the sacral segments 1 to 4 are affected, as so commonly is the case, partial or total paralysis of the pelvic floor, anal sphincter and the bladder occurs. Paralysis of the anal sphincter is heralded by a patulous anus and loss of the anal reflex; rectal prolapse sometimes occurs (Fig. 7.7). Paralysis of the bladder is recognized by constant dribbling of urine. Overflow incontinence is usually present, and is diagnosed clinically by palpating a round, tense mass above the symphysis pubis.

Sensory Loss

The level of sensory loss does not always correspond to the level of motor loss; often there is a difference of one to two segments. Trophic ulcers develop in the anesthetic areas (heel, knee, buttocks and perineum). Prevention of these chronic indolent trophic ulcers makes heavy demands on the nursing care.

Additional Malformations

The most common and severe malformation associated with myelo-meningocele is hydrocephalus, complicating about 80 % of all chil-dren with myelomeningocele. In some cases it occurs because of an associated anomaly (e. g. aqueduct stenosis), but more commonly hydrocephalus is caused by the so-called Arnold-Chiari malformation (Chapter 18). About 25 % of myelomeningocele patients are afflicted with malformations of the urogenital system (cystic kidneys, dys-plastic kidneys, urinary tract duplications, etc.). Most patients with myelomeningocele develop vesicoureteric reflux early, either as a separate anomaly (Chapter 18) or secondary to recurrent urinary infections triggered by the neurogenic bladder (Chapter 18). Addi-tional vertebral malformations are seen in about 40 % of the cases; wedge shaped vertebrae, hemi-vertebrae and fusions of vertebrae (Klippel-Feil syndrome) produce severe additional kyphosis and scoliosis (Fig. 7.9). Finally, children with myelomeningoceles often suffer from other deformities such as cardiac defects, omphaloceles, ectopic bladder, etc.

Treatment

Before satisfactory surgical treatment of hydrocephalus was devel-oped, no treatment for myelomeningocele was carried out. Even to-day, most experts agree that treatment should be withheld in those babies with severe deformities: complete paralysis of the pelvic floor and of the lower extremities, serious scoliosis and kyphosis, marked hydrocephalus present at birth and those with severe associated anomalies (cardiac defects, ectopic bladder, etc.) This pertains in about 1 out of 10 cases, who usually die during the first days or

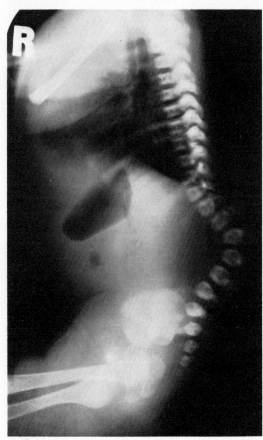

Fig. 7.9.
Newborn infant
with lumbosacral
myelomeningocele.
Marked kyphosis of
lower thoracic and
lumbar spine

weeks of life. When only the lower extremities are paralyzed, every case has to be judged individually as to the wisdom of surgical treatment.

Treatment by the Referring Physician

The decision concerning treatment must be made by a specialized team with experience in these matters at the appropriate referral center. The burden of making this decision rests solely on the shoulders of the parents. Every child born with a myelomeningocele should therefore be transferred to the nearest pediatric surgical center immediately after birth. The exposed neural plate must be covered with a damp, sterile dressing soaked in saline immediately after birth, and must be kept moist during transport to the hospital; alternatively it could be wrapped in a sterile bowel bag.

Treatment in Hospital

At the hospital a team of specialists should accept responsibility for the treatment of the child. If they decide that surgical treatment is justified, the myelomeningocele should be repaired during the first 24 hours of life. The neural plate must be covered by membrane and skin to avoid meningitis and desiccation of the exposed neural plate. At best this operation preserves the neural function which exists at birth; the hope that early operation would improve neural function has not materialized. If a hydrocephalus develops, a ventriculoatrial shunt is performed (see Chapter 8) after the myelomeningocele wound has healed. During the first hospitalization an intravenous pyelogram is performed to detect additional abnormalities of the kidneys; a radiograph of the hip documents hip dislocation, which is frequently present. In favorable cases, early bladder percussion training may prevent urinary infections by reducing the quantity of residual urine. Nevertheless, most patients sooner or later develop chronic urinary infections. Physiotherapy helps prevent secondary joint contractures.

With parenteral cooperation, a timetable for the many necessary therapeutic measures is arranged (fitting of orthopedic appliances, orthopedic operations, walking practice, operations for urinary diversion because of recurrent infections, incontinence and urinary tract dilatation, etc.). The aim of all these efforts is to offer these children a life in the community which is as normal as possible. The child should certainly be able to walk, at least with the aid of braces, he ought to be dry for at least 2 hours at a time (otherwise he will not be socially acceptable), and if possible he should be able to attend a normal school. Despite great efforts, this goal is unfortunately not frequently achieved.

Prognosis

About half of all children with myelomeningocele die during the first year of life, most during the first three months. The most common causes of death are meningitis or serious additional malformations. Only isolated cases die between the ages of one and four years, mostly of complications caused by hydrocephalus (acute intracranial pressure elevations, infections, etc.). About 50 % of the children live to the age of four to ten years. Over four years of age, life expectancy relates directly to the condition of the urinary tract. The I. Q. of the children depends on the gravity of the hydrocephalus and the time and success with which it has been relieved by operation. Children without hydrocephalus possess normal intelligence. About 40 % of children between the ages of five and ten years attend a normal school, 50 % attend a school for the physically handicapped and about 10 % are so severely handicapped that they cannot attend any school.

Sacral Agenesis

It is not uncommon to find agenesis of one or more sacral vertebrae on incidental radiographs of the spine. If only one or two vertebrae are missing this is of no importance. Agenesis of more than three sacral vertebrae causes severe disturbance in the innervation of the pelvic floor, with total or partial paralysis of the bladder and anus. Fig. 7.10 shows an example of sacral agenesis in a one-year-old boy

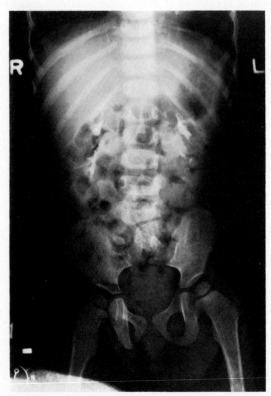

Fig. 7.10.
Sacral agenesis of 1-year-old boy; L$_5$ and S$_1$ are deformed; S$_2$ to S$_5$ are missing

with paralysis of the pelvic floor. The gaping anus and the absent anal reflex document the paralyzed external sphincter. A neurogenic bladder usually presents with incontinence and constant dribbling of urine. Overflow incontinence with all its later complications is usually present (Chapter 18). Sacral agenesis sometimes occurs together with anal or rectal atresia (Chapter 6) or with malformations of the urogenital system (Chapter 18).

Postural Deformities of the Spine

Anatomy

The posture of the spine shows marked variations in different age groups. At birth the spine is curved convexly from the occiput to the sacrum, resembling the shape of a banana. At about the age of two months when the child begins to lift his head while lying prone, physiological lordosis of the thoracic spine begins to develop. When sitting up at the age of six to eight months the spine straightens. At the age of ten to twelve months the child starts to stand and walk, which results in lumbar lordosis. This is most marked at the age of two to three years, but it decreases again afterwards. If it persists, it is usually a sign of general hypotony. The most common postural anomalies are discussed below (for details consult books on orthopedics).

Torticollis

Torticollis or wry neck is usually caused by fibrous contracture of the sternomastoid muscle. Rarely, a malformation of the cervical vertebrae (hemivertebrae, Klippel-Feil syndrome) causes torticollis.

The muscular type of torticollis is secondary to unilateral shortening of the sternomastoid muscle which is converted into fibrous tissue in its distal third. It is not certain whether this is caused by trauma, a true tumor (fibromatosis), a vascular accident or a local malformation.

Clinical Picture

Babies with torticollis often, but by no means always, are breech presentations. Shortly after birth the mother notices that the infant holds his head at an angle, or that there is a firm swelling on one side of the neck. Palpation reveals the typically olive-shaped, firm tumor in the lower third of the sternomastoid muscle. The head is inclined towards the affected side, but the face looks towards the opposite side. In severe cases it is impossible to rotate the face towards the affected side. In the majority of cases the tumor disappears spontaneously sometime during the first year of life.

If the torticollis remains until the second year of life, the clinical picture is quite typical (Fig. 7.11).

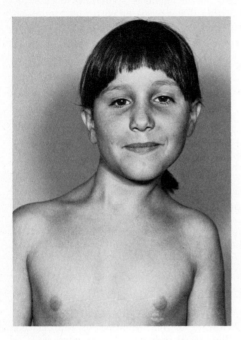

Fig. 7.11. Muscular torticollis of seven-year-old girl. The shortened muscle strand is clearly visible. The head is flexed towards the affected side and rotated towards the opposite side. Facial asymmetry

The shortened muscle strand is visible and palpable beneath the skin of the neck. The head is inclined towards the affected side and the shoulder on this side is slightly elevated. The child's face looks toward the unaffected side. In severe cases growth of the face on the affected side is retarded, the forehead appears flattened and the axes of the eyes are rotated. There is a postural scoliosis of the cervical spine with a compensatory curvature of the thoracic spine.

Treatment

During the first year of life parents administer physiotherapy which is designed to stretch and elongate the affected muscle; the baby is encouraged to look and sleep prone with his face turned toward the involved side. If the torticollis persists until the second year of life the shortened muscle is divided at its sternal and clavicular origin. This small operation is without any bad after-effects. After the operation the patient wears a light plastic collar for a number of weeks to accustom him to the new position of the head. Postoperative physiotherapy is necessary in neglected or especially severe cases. If the operation is carried out in time, the secondary deformities of the face and spine disappear spontaneously.

Postural Scoliosis of Infants

Infants occasionally have a lateral curve of the spine when lying supine. When a baby lifts his head while prone, or when one lifts up the child by placing his hands under the axilla, the scoliosis usually disappears. Neurological examination and spinal radiographs are normal. This type of scoliosis is usually within the normal physiological range and disappears spontaneously during the following months, with or without the help of physiotherapy. Nevertheless, these children must be watched at regular intervals for 1 to 2 years, because a few patients with postural scoliosis progress to idiopathic scoliosis, which is difficult to cure and requires lengthy orthopedic treatment (Fig. 7.12, 7.13).

Structural Scoliosis

There is a definite anatomical cause for structural scoliosis, which may be congenital or acquired. In the congenital type, hemivertebrae, wedge-shaped vertebrae and fused vertebrae (Klippel-Feil syndrome), etc. are found. Destruction of one or more vertebrae may cause an acquired structural scoliosis (osteomyelitis, neurofibromatosis, eosinophile granuloma, etc.).

Paralytic Scoliosis

Here scoliosis of the spine is caused by a neuromuscular disease, e. g. poliomyelitis, transverse myelitis, muscular dystrophy, etc.

Compensatory Scoliosis

This may occur due to unequal length of the lower limbs. In the standing patient it is easily recognized by noticing a pelvic tilt. In mild cases raising the heel of the shoe on the side of the short limb will equalize the length of the limbs sufficiently to cure the scoliosis. The most common cause of unequal length of the lower limbs is a badly united fracture (Chapter 22).

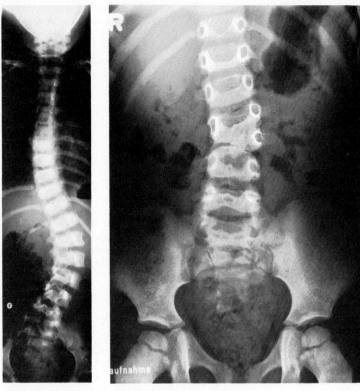

Fig. 7.12.   Fig. 7.13.

Fig. 7.12.   Idiopathic scoliosis of 7-year-old boy
Fig. 7.13.   Scoliosis secondary to hemivertebra convex towards the left in a 3-year-old boy

Scheuermann's Disease (Adolescent Kyphosis)

Scheuermann's disease generally afflicts adolescent males to produce marked kyphosis, especially in the upper thoracic spine. Many patients have bad posture and underdeveloped musculature in addition to their round back. The mobility of the thoracic spine is markedly reduced. The patient suffers back pain when he has to stand for long periods. On radiography flattened, partly wedge-shaped, deformed vertebrae are seen to cause the marked kyphosis of the thoracic spine. In mild cases, treatment consists mainly of postural exercises and physiotherapy, in serious cases in placing the patient in a plaster of Paris bed, etc. (For details see books on orthopedic surgery).

Dimples and Sacrococcygeal Sinuses

Many children have a small dimple or epithelium-lined tract superficial to the coccyx. Both these lesions give rise to little trouble. In the adult they may cause local infections secondary to sweating, seborrhea, growth of hair (infected sacral dermoid). If the dimple or sinus is relatively deep and narrow, it should be excised in childhood. If the dimple lies above the sacrum, it may be associated with spina bifida (Fig. 7.14). Very rarely there is a connection with the spinal

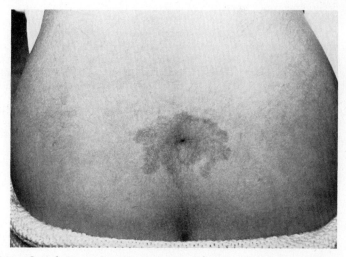

Fig. 7.14.   Sacral sinus of 10-year-old girl. The sinus is surrounded by a pale port wine stain. At operation it communicated with the subdural space

canal. If the bottom of such a dimple or sinus cannot be seen, or if it is very narrow, early careful excision is always indicated to prevent meningitis. In a child with recurrent meningitis of obscure origin the possibility of such a sacral sinus must be considered and the sacral region carefully examined.

8 Malformations and Surgical Diseases of Skull and Brain

U. G. STAUFFER

From the surgical point of view the most important deformities and diseases of the skull and brain are hydrocephalus, encephaloceles and craniosynostoses, which are discussed in this chapter. Tumors of the brain are not described here as they are generally treated by the neurosurgeon.

Hydrocephalus

Enlargement of the ventricles is referred to as *hydrocephalus internus* whereas enlargement of the subarachnoidal space is termed *hydrocephalus externus*. *Hydrocephalus externus* is usually caused by subarachnoid hemorrhage and is not discussed here. *Hydrocephalus internus* is usually caused by abnormal circulation of cerebrospinal fluid, more rarely it appears secondary to an atrophic process of the cerebrum. Cerebrospinal fluid is mainly produced in the choroid plexus within the ventricles, and to a lesser degree in the subarachnoid space. It circulates freely from the lateral ventricles through the third ventricle and the aqueduct to the fourth ventricle, from which it flows into the basal cysterns and the subarachnoid space around the cerebrum and spinal column. Absorption of cerebrospinal fluid into the blood occurs mainly in the subarachnoid and perineural spaces.

Congenital Hydrocephalus

Hydrocephalus occurs as an isolated event only once in 2000 births. However, it complicates about four-fifths of children with myelomeningocele as an additional problem (see Chapter 7). Therefore, overall it is a relatively common malformation.

Isolated Hydrocephalus

Isolated hydrocephalus is usually caused by a block in the area of the aqueduct of Sylvius (aqueduct stenosis). Accumulation of cerebrospinal fluid produces progressive enlargement of the lateral ventricles and of the third ventricle. Rarely isolated hydrocephalus results from stenosis of the foramen of Monro or of the foramina of Luschka and Magendie caused by a malformation or by pressure from a cyst or a tumor.

Hydranencephalus

The most severe (and fortunately rare) form of isolated hydrocephalus is hydranencephalus. In this condition both hemispheres of the cerebrum are partially or completely missing, replaced by a thin membrane consisting of some glial tissue and islands of undeveloped nerve tissue. The basal ganglia are normally developed. Etiology of hydranencephalus is obscure, perhaps resulting from faulty cerebral blood supply in its very early development. Although both lateral ventricles and the third ventricle are absent, children with hydranencephalus often have rapidly enlarging head circumferences. This must be due to additional disturbances in the flow of the cerebrospinal fluid.

Hydrocephalus and Myelomeningocele

Hydrocephalus often is associated with myelomeningocele. At times a stenosis of the aqueduct can be identified, but more commonly hydrocephalus results from an Arnold-Chiari malformation. The Arnold-Chiari malformation implies caudad displacement of the medulla and parts of the cerebellum through the foramen magnum. The tonsils of the cerebellum are pressed against the spinal cord, in this fashion blocking the flow of cerebrospinal fluid from the fourth ventricle to the basal cysterns and subarachnoid space.

Acquired Hydrocephalus

Hydrocephalus may be acquired at any age, often due to adhesions which form subsequent to a bout of meningitis and less frequently after a cerebral hemorrhage. Hydrocephalus secondary to toxoplasmosis is a classic example of an intrauterine acquired anomaly. In infancy, hydrocephalus occurs most commonly from adhesions generated by a coliform or hemophilus influenza meningitis. Hydrocephalus triggered by postpartum hemorrhage may manifest itself during the first few weeks of life. Rarely, hydrocephalus develops later in childhood following a traumatic intracranial hemorrhage. Hydrocephalus commonly develops secondary to cerebrospinal fluid flow occasioned by a cerebral tumor.

Clinical Features

Rarely, in true congenital hydrocephalus the head becomes markedly enlarged in utero, and may present an obstacle during labor; usually the head circumference is normal at birth. Fig. 8.1 illustrates an untreated hydrocephalus in a five-month-old boy. In such severe cases the diagnosis is obvious by the large head, separation of the

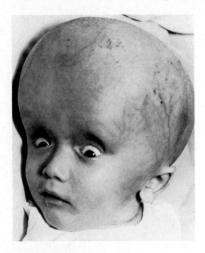

Fig. 8.1. Untreated hydrocephalus in a 5-month-old child

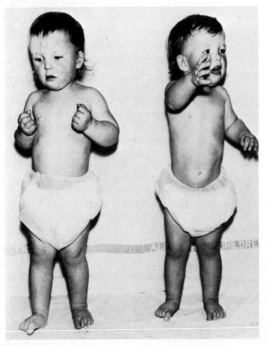

Fig. 8.2.
Three-year-old twins; one was operated upon for severe hydrocephalus at the age of two months

sutures, the wide anterior fontanelle, the comparatively small face with the eyes displaced downwards, etc. In these children, complications of marked cerebral pressure elevation are found: convulsions, opisthotonus, spasticity, internal strabismus, nystagmus and optic atrophy as well as other neurological symptoms. Treatment at such an advanced stage is impossible because the neurological damage is irreversible. The results of neglect, as depicted in Fig. 8.1, should not occur today. In contrast, Fig. 8.2 shows hydrocephalus in a three-year-old child which was diagnosed early and surgically corrected when the patient was two months old. Early diagnosis is therefore of great importance for the future development of these children. Physicians must be familiar with the early signs of hydrocephalus, which are discussed later.

Hydrocephalus in Neonates and Infants

Increase in the Circumference of the Head

Serial measurements of head circumference of neonates and infants is the most important clue to early diagnosis of hydrocephalus. If

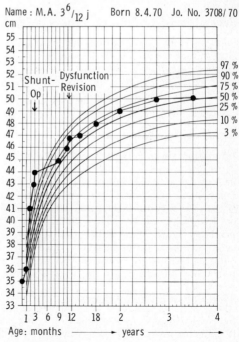

Fig. 8.3.
Head circumference curve in congenital hydrocephalus. The circumference has increased from the 25th to the 97th percentile. It normalizes after operation

the head is abnormally large at birth, or if it grows abnormally quickly during the first weeks of life it must be measured at least once a week and plotted on a curve (Fig. 8.3). If the growth of the head circumference deviates significantly from normal in either direction, the baby should be referred to a special center for a more sophisticated examination. In some infants the abnormal rate of growth of the head may be the only sign of hydrocephalus for some time. In contrast, when the fontanelles have closed later in childhood, head circumference is only of secondary importance; far more significant in these children are the signs of increased intracerebral pressure which rapidly develop (see below).

The "Setting-Sun" Sign

This describes a temporary or permanent downward displacement of the eyes, the sclera appearing as a white crescent above the iris (Fig. 8.1). The setting-sun sign is an early manifestation of hydrocephalus, probably caused by the pressure of the enlarged third ventricle on the oculomotor nerve. This phenomenon is occasionally seen in healthy infants.

Separation of the Sutures, Tense Fontanelle

Separation of the sutures implies rapid enlargement of the head, and is usually associated with a tense fontanelle as the classical sign of increased intracerebral pressure. However, since the skull bones separate relatively easily in infants and newborns, pathologically elevated intracerebral pressure need not be associated with a tense fontanelle in the very young.

Cranial Nerve Paralyses

Internal strabismus is commonly seen in babies with hydrocephalus, probably caused by compression of the sixth cranial nerve during its long intracranial course. The squint usually disappears after treatment when the cerebral pressure returns to normal. Sometimes paralysis of the recurrent laryngeal nerve and of the glossopharyngeal nerve is observed, or optic nerve atrophy occurs. These are probably primary disturbances rather than secondary to increase in intracerebral pressure. Papilledema, which is of diagnostic importance in older children with hydrocephalus, hardly ever occurs in newborn babies and infants.

Thinning of the Skull Bones

Severe hydrocephalus produces thinning of the skull bones which is detected radiographically (Lückenschädel). The "beaten silver" appearance on X-ray of skull bones which occasionally is seen in older children may not have the same significance, because it sometimes occurs in perfectly normal children as well as in children with raised intracerebral pressure.

Spasticity

Even in newborns and small infants increased muscle tone and reflexes secondary to increased intracranial pressure is detectable. This is perhaps best demonstrated when eliciting the patellar reflex. These neurological symptoms may precede clinically apparent hydrocephalus by days or weeks.

Transillumination

A strong light source applied to the skull of an infant with hydrocephalus in a darkened room will transilluminate brilliantly red those portions of the brain which are distended with cerebrospinal fluid. This simple test will document the extent of the hydrocephalus.

Hydrocephalus in the Older Child

Older children exhibit manifestations of increased intracranial pressure much more rapidly than infants because fontanelles have closed and the skull is less elastic. Symptoms are similar to those found in adults: headaches and nausea and vomiting. Percussion of the skull elicits the typical "cracked pot" sound in advanced cases. Radiography shows classical widening of the suture lines. Retinoscopy reveals papilledema secondary to compression of the central optic vein caused by the increased intracranial pressure.

Special Investigations

Radiography of the Skull

Anteroposterior and lateral X-rays document widening of the suture lines, the thinned skull bones exhibiting the typical "beaten silver" appearance. Intracranial calcifications are occasionally seen, indicative of a former meningitis (i. e. toxoplasmosis).

Serological Examinations

Blood is examined for antibodies against toxoplasmosis, cytomegalic inclusion bodies, etc.

Ventricular Puncture

Neonates and young infants should have the lateral ventricles punctured with a special needle inserted through the lateral angle of the anterior fontanelle to measure intracranial pressure and to analyze cerebrospinal fluid chemically and bacteriologically. A cerebrospinal fluid pressure which is over 120 mm of water is pathologically elevated for infants.

Air Encephalography

Radiographs taken after air has been injected into the lateral ventricle will define the severity of hydrocephalus, the thickness of the re-

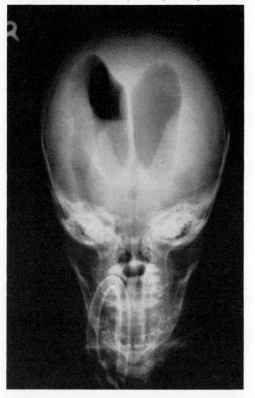

Fig. 8.4.   Air encephalography of hydrocephalus secondary to meningitis (a) AP, (b) lateral. Marked dilatation of lateral ventricles and 3rd ventricle. Air does not pass into 4th ventricle

maining pallium (cortex) and the shape and size of the ventricles. It also may uncover additional malformations such as porencephaly, absent corpus callosum, etc. (Fig. 8.4). Today treatment does not hinge upon precise differentiation between communicating hydro-cephalus (where the intracranial cerebrospinal fluid system com-municates with the subarachnoid spaces) and noncommunicating hydrocephalus (where there is a block in the ventricular system) (see below). It is therefore usually sufficient to inject 20 to 40 ml of air after aspirating double that amount of cerebrospinal fluid from the lateral ventricles. Fig. 8.4 shows an air encephalogram on a three-month-old infant with hydrocephalus secondary to stenosis of the aqueduct.

Differential Diagnosis

An abnormally large head is also found in children with so-called *macrocephaly*, a variant of normal in which the head is abnormally large but grows at the same rate as a normal head. The brain mass is increased, the ventricles are of normal size and the intracranial pressure is normal. It is interesting that patients with macrocephaly are usually below normal in intelligence and their development is retarded. An abnormally rapidly growing head is also found in children with chronic subdural hematoma and subdural hygroma (see Chapter 21).

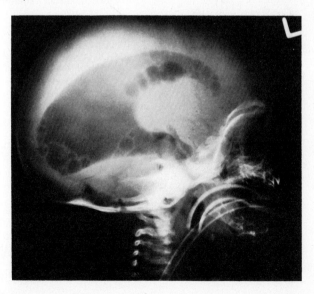

Fig. 8.4 b

Treatment

Treatment of hydrocephalus is surgical. The aim of the operation is to lower intracranial pressure to normal by shunting excess cerebrospinal fluid into the bloodstream, the pleura or the peritoneal cavity. A ventriculoatrial shunt is most commonly employed; we recommend the Holter valve. Fig. 8.5 shows the entire drainage system in situ. The cerebrospinal fluid flows through a catheter from the right lateral ventricle into a reservoir which is connected to the valve; the valve allows unhindered flow of cerebrospinal fluid downstream but prevents any reflux of blood. It opens at a pre-set pressure to allow cerebrospinal fluid to flow through the distal catheter via the internal jugular vein and superior vena cava into the right atrium.

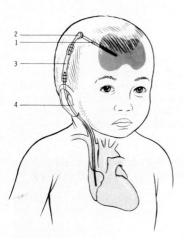

Fig. 8.5.   Schematic representation of ventriculoatrial shunt using the Holter valve:
1, ventricular catheter;
2, reservoir;
3, valve;
4, Distal catheter passed via internal jugular vein and superior vena cava into right atrium

Complications

The most common complication of all drainage operations for hydrocephalus is blockage of the system and infection.

Blockage of the Drainage System

The ventriculoatrial drainage system ultimately becomes blocked in nearly half of the cases. Most commonly the ventricular catheter becomes blocked by fibrin, choroid plexus or blood clot; percutaneous puncture of the reservoir and infection of saline down the proximal catheter will generally relieve this kind of block. Blockage of the distal catheter is less common, and must be surgically corrected.

The *symptoms* of a block in the drainage system are headache, vomiting, a bulging fontanelle, unexplained fever, occasionally neck rigidity or a sudden internal squint.

Infection

Infection complicates nearly a quarter of the cases and is extremely serious. It often forces the surgeon to temporarily remove the entire drainage system.

Prognosis

Prognosis depends on the severity of the hydrocephalus, its causative disease (toxoplasmosis, myelomeningocele) and the age at which treatment is begun. Most deaths are caused by associated malformations; less commonly infections or acute intracranial pressure crises will cause fatalities. The intelligence of the surviving children is at times surprisingly high. No correlation exists between the thickness of the remaining cerebral cortex and intelligence of the patient after operation. Children with a cerebral cortex only 10 mm thick may be normal or near normal in intelligence. About 50 % of the children who reach school age after early operation are of normal intelligence.

Encephalocele

An encephalocele is a sac-like protrusion of meninges and brain through a congenital defect in the skull, usually in the occipital region. Encephaloceles can be very large and contain the cerebellum and parts of the cerebrum; if so, there is usually an associated microcephaly (Fig. 8.6). More rarely only the meninges but not the brain protrude (occipital meningocele, Fig. 8.7). The skin over the encephalocele is often normal in texture but may be very thin and translucent. Less than 1 % of cases exhibit a so-called anterior meningocele, which is usually situated at the root of the nose. Radiographs pinpoint the size and precise location of the bony defect. The air encephalogram may reveal associated cerebral malformations, which not uncommonly co-exist with encephaloceles.

Treatment

Resection of the meningocele or encephalocele must be performed. It is impossible to replace protruded brain matter, as this produces a dangerous rise of intracranial pressure. The defect is closed by

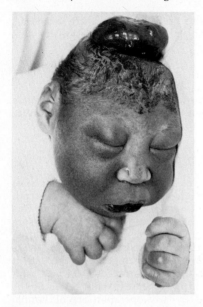

Fig. 8.6. Occipital encephalocele. The sac contains cerebellum and part of cerebrum. Microcephalus

dura. Children with severe encephaloceles usually survive for only a few months; however, the prognosis for occipital meningoceles is usually good, although some of them develop hydrocephalus postoperatively.

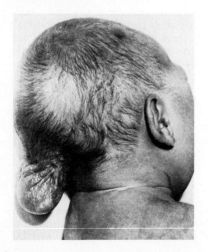

Fig. 8.7. Occipital meningocele. The sac contains no brain tissue

Craniosynostosis

In the skull, bone growth occurs only in the region of the sutures. Normally these sutures do not ossify until late in adult life; only the frontal cranial suture ossifies shortly before or after birth. Premature closure of cranial sutures leads to craniosynostosis. If one suture closes prematurely, compensatory overgrowth occurs in the vicinity of the remaining still-open sutures. This produces at times grotesque deformities of the skull. If several sutures unite prematurely, brain development is retarded. The etiology of craniosynostosis is unknown. Occasionally it occurs in families, but a definite inheritance has not been proved. Boys are more commonly affected than girls (4:1).

The prematurely closed suture is often palpable as a ridge beneath the scalp. Skull radiographs demonstrate the bony ridge along the suture line which can, however, still be recognized; bone bridges the suture at different places. Complete ossification of the suture only occurs after weeks or months. The other sutures are wide open. The degree of skull deformity can be objectively recorded according to the method described by Grob, which is calculated from the formula

$$\frac{\text{width (cm)} \times 100}{\text{length (cm)}} = \text{skull index}$$

The normal skull index is between 70 and 80.

Clinical Picture

The most common skull deformities are schematically illustrated in Fig. 8.8. Most commonly affected are the sagittal suture, then the bilateral coronal sutures, then the frontal and least commonly the unilateral coronal suture. The rarest malformation is premature closure of all sutures.

Premature Closure of the Sagittal Suture

(Fig. 8.8 a)

This produces a skull deformity referred to as *scaphocephaly*. There is compensatory growth at the coronal-lambdoid suture which results in a long and narrow head with a frontal prominence, resembling a turned-up boat. The skull index is between 60 and 70. Fig. 8.9 shows a four-month-old infant with scaphocephaly.

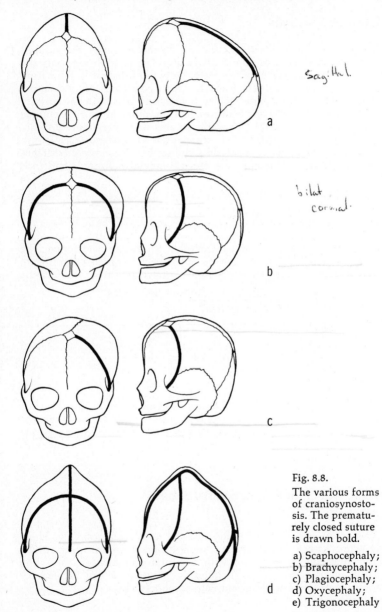

Sagittal.

bilat. coronal.

Fig. 8.8.
The various forms of craniosynostosis. The prematurely closed suture is drawn bold.

a) Scaphocephaly;
b) Brachycephaly;
c) Plagiocephaly;
d) Oxycephaly;
e) Trigonocephaly

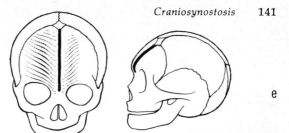

Fig. 8.8 e.

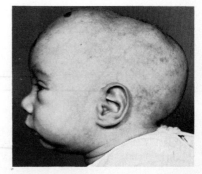

Fig. 8.9. Premature closure of sagittal suture (scaphocephaly) in three-month-old infant. The head is long and narrow

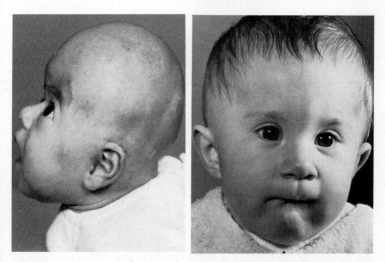

Fig. 8.10. Premature closure of coronal sutures (brachycephaly) in 4-month-old infant. The head is broad and short

Fig. 8.11. Premature closure of frontal suture (trigonocephaly) in one-year-old girl

Premature Bilateral Closure of the Coronal Suture

(Fig. 8.8 b)

The result here is *brachycephaly*. The head grows compensatorily at the sagittal suture and is high, broad and short (Fig. 8.10). The skull index is usually over 90.

Premature Unilateral Closure of the Coronal Suture

(Fig. 8.8 c)

This results in asymmetrical *plagiocephalus.* The forehead on the affected side is flattened, the orbital arch pulled upward and the palpebral fissure appears to be enlarged. The actually normal opposite side appears to bulge. Sometimes the expression plagiocephalus is also used for children with congenital torticollis (see Chapter 11), but in the latter condition the whole skull is affected with actual flattening on one side and bulging on the other.

Synostosis of the coronal suture is often combined with other malformations; when combined with syndactyly, it is called *Crouzon's syndrome.* Here the malformation is more complicated as the skull

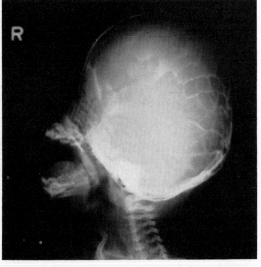

a) Radiograph when three months old. Thinned skull bones with "beaten silver" appearance, short, high skull.

Fig. 8.12.   Premature closure of all skull sutures

base is short and thick and the orbits are frequently underdeveloped, causing exophthalmos and occasionally primary optic atrophy because of narrowing of the optic foramina.

There is frequently associated mental retardation. The prognosis of Crouzon's disease is less favorable than that of simple unilateral closure of the coronal suture.

Premature Closure of All Sutures

(Fig. 8.8 d)

This produces *oxycephalus,* in which the head can only grow upward in the region of the anterior fontanelle (Fig. 8.12). Brain development is markedly restricted.

Premature Closure of the Frontal Suture

(Fig. 8.8 e)

The result here is *trigonocephaly,* in which the forehead is narrow, resembling the keel of a ship (Fig. 8.11). This deformity usually requires no treatment. Operation is only indicated in very severe cases.

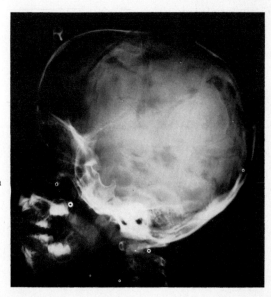

b) Radiograph when two years old. One can still recognize the linear craniectomy along the coronal and sagittal sutures. Skull deformity less marked

Diagnosis and Differential Diagnosis

Characteristic skull deformity and typical radiographs usually leave little doubt about the diagnosis. Occasionally, primary microcephaly may be mistaken for premature closure of several sutures, but the radiograph shows open sutures throughout.

Treatment

Treatment consists of excising a strip of bone parallel to the affected suture and enveloping the raw bone edges in a silicone sheath to prevent renewed premature closure. Indication for operation is mainly cosmetic. Only if several sutures are affected is there danger of retardation of brain development. The earlier the operation, the better the results. If operation is carried out at the age of two to four months, the shape of the skull should normalize during the next two to three years (Fig. 8.12).

9 Constipation

R. T. SOPER

General

Constipation is rare in the very young but is a common complaint during older infancy and childhood, at one time or another likely to affect almost every child. About 5 % of school children have chronic and often recurrent bouts of constipation as a significant complaint bringing them to the physician.

A brief classification of constipation problems in childhood would include certain metabolic disturbances such as hypothyroidism and hyperparathyroidism, which have as part of their clinical picture chronic constipation. Both of these metabolic disorders have other distinctive stigmata that allow identification of the primary disease, correction of which relieves the constipation.

Certain neurological disorders are frequently associated with constipation. Paraplegic babies with myelomeningocele have constipation as one of their numerous problems, likely from paralysis of abdominal wall muscles. Babies born with a congenital absence of abdominal wall musculature, the so-called "prune belly syndrome" (Chapter 19), also have difficulty in both bowel and bladder function, signifying the importance of voluntary abdominal wall contraction for normal defecation and urination. Children with cerebral palsy or mental retardation have a higher than expected incidence of constipation, for reasons which are less clear. Diagnosis of these neurological conditions which predispose to constipation are generally self-evident. The constipation is a minor part of their overall problem and is treated symptomatically.

Primary intestinal causes for obstipation include ileus of both paralytic and mechanical origin: the temporary and acute nature of the constipation plus the associated findings clearly separate these problems (Chapter 5) from ordinary constipation. When intake of food is curtailed, whatever the reason, constipation ensues; this is a common complaint in babies with pyloric stenosis, for example. Anything which produces anal or perianal pain makes defecation a painful and unhappy experience, leading to withholding of stool. Fissures, perianal fistulae and perianal abscess are the most common examples.

There is a fairly large number of children with unknown causes for their constipation, variously termed "acquired constipation", "psychogenic constipation" or "habit constipation". In many of these children constipation originates near the toilet training period of life (generally during the second year), the voluntarily withheld stool acting as a psychological weapon demanding more parental attention. This variety of constipation is associated with frequent fecal soiling, social ostracization and a remarkable amount of parental concern, which may simply perpetuate the problem. Abrupt, traumatic or premature attempts at toilet training on the part of the parents often trigger this cycle. Psychogenic overtones are quickly acquired in these patients, whether or not they exist at the onset.

There is a relatively smaller group of patients who become constipated during preschool or early school years simply because they develop bad bowel habits. Because of play activities or other current interests, they resist the natural urges to defecate and ultimately end up with a dilated, stool-filled rectum and sigmoid which is relatively atonic. If these children are psychologically normal, they respond well to symptomatic treatment which will be discussed later.

Constipation Related to Age

Infancy

Constipation that begins during the first year of life, after an initial period of several weeks or several months of normal bowel movements, is likely to be secondary to acute anal fissure.

This type of constipation results from a vicious cycle: an acute linear tear in the anal mucosa produces exquisite pain during the passage of an unusually firm or bulky stool (often accompanied by blood streaking or following the stool), which then triggers reflex anal sphincter spasm; memory of the painful defecation induces the baby to voluntarily withhold stool for several days, while the fecal material becomes more firm, dehydrated and larger in diameter in the now dilated rectal ampulla. When it becomes impossible to resist defecation, this large and hard stool is passed which reopens the fissure and again triggers exquisite pain to rekindle the cycle. Constipation on this basis can either be intermittent or continuous and progressive.

During the acute stage of the fissure, diagnosis is easily confirmed by inspecting the anal canal which is everted when the buttocks are spread apart. Treatment includes glycerine suppositories to lubricate the anal canal and trigger a daily bowel movement, the stool consistency being altered by a softener such as mineral oil or Colace. The daily bowel movement of soft, easy to pass stool through a well lubricated anal canal quickly heals the fissure and in a short time spontaneous and pain-free bowel movements are restored. Treatment is tapered and ultimately discontinued.

If the patient does not come to diagnosis until after several weeks of this cycle, the anal fissure which triggered the episode initially or which served to perpetuate it from time to time, may have healed long since. Inspection of the anal canal is normal at this time, with generally no trace of the previous fissure. The diagnosis is suspected by the history, however, and is confirmed by digital examination of an unusually tight anal sphincter spasm and a commodious rectal ampulla filled with hard stool, often with residual firm stool palpable in the sigmoid colon. Treatment begins by evacuating all the residual stool by oil retention enemas followed by cleansing saline enemas. Once the lower colon is emptied of stool, treatment is shifted to a daily glycerine or medicated (Dulcolax) suppository while the stool consistency is softened by dietary manipulation and/or stool softeners. The dosage of the stool softener is tailored to produce a soft-formed or slightly unformed stool. After the bowel movements have been controlled on a daily basis in this manner for two or three weeks, treatment is gradually tapered and diminished with the expectation that the youngster will resume normal bowel habits spontaneously. There is rarely any need to consider sigmoidoscopy, barium enema studies or more sophisticated investigation of this kind of constipation.

Constipation Originating During the Second Year of Life

Constipation onsetting during the second year of life, after previously normal bowel habits, often centers around toilet training. Careful history reveals that the toilet training was abrupt, punitive, rigidly enforced or begun at too early an age to expect patient cooperation. These children voluntarily withhold stool, often in a manner which is misconstrued by parents as an attempt to **have** a bowel movement. The child quickly learns that the longer he withholds stool the more concerned the parents become and the more attention they pay to him, even though the attention is commonly traumatic. When stool is withheld for several days, the rectal ampulla dilates and the sigmoid colon fills with palpable lumps of firm stool. These children frequently soil their underpants with liquid stool ("paradoxical diarrhea"). The incontinence of stool is best explained by constant pressure on the levator sling musculature of the wedge-like bolus of firm stool which is almost constantly resident within the rectal ampulla. Because skeletal muscle ultimately tires, the puborectalis gradually becomes more and more lax and ultimately a wedge of stool is driven down into the terminal rectum. When the external anal sphincter fatigues, the tip of this firm stool is often visible upon spreading the buttocks. As fermented and much more liquefied stool is brought to the distal bowel by peristaltic activity, it commonly flows around the impacted ampullary stool and leaks through the now-patulous sphincter to stain the underpants. Because of the patulous anus, the visible firm stool in the anal canal and the constant soiling, these children are often referred to diagnostic centers because of presumed neuromuscular disability.

Physical examination reveals the rectal ampulla dilated with hard stool, a rather lax puborectalis-levator sling and palpable stool in the sigmoid colon. Neurological examination is normal.

Treatment of the problem begins with getting rid of all the residual stool in the lower bowel by the methods previously mentioned. Once residual stool is gone, bowel movements are controlled by daily use of medicated Dulcolax suppositories, while the stool consistency is controlled by dietary changes and stool softeners. Part of the treatment is to initiate good bowel habit patterns, preferably having a stool at the same time each day. To this end, mothers should be instructed to insert the medicated suppository into the rectum just before the youngster sits down to breakfast each morning. After three or four weeks of treatment, the rectal ampulla shrinks to a normal size and the levators ani regain tonicity. The children appreciate that they feel better when their bowels are emptied daily and they are no longer socially ostracized. Gradually the doses of drugs are reduced, and ultimately treatment is discontinued, with full expectation that normal bowel habits will be maintained spontaneously. Sigmoidoscopy, barium enema and rectal biopsy can be avoided in most of these children by careful history and physical examination.

Psychogenic problems sometimes underlie and trigger the constipation-soiling problem. Further, ostracism from the family and peer group adds to the psychological problems of the patient, and often in time psychogenic problems dominate the picture, even if they were absent or minimal at onset. Psychiatric help is rarely necessary or helpful, since the psychogenic problems begin to disappear as the constipation comes under control.

Constipation Beginning in Older Childhood

Sometimes constipation begins in preschool years or in the young school child who is unwilling to have a bowel movement when the urge comes simply because his attention and interest are directed at some play or school activity. This, too, can lead to a semivicious cycle since the more these defecatory urges are resisted, the more the rectum becomes dilated and filled with firm, dehydrated stool (Fig. 9.1). In time, the rectal tone diminishes and residual stool increases. The same kind of anatomic changes now occur as we previously described in the two-year-old constipated child: laxity of the striated sphincter muscle, frequent soiling, paradoxical diarrhea and social ostracism with its psychogenic overtones.

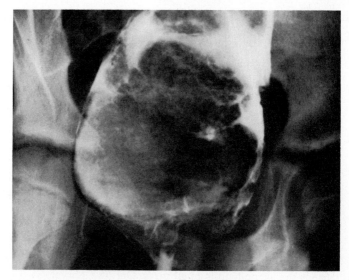

Fig. 9.1. Barium outlining a hard bolus of retained stool in the dilated rectum of a child with acquired constipation and encopresis

Diagnosis and management are identical to those described above. Again, sophisticated evaluation is not often required for proper diagnosis and treatment.

Hirschsprung's Disease

Hirschsprung's disease (congenital aganglionosis coli) is the most common congenital, non-mechanical cause of intestinal obstruction. It occurs somewhere between 1 in 2000 and 1 in 5000 live births. For unknown reasons, it is more common in the male than in the female by a factor of 4:1. Curiously, greater lengths of bowel are involved when it does occur in females. Siblings or blood relatives also have Hirschsprung's disease in about 5 % of patients, and there is a statistically significant correlation with mongolism, as well.

The basic pathophysiology of Hirschsprung's disease is absence of ganglion cells of the autonomic nervous plexus in the involved bowel. Ganglion cells normally lie in the submucosal (Meissner's plexus) and intermuscular (Auerbach's plexus) plane throughout the entire gastrointestinal tract. They serve to propagate coordinated peristaltic waves in an aboral direction (from mouth to anus) which move the succus entericus and stool in an orderly manner downstream for evacuation per anus.

In Hirschsprung's disease, lack of ganglion cells in the involved bowel dampens out the peristaltic wave propagated from above, resulting in stasis and collection of stool just proximal to the junction between ganglionated and aganglionic bowel. Megacolon occurs proximal to this "transition zone". The aganglionic distal bowel remains contracted with a narrow lumen, in sharp contrast to the dilated bowel just upstream from the transition zone. In about 20 % of patients, the agangionosis is limited to the extraperitoneal rectum. In 1 % of patients there are no ganglion cells throughout the entire gastrointestinal tract. The aganglionosis in an additional 10—15 % extends proximally to involve varying lengths of intra-abdominal colon above the sigmoid, and in another 5 % there are no ganglion cells within the entire colon. In the remainder (about 60 %), the transition zone lies somewhere in the sigmoid or rectosigmoid.

Regardless of where the aganglionosis begins, it invariably continues distally from that point to involve the internal anal sphincter, thereby allowing transanal rectal wall biopsy to histologically document the aganglionosis in all cases. During embryologic life, ganglion cells appear first in the mouth, then the esophagus, then the stomach and on downstream in an orderly aboral manner. It is clear that whatever the basic etiology of Hirschsprung's disease, it arrests the propagation of these ganglion cells at some point in the intestine, producing this interesting consistency in the aganglionic pattern. There is no good explanation for this failure of propagation of ganglion cells, nor why in the majority of patients the transition zone lies in the rectosigmoidal area.

Signs and Symptoms

The clinical symptoms of Hirschsprung's disease are those of partial bowel obstruction at the transition zone, and therefore are somewhat related to the length of bowel involved. In general, children with longer lengths of aganglionic distal bowel are more symptomatic and come to diagnosis earlier in life than those with shorter segments of involved bowel.

The most common symptom is constipation associated with abdominal distention, present to some degree since birth. However, patients symptomatic enough to require hospitalization during the first three months of life exhibit more severe and non-specific symptoms of partial intestinal obstruction: vomiting, failure to thrive, episodic diarrhea, feeding problems, etc. This is an important element in prognosis, since almost all deaths from this disease occur during the first few months of life. The older the child at diagnosis, the more likely he is to fall into the classical prototype of constipation, abdominal distention, and mild malnutrition, and the less likely is life to be threatened by the disease.

Complications

Approximately one-third of patients with Hirschsprung's disease develop complications of the obstruction by the time diagnosis is established. Non-specific enterocolitis occurs frequently in a mild form, but is acute, severe and fulminating in an appreciable number of young infants, about half of whom die from this severe complication. Enterocolitis is heralded by diarrhea, increasing abdominal distention, anemia, dehydration and fluid and electrolyte depletion, leading to shock. The diagnosis of acute enterocolitis is largely clinical. Edema, superficial mucosal ulceration and marked inflammation with areas of necrosis involve the bowel proximal to the transition zone (Fig. 9.2). Specific bacteria are not consistently cultured from the stool or blood. Treatment is largely supportive (nasogastric suction, antibiotics, parenteral fluids and electrolytes); saline washouts of the colon and colostomy to disobstruct the bowel are the only definitive measures to arrest this complication.

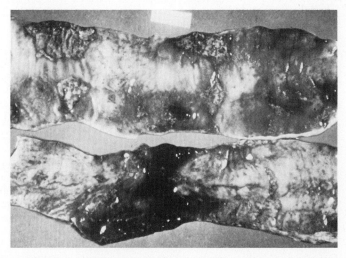

Fig. 9.2. Autopsy specimen of colon from an infant with severe enterocolitis complicating Hirschsprung's disease; note the bowel edema, hemorrhage and ulceration (from: R. D. Liechty and R. T. Soper: Synopsis of Surgery. Mosby, St. Louis, Mo., 1972)

Rarely, patients with Hirschsprung's disease have a sufficiently high grade obstruction to perforate the bowel somewhere within the mega-colon proximal to the transition zone. This catastrophic complication is likewise limited almost exclusively to the neonatal period of life. Emergency exploration to exteriorize the perforated bowel is the preferred treatment, salvaging perhaps one-half of these patients.

Most patients diagnosed beyond the neonatal period of life are below normal in height and weight. Nutrition invariably improves when the intestinal obstruction is relieved, either by definitive surgical treatment or by colostomy.

Mortality

The overall mortality rate for Hirschsprung's disease is 20 %, the deaths occurring almost exclusively in young infants. Deaths are occasioned by the above-described complications of the disease, enterocolitis and bowel perforation being the two major killers.

Physical Examination

A somewhat undernourished youngster is revealed with some degree of abdominal distention, mainly gaseous but often with palpable masses of retained feces in the abdomen. Rectal digital examination characteristically reveals a small, empty rectum which snugs itself around the examining finger. In patients with only rectal or recto-sigmoidal involvement, the finger can often be advanced past the transition zone into the acutely dilated (but normally ganglionated) megacolon just proximally. Withdrawal of the finger is often followed by an explosive decompression of gas and liquid stool.

Barium Enema

This is diagnostic in patients who are old enough to have developed the classical differentiation in bowel size on which radiographic diagnosis rests: a narrowed distal colon which funnels into a mega-colon at the point of transition (Figs. 9.3, 9.4, 9.5, 9.6). Commonly this size distinction does not occur for the first two to three weeks of life. Delayed expulsion of the barium from the dilated bowel is always found, even in neonates.

Definitive diagnosis rests with transanal rectal wall biopsy documenting the lack of ganglion cells. If the ganglion cells are absent in the submucosa, they are also absent in the intermuscular plane, making biopsy of either mucosa or muscularis diagnostic. Recently, histochemical studies have consistently shown an increase in parasympathetic nerves with acetylcholinesterase activity within aganglionic bowel; this may supplant the currently used biopsy techniques

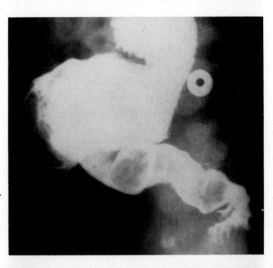

Fig. 9.3.
Lateral view of narrowed rectum which changes abruptly into an enlarged sigmoid colon (megacolon) in a baby with Hirschsprung's disease (from: R. D. Liechty and R. T. Soper: Synopsis of Surgery. Mosby, St. Louis, Mo., 1972)

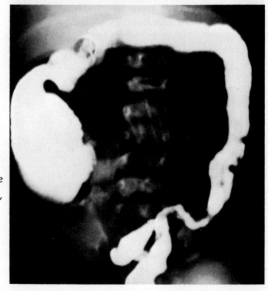

Fig. 9.4.
Barium enema on newborn with aganglionosis of the entire colon; note the "picture-frame" foreshortened colon and the dilated, gas-filled obstructed small bowel loops (the megabowel) centrally

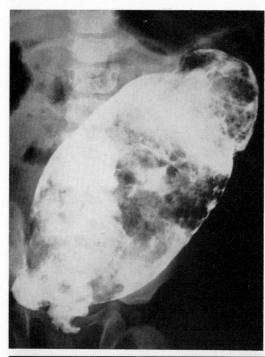

Fig. 9.5.
Barium enema in
older child with
neglected Hirsch-
sprung's disease;
note the enormous
megasigmoid filled
with old stool

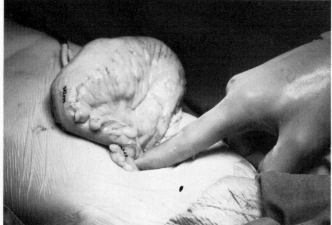

Fig. 9.6. Operative photography of narrow rectosigmoid (at tip of surgeon's finger) and dilated megasigmoid proximally

to confirm the diagnosis of Hirschsprung's disease. Manometric studies carried out with anorectal balloons show absence of peristaltic propagation and failure of relaxation of the internal anal sphincter (smooth muscle).

Surgical treatment is recommended at virtually any age to forestall potential complications, and to relieve the patient of the discomfort of the disease or its medical management. Staged surgical treatment of most patients with Hirschsprung's disease is preferred, starting with colostomy performed in ganglionated bowel. Colostomy relieves colonic hypertrophy and dilatation, treats or prevents the catastrophic complications of enterocolitis and perforation and improves the patient's nutritional status so that he comes to definitive surgery a better operative risk. Definitive operation involves resecting and/or bypassing aganglionic bowel, bringing normally innervated intestine near to the anus.

10 Malformations of the Mouth

M. Perko

Harelip and Cleft Palate

Introduction

Harelip and cleft palate are two of the most common malformations. Their number is increasing and the frequency has reached 0.194 % in Europe, i. e. one child with harelip or cleft palate is born for every 500 live births. There are considerable geographical, racial and sexual variations in the incidence. In the North of Europe and in the mountains these malformations are more common than in the South and in the lowlands. They are less common in Negrids than in Europids, though more common in American Indians than in Europids. Boys are slightly more affected by these malformations than girls. During the last 20 years the incidence of harelip and cleft palate has nearly doubled. This is mainly due to the fact that the stillbirth rate and neonatal mortality have decreased by virtue of improved obstetrical pediatric and pediatric surgical care. Since this trend will predictably continue, we can expect further increases in the incidence of harelip and cleft palate in the future.

Etiology

Harelip and cleft palate have both genetic and exogenetic factors of etiology. The exogenetic factors include the following:

1) ionizing and radioactive rays
2) virus infection
3) toxoplasmosis
4) various drugs and hormones (Aminopetrin, Cortisone, etc.).

Experimentally, exposure of the fetus to these exogenetic factors may cause harelip and cleft palate up to the fifth week of intrauterine life. Isolated cleft palates may theoretically be produced as late as the twelfth intrauterine week. Exogenous factors introduced later than this period cannot be the cause of such deformities.

Development of Harelip and Cleft Palate

Facial clefts are probably caused by a deficient union of the facial bones during intrauterine development. In the normal embryo the so-called ectodermal epithelial walls of the facial bones dissolve to be replaced by mesenchymal connective tissue. If this epithelial wall remains intact a cleft results. This best explains the development of harelips. Harelips and cleft palates do not develop during the same period of intrauterine life.

Types of Facial Clefts

We distinguish between isolated harelip, harelip associated with a cleft palate and isolated cleft palate. All degrees of severity may occur from the small notch in the lip to the complete cleft of lip, alveolar margin and hard and soft palate.

Anatomy of Harelip and Cleft Palate

The Harelip

This is usually situated beneath either the left or the right nostril. A cleft which extends into the nostril is called a "total cleft", which is usually associated with a deformed ala nasi (which is widened and flattened). The nasal septum is not midline, but deviates toward the normal side. The red margin of the lip is pulled into the nostrils and the two segments of the upper lip therefore appear foreshortened. If the harelip is associated with a cleft palate, the upper jaw is even more deformed and there is increased facial asymmetry.

The Cleft Palate

This is situated between the lateral incisor tooth and the canine tooth. Cleft palates vary according to the relative position of the two segments of the palate, the width of the cleft and the position of the nasal septum.

Bilateral Cleft Palate

The upper lip and the alveola are divided into three parts, the middle segment corresponding to the premaxilla. This segment is isolated and appears to be suspended from the vomer. The width of the premaxilla varies, and the bone often projects far forward. The glabella is not developed and one has the impression that the premaxilla is only a continuation of the tip of the nose.

Incomplete, Unilateral Cleft Palates

The cleft is situated lateral to the nasal septum, with a more or less wide connection between the oral and the nasal cavity. As the lateral cleft runs posterior it approaches the midline, which it reaches at the soft palate (Fig. 10.1).

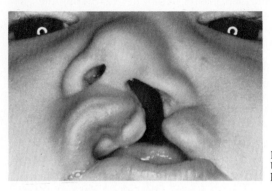

Fig. 10.1.
Unilateral total cleft lip and palate

Bilateral, Total Cleft Palate

There is a cleft on each side of the nasal septum. The lateral part of the palate may be displaced medially so that the premaxilla cannot find a place between the two lateral segments and is pushed forward. These anatomical peculiaritis cause great difficulties in surgical orthodontic therapy (Fig. 10.2).

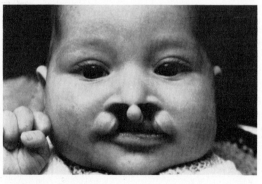

Fig. 10.2.
Bilateral total cleft lip and palate

Isolated Cleft Palates

Isolated cleft palates are nearly always situated in the midline, and there are several varieties. The simplest deformity is the split uvula (uvula bifida). The cleft can extend as far forward as foramen incisivum, which we call a *total isolated cleft palate*. In these cases the alveolus is normally formed (Fig. 10.3).

A special form of cleft palate is the so-called *submucous cleft*. Here the mucosa has united, but there is failure of union of the soft palate musculature, which produces disturbance of function of the

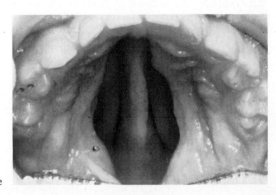

Fig. 10.3.
Isolated cleft palate

palate. Although the palate is intact, the child speaks with a typical "nasal twang" of a cleft palate patient.

Other rare forms of facial clefts do exist, such as median harelips, clefts lateral to the mouth, the very rare cleft of the lower lip, etc. Children with harelip and cleft palate often suffer from other mal-formations.

Problems of Treatment

In treating patients with these malformations, the following problems are encountered:

1) esthetic
2) functional
3) speech
4) psychologic

In order to solve these problems, a number of experts from different fields must work together as a team: pediatricians, surgeons, ortho-dontists, speech therapists, psychologists and otonasolaryngologists. The surgeon is not capable of complete care of these patients.

The treatment of harelip and cleft palate starts immediately after birth. The newborn cannot suck if the upper lip is not complete. The gap in the palate, i.e. the communication between oral and nasal cavities, makes swallowing very difficult.

Feeding is relatively easy, and is best carried out with the child tilted upwards at an angle of 45 degrees. Many children are successfully fed with a nipple which is especialy long and has a large orifice; the end of the nipple is inserted as deeply as possible into the mouth. If this method is unsatisfactory, the formula is delivered either by pipette or by a teaspoon. In the vast majority of cases feeding by gavage is not necessary.

In children with cleft palate it is impossible for the soft palate to close off the oropharynx from the nasopharynx. They therefore speak with a nasal twang. Many of these children have hearing defects which further hampers speech training. The hearing problems are best explained by their predilection for middle ear infections.

Treatment

Immediately after birth the child is fitted with a plate constructed by the orthodontist which occludes the gap in the cleft palate. This plate greatly facilitates feeding, and also prevents progessive deformity of the upper jaw by external influences, such as the pull of the muscles or the cheek and lip, protrusion of the tongue into the gap between the two halves of the cleft palate, etc. As the child grows, this plate has to be changed a number of times until operative repair is carried out. This plate is well tolerated by most children.

The cleft lip is repaired by operation between the fourth and sixth month of life.

The surgical treatment of cleft lip and palate is carried out as follows:

Unilateral Cleft Lip

A unilateral cleft lip is closed when the child is about six months old, or when he weighs about 6 kg. At the same time the cleft in the alveola is closed with soft tissue.

Bilateral Cleft Lips

Bilateral cleft lips are usually repaired in two stages. When the child is four months old, the nasal floor and the anterior nares are repaired. This changes the total bilateral cleft to a partial bilateral cleft. At the second operation, carried out when the child is about six months old, the lip is repaired. The palatal plate is reinserted after lip repair, and is worn until the cleft palate is surgically corrected.

Cleft Palate

The cleft palate is also usually repaired in two stages. In order to encourage proper speech, the soft palate is repaired at about 18

Table 10.1. **Timetable for Treatment of Cleft Lip and Palate**

Age	Orthodontic Treatment	Speech Therapy	Surgery
After birth	Palatal plate		
4 months			First operation of bilateral cleft lip
6 months			Operation of uni-lateral cleft lip, second operation of bilateral cleft lip
18 months			Repair of soft palate
3—5 years	Occlusion plate of hard palate to allow for speech		
3—9 years		Speech therapy	
6 years			Repair of unilateral cleft and hard palate
7—9 years	Orthodontic interim treatment		
8 years			Repair of bilateral hard palate
9—13 years			Possible second-ary surgical treat-ment: further correction of lip and alveolus columella
11—15 years	Final orthodontic treatment		

months of age. By this time the palate has already achieved about
80 %/o of its growth potential, and surgical detachment of the periosteum or cicatrization is then negligible. After the palate has been
closed, the child is followed up by the orthodontist. Table 10.1 summarizes the optimum times for treatment.

The great anatomical variations encountered in harelips makes individual treatment necessary. It is impossible to close all lips in the
same way. Width and position of the gap, development of the muscles, and position and shape of the maxilla all must be considered.
When choosing a definite method of operation, the most important
point is to consider the optimum repair of the muscles (Figs. 10.4 a, b
and 10.5 a, b).

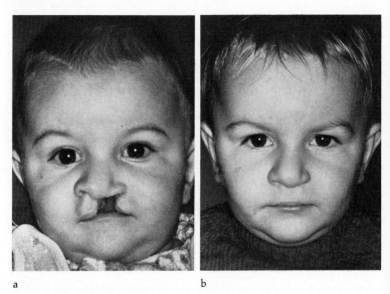

a   b

Fig. 10.4a, b.   Total cleft lip and palate before and after operation

If the palate is closed too early, preparation of the periosteum and
formation of scar tissue postoperatively may later lead to gross disturbances and deformities of the jaw. To avoid these deformities,
orthodontic treatment is absolutely necessary, both before and after
operation. An operative method is chosen which will disturb the
subsequent development of the jaw as little as possible. Since the
hard palate is closed only when it has realized most of its growth

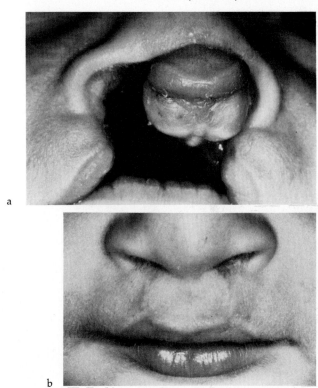

a

b

Fig. 10.5a, b. Bilateral cleft lip and palate before and after operation

potential (6—8 years), subsequent deformities of the jaw are minimized (Fig. 10.6 a, b).

Secondary Surgical Treatment

When closing a bilateral harelip it is usually impossible to lengthen the columella at the same time. This operation is therefore usually delayed until the child is about seven years old. In some cases a bridging of the gap with the aid of a bone graft may be necessary later on.

In many patients with cleft lip and palate, later correction of the nose is necessary. This correction should be carried out when the patient is about 18 years of age.

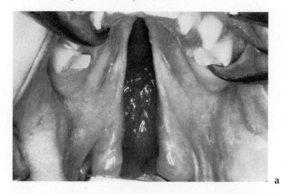

a

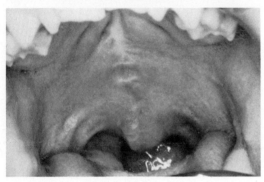

b

Fig. 10.6a, b.
Isolated cleft palate
before and after
operation

Other Malformations

Ranula

Ranula is a cystic structure, usually 2 to 4 cm in size, which underlies the mucosa at the floor of the mouth. When the tongue is
protruded the bluish, soft and fluctuant mass becomes easily visible.
The swelling may disturb the child when speaking or swallowing,
but it has no connection with the salivary glands. Ordinarily a
ranula lies just lateral to the frenulum of the tongue, but large
ranulas may extend across the midline. Upon rupture a clear, viscid
mucus exudes; in most cases the ranula fills again during the next
few days. The cause of ranula is not known. Differential diagnosis
includes dermoid cysts, hemangiomas and lymphangiomas occupying
the same site, but these can usually be excluded on examination.
Treatment consists of complete resection of the cyst; incision alone
will certainly lead to later recurrence.

The Lingual Frenulum

The lingual frenulum is occasionally somewhat short and attached toward the tip of the tongue. Contrary to popular teaching, this does not interfere with tongue motility with sucking and later on with speech and treatment is therefore unnecessary. Occasionally in very severe cases the frenulum is divided without anesthesia.

Macrostomia

This is a relatively rare malformation which can be either unilateral or bilateral. The involved angle of the mouth continues in a narrow, elongated manner obliquely downward and laterally (Fig. 10.7). It is likely that macrostomia is caused by an early arrest in the embryonic development of the face.

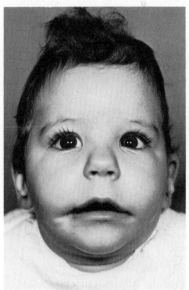

Fig. 10.7.   Macrostomia

Treatment

Macrostomia is corrected by a plastic operation which is undertaken at some elective pre-school age. The margins of the gap are excised, the circumoral muscles are sutured together and the wound is closed in layers so as to restore the normal angle between upper and lower lip.

11 Deformities and Masses of the Neck

R. T. SOPER

General

Masses of the neck occur throughout infancy and childhood. Careful palpation of school children often reveals multiple, often bilateral, movable and slightly tender masses comprising hyperplasia of jugulodigastric lymph nodes in response to infections originating in the pharynx and tonsillar regions. In the majority of cases, this completely benign adenopathy regresses and disappears shortly after the infection has run its course. At the other end of the spectrum are cervical masses representing either primary or metastatic malignancies, which carry very serious portent. Neck masses also are extremely varied in terms of etiology: remnants of vestigial embryologic structures (thyroglossal cysts, branchial cysts and sinuses), simple adenopathy already mentioned, suppurative adenitis (bacterial and tuberculous origin), neurogenic elements (neurofibroma), hamartomas (cystic hygroma, hemangioma), neoplasms (neuroblastoma, carcinoma of the thyroid), metabolic disturbances (goiters, hyperthyroidism), and salivary gland abnormalities (tumors, inflammation). Although neck masses are more common during the middle years of childhood, no age is immune from the newly born to the late adolescent.

At times the diagnosis of neck masses requires only inspection, physical examination and simple bedside tests (cystic hygroma, hemangioma, cervical adenitis) whereas on other occasions diagnosis can defy even the most extensive and sophisticated of workups short of biopsy. It is in hopes of clarifying this sometimes bewildering panorama of neck masses in infants and children that this chapter is written.

The Thyroid Gland

The thyroid gland and its embryologic *anlage* account for most of the midline neck masses of childhood. The simplest abnormality is thyroglossal duct cyst (Fig. 11.1) which is simply a retention of some part of the epithelial-lined thyroglossal tract, an embryologic structure tracing the development and descent of the thyroid gland.

Normally, all remnants of the thyroglossal duct disappear during the second month of gestation. If any portion of this duct remains, its columnar or squamous epithelium secretes mucus which collects and expands into a cyst. The cyst gradually enlarges, generally becoming

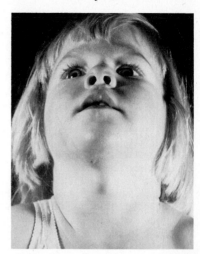

Fig. 11.1. Asymptomatic midline upper neck mass in a 5-year-old girl which elevated upon protrusion of tongue: classical thyroglossal duct cyst (from: R. D. Liechty and R. T. Soper: Synopsis of Surgery. Mosby, St. Louis, Mo., 1972)

apparent during the first four or five years of life. The majority lie at or adjacent to the body of the hyoid bone in the midline, rarely taking an eccentric position just off the midline. For some unknown reason, that part of the thyroglossal duct cephalad to the cyst is generally retained, oral bacteria occasionally invading this connection to set up recurrent bouts of inflammation in the cyst. Although thyroglossal remnants never have preformed fistulas draining to the skin, inflammation may produce an abscess which dissects to the skin of the neck and spontaneously discharges its contents, from whence mucopurulent material subsequently drains. If the abscess is incised and drained, subsequent periodic mucopurulent drainage is also the rule.

Physical examination of the thyroglossal cyst (Fig. 11.1) reveals a 1—2 cm soft, generally non-tender mass at the level of the hyoid bone. Protruding the tongue and swallowing characteristically elevate the mass, signifying its proximal attachment to hyoid bone and foramen cecum. Inflammation lends degrees of tenderness, erythema and fluctuance to the cyst. Thyroglossal cysts never become malignant, but because of their cosmetic defect and infection potential should be surgically excised. Complete surgical removal of a thyroglossal duct cyst requires en bloc removal of the cyst, the midpoint of the body of the hyoid bone and the cephalad extension of the tract up to the foramen cecum of the tongue.

Important in the differential diagnosis of thyroglossal duct cyst are simple dermoid cysts; they are located in the cervical midline from the floor of the mouth down to the suprasternal notch, do not characteristically become inflamed nor do they usually move with protrusion of the tongue. At surgical excision, they are clearly distinguished from thyroglossal cyst because they lack a cephalad tract through the hyoid bone to the base of the tongue.

The ectopic or aberrant thyroid gland represents simply a failure of normal descent of at least a portion of the thyroid gland, with a solid mass of thyroid tissue located somewhere along the thyroglossal tract. Thyroid scans quickly establish the thyroidal nature of this mass, in distinction to the thyroglossal cyst which does not entrap radioiodine, and also determines whether this aberrant thyroid is the only thyroid the patient possesses. If so, it should be preserved by splitting the gland vertically in its midportion to preserve the blood supply coming in laterally, rotating the thyroid halves laterally under the sternocleidomastoid muscle to render them less cosmetically conspicuous. In the presence of a normal thyroid gland, they are completely excised with impunity. The lingual thyroid is characterized by a purplish mass visible at the base of the tongue which protrudes into the pharynx and may produce dysphagia or respiratory distress; further, it is subject to the same diseases as the normal thyroid gland such as hyperthyroidism, adenoma and even malignancy. Total excision transorally is the treatment of choice; if this constitutes the patient's only thyroid gland, replacement therapy is necessary for the rest of his life.

Goiter

The word **goiter** means enlargement of the thyroid gland, regardless of cause. Thus, enlargement of the thyroid due to neoplasm, hyperplasia and hypothyroidism is encompassed by this term. Without question, the most immediate threat to life is the thyroid which is enlarged at the time of birth (Fig. 11.2). The neonatal trachea is very malleable and is easily compressed or distorted by any adjacent mass. Since the thyroid surrounds three-quarters of the tracheal circumference, its enlargement immediately threatens the airway. The most common causes for neonatal thyroid enlargement are hyperplasia due to some maternal stimulus to the fetal thyroid, congenital myxedema and the rare tumors of (teratoma) or near (hemangioma) the thyroid gland. If the airway is severely compromised, surgical exploration must be carried out: the teratoma and hemangioma are totally resected and the goiter should have its circumferential grip on the trachea relieved by isthmusectomy. If the airway is not threatened, watchful waiting suffices. Congenital thyroid hyperplasia due to maternal stimuli transmitted transplacentally (maternal hypothyroidism, ingestion of potassium iodide, iodine deficiency, anti-

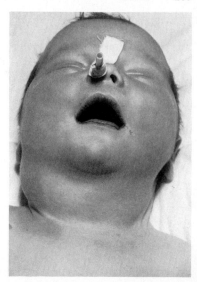

Fig. 11.2. Newborn with thyroid hyperplasia producing severe airway (tracheal) obstruction relieved temporarily by nasotracheal tube (from: R. T. Soper: J. Iowa St. med. Soc., 329—336, June 1962)

thyroid drugs, maternal diets high in thiouracil compounds such as rutabagas and soybeans) are withdrawn from the baby at delivery, and with the passage of time the goiter predictably regresses. If the goiter is due to an inborn error of fetal thyroid metabolism, neonatal hypothyroidism should be looked for and appropriately treated with replacement thyroid extract, which should diminish the size of the gland.

Goiter in the Adolescent Patient

In adolescence, goiter is generally due to iodine deficiency, thyroiditis or hyperthyroidism. Dietary iodine supplements produce goiter regression when it is due to iodine lack, and no surgical treatment is indicated. Metabolic thyroidal defects occasionally stimulate TSH enlargement of the gland which generally regress with thyroid replacement therapy; if not, subtotal thyroidectomy is carried out for cosmetic reasons. Thyroiditis is confirmed by needle biopsy.

Goiter Arising During Puberty

This is so common, especially in females, that it might be considered almost physiologic for this age. It is related to the increased metabolic demands of this period of life characterized by rapid body growth and hormonal and physiological changes. Most spontaneously regress when young adulthood is achieved. Aggressive treatment, particularly thyroidectomy, is never indicated. In those that produce alarming enlargement, small doses of desiccated thyroid generally induce a prompt regression in size.

Hyperthyroidism

The condition is rare in children, about two-thirds of the reported cases occurring in adolescent females. Childhood hyperthyroidism is almost always associated with high TSH levels, signifying an apparent absence of the normal inhibitory feedback mechanism of increasing thyroxine levels. The thyroid gland is diffusely enlarged, and histologically shows proliferation and cellular hyperplasia of the acini. Clinically, the signs and symptoms of hyperthyroidism in children are identical to those in adults: nervousness, hyperactivity, irritability, increase in appetite, exophthalmos, heat intolerance and tachycardia. Diagnosis is confirmed by appropriate tests of thyroid function. Initial treatment consists of antithyroid agents (thiouracil, propylthiouracil) which at least temporarily control the hypermetabolism. Should the child become sensitive to the drug (leukopenia, skin reactions) or should relapses occur after treatment is discontinued, subtotal thyroidectomy should be the next line of treatment. Radioiodine will indeed control hyperthyroidism, but is dangerous because of the unknown long-term effects of thyroid irradiation.

Carcinoma of the Thyroid

This is the only carcinoma (as distinct from sarcoma or other malignancies arising from mesenchymal or embryonal tissues) fairly common to the pediatric age patient. It is rare below the age of 7 years and is most common about the age of 10 years. The male: female ratio is 1 : 2—3. One percent of all carcinomas of the thyroid occur in children. Interestingly, the majority of children with thyroid carcinoma have been subjected to irradiation of the chest, head or neck (for an enlarged thymus, suppurative adenitis) averaging from 5—10 years prior to developing their thyroid malignancy. The apparent causal relationship between prior irradiation and thyroid carcinoma accounts for the recent increase in incidence of this neoplasm.

About 90 % of childhood thyroid carcinomas contain papillary features and are well differentiated, with a relatively slow rate of growth and good prognosis. The disease is often heralded by asymptomatic, slowly enlarging lateral neck masses which represent neoplasm metastatic to lower cervical lymph nodes. The neck masses have generally been present for several months or even years before diagnosis is established. The nodes are discrete, smooth, firm, non-tender and movable. The thyroidal primary is irregular and rock-hard and is located in one lateral lobe. It is extremely rare for children with thyroid carcinoma to present with distant metastases (lungs, bone marrow), attesting to its relatively slow growth rate.

Diagnosis

Diagnosis of thyroid carcinoma depends upon biopsy performed either percutaneously with a needle or at open operation. The children are generally euthyroid and preoperative laboratory studies hardly ever establish diagnosis. Radioiodine scans may show a "cold" spot (no uptake) in that part of the gland bearing the primary neoplasm.

Treatment

The treatment of thyroid cancer includes removing the entire involved lobe from which the primary arises plus the isthmus of the gland and a near-total resection of the contralateral lobe. A small amount of posterior thyroid capsule is preserved on the contralateral side to protect the parathyroid glands. Near-total thyroidectomy is indicated because of the common finding of occult neoplasm within the contralateral lobe, as well as to get rid of all competing thyroid to facilitate subsequent radioiodine therapy of residual or recurrent neoplasm. A conservative resection of lymph nodes involved by tumor should be carried out at the same surgical sitting. This modified neck dissection removes all grossly enlarged and involved lymph nodes from either or both cervical chains.

Postoperatively, the patient is treated with high doses of thyroid extract (3—5 grains daily), since many of the tumors are repressed by thyroid extract; further, the patients are metabolically hypothyroid and need thyroid replacement. Periodically, the thyroid extract is discontinued for three weeks before radioactive iodine uptake study, whole body scan and chest x-ray, looking for metastatic disease. If metastatic thyroid neoplasm is found and if it takes up iodine, radioiodine is administered in large therapeutic doses; high-dose thyroid extract replacement is then resumed. Residual or recurrent neoplasm which does not take up radioactive iodine should be externally irradiated, but response to this treatment is generally poor. No chemotherapy is currently available for thyroid carcinoma.

Acute Suppurative Thyroiditis

It is likely that this condition represents metastatic infection to the thyroid from an upper respiratory tract infection or abscessed tooth.

The disease is heralded by striking elevation in temperature and the appearance of an erythematous, exquisitely tender thyroid enlargement. Antibiotics, local warm, moist soaks and surgical drainage of pus constitute adequate treatment.

Subacute Viral Thyroiditis

Mild low anterior neck pain worsened with swallowing, associated with a slightly tender and mildly enlarged thyroid gland herald the disease. Mild fever, malaise and an elevated sedimentation rate complete the clinical picture. Needle biopsy confirms diagnosis. Treatment with bedrest, sedation and aspirin usually suffices.

Chronic Lymphocytic Thyroiditis

Ten times more common than viral thyroiditis is chronic lymphocytic thyroiditis. As with most thyroid abnormalities, there is a strong predisposition in the female over 10 years of age. A mild swelling of the gland usually brings the patient to the physician. The gland is diffusely and symmetrically enlarged, firm, non-tender and, in later stages, hard enough to suggest thyroid cancer. In the late stages, hypothyroidism gradually develops with a decrease in the radioiodine uptake of the gland. The disease is likely autoimmune in nature, the thyroid tissue becoming sensitized to its own hormone, with invasion of the gland by lymphocytes and fibrous tissue. Again, diagnosis is confirmed by needle biopsy. Treatment consists of thyroid extract in replacement dosages, with ensuing gradual return of the thyroid gland to normal or near normal size. Thyroid replacement generally is continued for life.

Diseases of the Cervical Lymph Nodes

Lymphadenitis

Acute Cervical Lymphadenitis

This is most commonly secondary to bacterial or viral infection in the nasopharyngeal area. The upper jugulodigastric cervical chain of lymph nodes waxes and wanes in size in response to upper respiratory infections of this kind; occasionally, the lymph nodes remain palpably enlarged for several weeks.

Particularly with infection caused by staphylococci, the cervical lymphadenitis may gradually develop signs of suppuration: recrudescence of a low-grade fever, tenderness and gradually enlarging nodes, and subtile erythema. If inadequate antibiotics were administered during the course of the upper respiratory infection, this kind of reaction may be delayed and modified considerably. Warm, moist soaks applied locally often speed resolution of the phlegmonous lymphadenitis, or hasten fluctuation in others. Once fluctuation develops, incision and drainage is promptly carried out under sedation and local anesthesia. A transverse incision is made in an overlying skin crease, the pus cultured and drained and the finger inserted to break down all loculations. A pack is placed in the depths of the wound, which is gradually withdrawn over the next few days while warm moist soaks are resumed. With this treatment, the abscess wall fills in from the bottom up with granulation tissue and quickly resolves the inflammation.

Chronic Cervical Lymphadenitis

Here the condition is generally due to one of four causes: cervical tuberculosis (scrofula), atypical Mycobacterium, secondary to the disease referred to as "cat-scratch fever" or fungal diseases. Tuberculous cervical adenitis is much less common in countries with pasteurization of milk and where antibiotics and public health measures have drastically lowered the incidence of tuberculosis. The entry point for the organisms is generally either the tonsil or the nasopharynx, but scrofula also occurs in conjunction with pulmonary tuberculosis. Children with cervical tuberculosis are eminently well in most instances, and come in because of chronic, gradually enlarging neck nodes on one or both sides; initially the nodes are firm, non-tender and matted but as the disease evolves the overlying skin assumes a shiny, erythematous and thinned-out appearance until finally spontaneous and chronic drainage of pus occurs.

The diagnosis of cervical tuberculosis rests on finding slowly enlarging cervical lymph nodes in a child with a positive tuberculin test and often a history of either ingesting raw milk or of contact with a known tuberculosis patient, usually within the close family. Chest x-ray is taken, looking for active pulmonary tuberculosis.

The treatment of cervical tuberculous adenitis is that of the generalized disease itself, administering the best drugs currently available for a two-year period. If breakdown of the erythematous, shiny skin overlying the nodes seems imminent, surgical drainage with curettage of the abscess should be carried out, with acid-fast stains and cultures of the purulent matter confirming diagnosis. Adequate drug therapy generally arrests the progression of cervical adenitis with gradual resolution of the signs of inflammation. Needle aspiration of the pus for stain and culture may forestall spontaneous perforation. Should residually enlarged lymph nodes persist after appropriate drug therapy, excision of the nodes allows confirmation of diagnosis and expedites resolution.

Atypical Mycobacterium

Very similar in its clinical evolution to cervical tuberculosis, and much more common in Western countries, is chronic cervical adenitis secondary to atypical Mycobacterium. This disease arises during the first few years of life and produces unilateral chronic, progressive adenopathy generally in the submaxillary area with few systemic signs of illness. In time, the nodes may become fluctuant and drain purulent matter intermittently. Chest x-ray is normal and there usually is no history of contact with a person harboring active tuberculosis. Tuberculin skin tests are usually weakly positive, and diagnosis rests on a much more brisk skin response when the atypical Mycobacterium antigens are injected. Culture of atypical Mycobacteria from the pus of an involved node confirms diagnosis.

Treatment consists of excising involved nodes, hopefully prior to suppuration or sinus formation; simple incision and drainage favors chronic purulent drainage. The role of chemotherapy in this disease is unclear; although in vitro resistance to Isoniazid and/or Streptomycin is often demonstrated, patients seem to fare better with chemotherapy plus surgery than those who are treated surgically alone. Para-aminosalicylic acid and Isoniazid in combination are the treatment agents of choice, administered for one to two years.

Cat-Scratch Disease

The disease is preceded by the scratch of a cat three to six weeks prior to adenopathy. Regional adenopathy is the rule, so that cat scratches of the upper extremity produce axillary adenopathy, and of the lower extremities inguinal adenopathy. Children who are scratched on the head or neck develop chronic cervical adenopathy. The disease is most likely caused by a microorganism of the psittacosis-lymphogranuloma group. Cat-scratch disease is heralded by fever and chronic regional adenopathy with tenderness and fluctuation. The pus from an abscess is generally sterile on ordinary culture. Diagnosis is confirmed by a positive skin test reaction with an antigen specific for the disease, negative skin tests to tuberculin and atypical Mycobacteria and a negative culture of the pus.

Treatment of cat-scratch disease is largely expectant, lacking a specific chemotherapeutic agent. Biopsy and culture of an involved lymph node exclude other forms of chronic lymphadenitis and malignant disease, and might indeed speed resolution of the process. Needle aspiration of pus is recommended before a sinus and chronic drainage occur. Conventional antibiotics are of little use. Rarely, complications of the disease occur including oculoglandular fever, thrombocytopenic purpura and encephalitis.

Fungi

Rarely, *fungi* produce chronic cervical lymphadenitis in children: coccidiomycosis, actinomycosis, histoplasmosis and blastomycosis. Usually this is simply part of a generalized disease, with adenopathy elsewhere and positive chest x-rays. Positive skin tests and rising antibody titers to the specific fungus plus biopsy and culture of an involved node confirm diagnosis. Antifungal drugs are the treatment of choice.

Cervical Node Neoplasms

Neoplasms of the Cervical Lymph Nodes

In children, these are generally primary neoplasms of the lymphosarcoma-Hodgkin's type, but occasionally are metastatic from carcinoma of the thyroid or malignancies originating in the nasopharynx. Since systemic symptoms are often absent, the presenting complaint is commonly that of progressive enlargement of a nontender lateral cervical lymph node or chain. First in consideration in the differential diagnosis must be chronic lymphadenitis; no recent upper respiratory infection, negative skin tests and chest x-rays and absence of tenderness, erythema or fluctuance rule against chronic lymphadenitis. After careful examination for a primary neoplasm of the head or neck, the next step in diagnosis should be excisional biopsy with culture.

The lymphoma group of neoplasms: cervical lymph nodes are enlarged in leukemia, the various types of lymphosarcoma and Hodgkin's disease. Appropriate bone marrow and peripheral blood studies quickly identify patients with leukemia, and node biopsy confirms Hodgkin's disease or one of the varieties of lymphosarcoma seen in children.

Hodgkin's Disease

Ten percent of the total incidence of Hodgkin's disease originates in childhood, generally heralded by cervical gland enlargement before any systemic symptoms or other adenopathy occur. Biopsy of the enlarged lymph nodes shows pleomorphism and large or giant cells with large nuclei, known as the Sternberg-Reed cells.

Since treatment of Hodgkin's disease is non-surgical (x-irradiation and chemotherapy), the next step is to establish as precisely as possible the degree of spread to the disease: chest x-ray, bone marrow biopsy, intravenous pyelography, careful palpation for lymphadenopathy elsewhere and for splenomegaly or hepatomegaly and perhaps lower extremity lymphangiography are in order. Recently, these attempts to precisely "stage" the disease have been augmented by laparotomy for splenectomy and biopsy of the liver and nodes from the periaortic, iliac and mesenteric chains. Once the extent of the disease has been precisely mapped out in this manner, the radiotherapist can treat all involved areas and exclude all uninvolved areas of the body. Particularly in children who are still growing, radiation of uninvolved tissues is dangerous.

Lymphosarcoma

Less common than Hodgkin's disease, and with a much poorer prognosis, is lymphosarcoma. Further, only about one-third of children have initial cervical involvement with lymphosarcoma, the remainder originating in other nodal groups throughout the body. Diagnosis is again dependent upon biopsy to exclude Hodgkin's disease, chronic lymphadenitis and metastatic malignancy. Irradiation and chemotherapy are the hallmarks of treatment, with generally a much more rapid and fatal progression than with lymphosarcoma of adulthood or Hodgkin's disease of childhood.

Cervical Lymph Nodes Enlarged by Metastatic Neoplasm

These are unusual in childhood. As we have seen, lower cervical lymph nodes are generally the ones involved with metastatic thyroid carcinoma. Upper cervical nodes are involved in metastases of tumors originating in the nasopharynx or head (rhabdomyosarcomas). A careful search of the nasopharynx and head should detect the primary neoplasm, and appropriate treatment (generally combined surgery and irradiation) can be planned.

Cystic Hygroma

Cystic hygroma is the most common lateral cervical mass developing during the first year or two of life (Fig. 11.3). Loculated collections of tissue fluid within endothelial-lined lymphatic spaces characterize cystic hygromas. Eighty percent occur in the neck, about 10 % in the axilla and the remainder are scattered elsewhere in the body, whereever there are lymphatics. About 5 % extend through the thoracic inlet into the superior mediastinum. 70 % of cystic hygromas are present at birth, and fully 90 % have made their presence known by a mass before the second birthday.

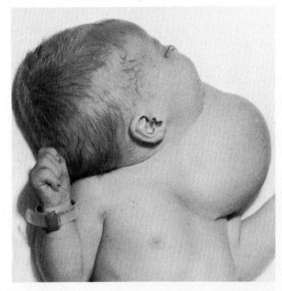

Fig. 11.3. Newborn with huge cystic hygroma producing some airway obstruction from tracheal deviation

Although the exact cause for cystic hygroma is not known, their locations suggest that faulty lymphatic coalescence might play a role. Further, it is also clear that while retaining the ability to accept more tissue fluid through afferent lymphatic channels, they have lost normal downstream or efferent connections to drain the lymph back into the venous system. Thus, infection in the area drained by the cystic hygroma results in temporary increase in size of the lesion, which then may diminish somewhat as the infection subsides.

The growth rate of cystic hygromas is unpredictable, at times influenced by regional infections, as mentioned. Cystic hygromas hardly ever disappear spontaneously, except occasionally following an infection of the cystic hygroma itself. Much more commonly, the cystic hygromas remain unchanged or periodically increase in size.

Cystic hygromas are not neoplasms, but do possess the ability to involve adjacent structures such as fascial planes, muscles and veins.

They are almost always multiloculated. The size of the locules varies, being large and macroscopic in areas and tiny and microscopic in other portions of the same lesion. Occasionally, nerves and strands of muscle pass through the cystic hygroma, having been surrounded by the enlarging hamartoma-like growth.

Cystic hygroma presents as a soft mass in the posterior triangle of the neck which is subcutaneous in location, non-tender and fluctuant. There is no overlying vascular pattern or color change to the skin. The most diagnostic feature of cystic hygroma is its brilliant transillumination (Fig. 11.4). When traumatized, blood may discolor the cyst contents to render them opaque, lending a bluish discoloration to that segment of the lesion. If the lesion lies in the lower portion of the neck it might well extend through the thoracic inlet to the mediastinum or under the clavicle following the brachial plexus into the axilla. Cystic hygromas of the anterior triangle of the neck are generally located in the submandibular region, often associated with intraoral lymphangiomas which elevate the tongue and impair both airway and feeding.

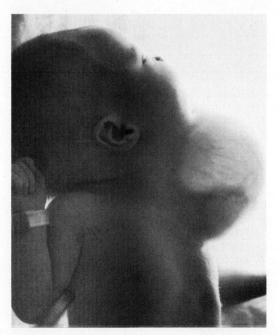

Fig. 11.4.   Transillumination of cystic hygroma

Cystic hygromas generally are asymptomatic except for the cosmetic disturbance of the mass itself. The large cystic hygroma, particularly in the newborn, may elevate the tongue or displace the trachea enough to produce serious respiratory obstruction (Figs. 11.3 and 11.4). Slight dysphagia and associated feeding problems may co-exist, but are not generally a threat to life.

Surgical excision is the treatment of choice for cystic hygromas. Irradiation, incision and drainage, sclerosing agents and periodic aspiration are older treatments which are largely ineffective, at times dangerous and are mentioned only in condemnation. If the lesion produces significant airway obstruction, emergency resection is indicated; otherwise, they can be observed for several weeks or months and electively removed at a convenient time.

The smaller cystic hygromas can be easily dissected away from the normal neck structures and totally excised, with a 100 % cure rate. The larger lesions often surround and involve many of the important anatomic structures of the neck, making their complete excision either difficult or dangerous. In this case, caution is the order of the day; the bulk of the tumor can always be safely resected, the peripheral extensions involving vital structures either being left alone (if their loculations are tiny) or simply opened to allow release of their entrapped fluid (if the locules are large). Suction catheter drainage postoperatively collapses residual locules that have been drained rather than excised, with an acceptably low recurrence rate. Radical resection at the expense of important neck structures is never justified. Recurrence of 10—15 % may be anticipated if gross portions of the lesion are left behind, but often it takes years for them to achieve sufficient size to require reoperation.

Branchial Remnants

Remnants of the embryologic branchial apparatus which persist into postnatal life produce an array of abnormalities in and around the ear and along the anterior border of the sternocleidomastoid muscle. Sinuses, cysts, fistulae and cartilaginous remnants are the most common manifestations of these interesting anomalies. The sinuses, fistulae and cartilaginous remnants are diagnosed in infancy and young childhood, whereas cysts take time to fill with secretions sufficient to produce a visible mass, often not coming to light until older childhood, adolescence or young adulthood. Overall, branchial remnants are slightly more common than cystic hygromas.

Considering the paired nature of the branchial apparatus, it is understandable that 10—15 % of their remnants are bilateral. Another 15 % of patients give a family history of similar remnants.

Diagnosis

Diagnosis of branchial remnants is generally not difficult. Inspection of sinuses, skin tags and cartilaginous remnants in characteristic locations often suffices. Probing and injection of radiocontrast material into the sinuses and fistulae are sometimes helpful. Branchial cysts are distinguished from cystic hygromas by their location deep to the sternocleidomastoid muscle and the fact that they do not brilliantly transilluminate.

Remnants of the First Branchial Apparatus

These present as external ostia, collections of cartilage, skin tags, appendages or cysts which lie in and around the external ear. The most common is the preauricular sinus. Most of them are externally visible and therefore are diagnosed in the first few years of life. Sinuses, cysts and fistulae have a disturbing tendency to develop recurrent infection and therefore should be surgically removed. Branchial remnants are removed in the operating room with good light and assistants, since they often travel close to the facial nerve and require meticulous dissection to preserve the nerve and yet totally remove the lesion.

Remnants of the Second Branchial Apparatus

The incidence is six times as high as that of remnants of the first branchial apparatus. Again, because of external manifestations, the fistulae and external sinuses (Fig. 11.5) are diagnosed during the

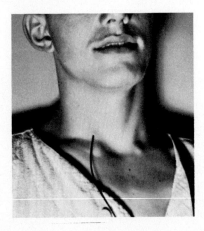

Fig. 11.5. Catheter inserted into a mucus-draining lower cervical ostium in an adolescent male: injected dye entered the tonsillar fossa on that side, characteristic of a second branchial fistula (from: R. D. Liechty and R. T. Soper: Synopsis of Surgery. Mosby, St. Louis, Mo., 1972)

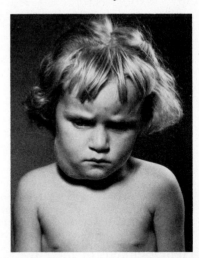

Fig. 11.6. Right cervical mass deep to sternocleidomastoid muscle characteristic of a second branchial cyst

early years of childhood, whereas cysts (Fig. 11.6) become evident as gradually enlarging masses, generally deep to the anterior border of the sternocleidomastoid muscle in the upper two-thirds of the neck, in later childhood or adolescence. Mucus drains from the external ostiae which lie along the anterior border of the sternocleidomastoid muscle in its middle to lower third. The mucoid drainage is secreted by the epithelial cells lining the tracts.

Second branchial remnants are removed in their entirety at some elective time, preferably before inflammation occurs. Since fistulae may span the distance from the lower third of the sternocleidomastoid muscle up to the supratonsillar fossa, two parallel incisions are commonly required for complete excision. The cysts are excised through an overlying transverse incision, with careful dissection of the cephalad tract which invariably leads between the two carotid arteries, behind the posterior belly of the digastric muscle to the supratonsillar fossa.

Recurrence is invariable if any part of the epithelial-lined tract is left behind. Neoplastic degeneration has not been reported in childhood, but occasional case reports in adults suggest this potential in a dormant branchial remnant.

Salivary Gland

Diseases of the major salivary glands (parotid and submaxillary glands) occasionally produce neck masses in children which occur in characteristic anatomic positions related to their gland of origin. The parotid swellings occupy the preauricular area superficial to the ramus of the mandible, the submaxillary masses occurring in the submaxillary triangle deep to the body of the mandible.

Sialadenitis

Recurrent inflammation of the major salivary glands, occasionally triggered by stones in the drainage ducts or other impediments to the normal outflow of saliva, is described as sialadenitis. Recurrent bouts of tender swelling associated with mild local discomfort is the rule. Occasionally inflammation is absent, and the swelling occurs promptly during mastication. Radiocontrast material injected into the salivary duct outlines the duct system and may reveal saccular dilatations, puddling of dye or displacement of the gland. If symptoms are recurrent and severe enough, surgical excision is justified.

Hemangiomas of the Parotid Gland

These occasionally produce a preauricular swelling which, because of its deep-seated nature, often is not heralded by overlying vascular markings or color changes which allow one clinically to make the correct diagnosis. These swellings tend to fluctuate from time to time, gradually enlarging but producing few symptoms. Their true nature is disclosed at the time of surgical excision undertaken for an unknown parotid mass. As in any parotid operation, precise identification and protection of the facial nerve are imperative, the operation being tedious and difficult.

The hemangioma should be excised.

Solid Tumors of the Salivary Glands

The same solid tumors of the salivary glands that occur in adults have been reported in children, but are so rare as to be worthy of little comment in a textbook such as this: mixed tumors, cylindroma, cystadenoma lymphomatosum and even the occasional carcinoma. For this reason, all parotid masses in children should be followed closely, and diagnosed by biopsy if they persist.

Neural Tumors

About 2—3 % of neuroblastomas of childhood arise from the sympathetic tissues of the neck in the form of a solid lateral neck mass which gradually enlarges. The fact that it is unilateral, free of any inflammatory elements and slowly but progressively enlarges tends to separate it from cervical lymphadenitis. Its true nature is discovered only at neck exploration undertaken for excisional biopsy. Most cervical neuroblastomas contain ganglion cells and other evidence of maturity. Perhaps related to this is the much better prognosis of cervical neuroblastoma as compared with primary abdominal neuroblastoma. Complete surgical excision should suffice as treatment. Following these treatment principles a 75 % cure rate is anticipated, far better than for abdominal primary neuroblastoma.

Occasionally, neurofibromas occur in nerves of the neck to produce a lateral cervical mass. They arise from the sheaths of peripheral nerves, varying from pea-sized to large growths. Their discreteness and firmness, plus associated café au lait spots or neurofibromas elsewhere, generally allow a correct clinical diagnosis. Cervical neurofibromas are removed to confirm diagnosis or for cosmetic reasons.

12 Abdominal Pain

R. T. SOPER

All children at times have abdominal pain. Fortunately most of the episodes are short-lived, relatively minor and are easily separated from significant attacks due to surgical disease. Only a minority of children with abdominal pain are even brought to the physician. The causes of these pain attacks are as variable as their number, ranging from the very minor intestinal colic associated with enteritis or dietary indiscretions to the life-threatening abdominal pain of perforating appendicitis. It is our purpose in this chapter to concentrate on the more common, significant and severe types of abdominal pain in infants and children.

Relationship to Age

Age is important when studying abdominal pain in children: infants and young children cannot give an accurate history or cooperate during the examination, rendering these important diagnostic measures less helpful than in the older child. Also causes of abdominal pain differ according to the age of the child.

Neonatal. The diseases causing abdominal pain in the newly born are associated with vomiting, and have been discussed in Chapter 5.

3—18 months of age. Nonspecific enterocolitis, constipation with fissures, intussusception, rarely appendicitis.

18 months—five years of age. Nonspecific gastroenteritis, Meckel's diverticulum complications, constipation, occasional appendicitis.

5—12 years of age. Nonspecific gastroenteritis, constipation, appendicitis, functional causes.

Adolescence. The same as for the 5—12-year-old age group, plus menstrual and internal genitalia problems in girls.

Pattern of Pain

Chronic (often recurrent) pain in the abdomen is generally limited to older children; life is not threatened, time is not a crucial element, and the workup can be leisurely and complete.

In contrast, the acute, generally nonrecurrent, abdominal pain of infancy and childhood is sometimes life-threatening. Time is important, and the workup needs to be simple and yet expedient enough for a correct decision to be made concerning the need for laparotomy within one or two hours. One of three decisions is made: 1) immediate laparotomy is necessary, 2) the patient needs further observation, 3) the condition is definitely nonsurgical.

Location of Pain

Visceral pain is carried by automatic afferents and tends to be vague, difficult for even the older cooperative child to describe, and centrally located in the abdomen. In contrast, pain of parietal peritoneal origin is carried by somatic afferents, is generally peripheral in location, and can be accurately described and well localized by the older child.

Referred Pain

Pain can be referred to the abdomen from adjacent body cavities or structures, as well as radiating from the abdomen to uninvolved areas. Lobar pneumonia can produce pain and abdominal rigidity on the ipsilateral side, ureteral colic can radiate to the ipsilateral groin or upper medial thigh, rheumatic endocarditis or pericarditis can produce epigastric discomfort and some migraine equivalents are associated with vague and recurrent epigastric abdominal pain. In the younger child, otitis media, tonsillitis, or simply hyperthermia are often associated with abdominal pain of a vague type, for reasons that are unclear.

Further, an irritated psoas muscle produces pain experienced in the medial thigh on the same side, pancreatitis pain classically bores straight through to the lower thoracic or upper lumbar back, cholecystitis pain commonly is experienced in the right scapular tip, and an irritated respiratory diaphragm produces pain radiating to the ipsilateral shoulder tip with inspiration or cough.

Physical Examination

Of special importance in the youngster with acute abdominal pain is a careful general examination to detect middle ear infection, tonsillitis, pharyngitis and nuchal rigidity. The general hydrational status is assessed, and the tongue inspected to see if it is coated. The lungs and heart are examined to rule out pneumonia, endocarditis, or pericarditis. The skin is inspected for ecchymoses, petechiae, or a rash.

The abdominal examination begins with evaluating its contour to note asymmetry, distention, or a scaphoid or even sunken abdomen. Abdominal wall muscle guarding should be evaluated as voluntary (in response to palpation) or involuntary (spasm even when the patient's attention is distracted or he is inspiring); involuntary guarding needs to be pinpointed as to location and quantitated for severity. The bowel sounds are evaluated as the examiner sits comfortably at the bedside and listens for 5—10 minutes. Percussion dullness which does not shift often indicates an underlying mass, while shifting dullness signifies free intraperitoneal fluid. Hypertympany suggests air within or outside of intestine. Finally, palpation for masses should be carried out gently with the flat part of the warm hand, and while the patient's attention is distracted as much as possible. The tender parts of the abdomen are palpated last. Tenderness should be quantitated and a decision made as to whether it is direct, indirect, or. rebound. The groins are evaluated for hernia masses.

The psoas muscle goes into spasm (producing hip flexion) in response to adjacent pus or inflammation, as with a retrocecal appendicitis or terminal ileitis. External rotation or extension of the hip produces pain and is therefore resisted by these patients, giving a positive "psoas sign". Plain radiographs of the abdomen commonly reveal a blurring or obliteration of the involved psoas shadow in these patients.

Laboratory Tests Commonly Needed

Nasogastric tube: often helpful to assess stomach contents for volume, blood, or bile, and to begin decompression.

Blood: a complete blood count should always be made. Serum electrolytes are often helpful. Additional studies occasionally needed include serum amylase, SGOT, urea nitrogen, blood pH, blood gases, and serum bilirubin.

Urine: especially helpful are the urine pH, acetone, sugar, and cells.

Radiography: plain films of the chest and abdomen, supine and upright.

In the acutely ill patient, supportive care is administered coincident with workup. Nasogastric suction begins to decompress the gastrointestinal tract, parenteral fluids, electrolytes, pH modifiers and vitamins begin the rehydrational process, intravenous antibiotics are administered when infection seems likely. If these supportive measures are carried out aggressively, the patient commonly will be ready to go to the operating room by the time the decision is made concerning laparotomy.

Factors Favoring Laparotomy

Pain: acute, colicky, peripheral, localized, worsened by motion.

Abdominal exam: distention, abnormal or absent bowel sounds, mass, localized tenderness, involuntary spasm, rebound tenderness, positive psoas sign.

Rectal exam: stool absent or bloody, cul-de-sac tenderness or mass.

Plain abdominal radiograph: gallstones, appendolith, small bowel gas, air-fluid levels, dilated single (so-called sentinel) loop of intestine, free air in the peritoneal cavity, obliteration of the retroperitoneal shadows (psoas muscle, kidney).

Differential Diagnosis

In terms of differential diagnosis, three categories are identified:

1) **Surgery clearly indicated,** so precise distinction is unnecessary: appendicitis, complication of Meckel's diverticulum, twisted ovarian cyst, acute cholecystitis, gastrointestinal perforation, mechanical intestinal obstruction, tumor, major visceral trauma, intussusception.

2) **Laparotomy not necessary, but not particularly harmful** in the doubtful case: mesenteric lymphadenitis, Crohn's disease (transmural enterocolitis), acute nonspecific gastroenteritis.

3) **Surgery contraindicated:**

Diabetic keto-acidosis. History of polydipsia, polyuria, and weight loss; urine is acid, and contains sugar and acetone.

Acute rheumatic fever. Temperature greater than 38.5° C. for several days, recent sore throat, heart murmur, skin rash, no nausea or vomiting, and high ASO titer, C-reactive proteins and sedimentation rate.

Primary peritonitis. Metastatic infection to the peritoneum, generally pneumococcal or streptococcal in origin, often from ENT primary source. Patients with nephrosis or who are on steroids for some reason are predisposed. Patients have decreased appetites with high fever and diffuse abdominal pain *from the beginning of their illness.* Abdominal paracentesis yields syrupy mucoid purulent fluid which contains gram-positive cocci. If diagnosis uncertain, laparotomy is justified; however, intravenous fluids and penicillin produce a rapid reversal of the signs of primary peritonitis.

Sickle Cell Anemia. In Negrids with palpable spleen and anemia; develops abdominal pain and ileus when splanchnic circulation is partially occluded by sickle cells, producing localized, relative visceral ischemia, attacks often triggered by dehydration. Blood shows anemia with sickle cells on smear.

Lobar Pneumonia. Cough, rales, dyspnea, reduced breath sounds, positive chest x-ray. Abdominal pain and spasm limited to the hemi-abdomen on that side, not aggravated by abdominal pressure.

Pancreatitis. See Chapter 15.

Herpes Zoster. Occurs in teenagers, not younger children. Pain is boring in nature, originates in lumbar or low thoracic region, and may radiate unilaterally. Abdominal muscles are tense, but there is no true tenderness. Hyperesthesia is found over the afflicted dermatome.

Lead poisoning (pica). Symptoms generally arise in the summertime when the patient has been in the sun. The pain is colicky, and is associated with constipation and vomiting. No localized findings on abdominal examination. Blood shows anemia with basophilic stippling of the red blood cells; abdominal x-rays reveal scattered flecks of plaster in the intestine, and long-bone x-rays show "lead lines".

Abdominal epilepsy. Abrupt onset, localized in the mid or upper abdomen, uncommonly lasting longer than a few minutes, and often recurring periodically. May be accompanied by nausea and vomiting, often with disorientation or confusion and generally followed by sleep. Few objective findings on abdominal examination. Electroencephalogram is usually abnormal, but changes are nonspecific. Pain attacks cease with Diphenylhydantoin, serving to reinforce the diagnosis.

Henoch-Schönlein Purpura (Acute Vasculitis). Pain is colicky and often associated with mild GI bleeding. Often there is a skin rash over the lower extremities which is flat, sharply defined, purplish, and does not blanch with pressure; edema, arthralgia and hematuria are commonly seen. Two to three percent of patients will have bleeding occur intramurally and induce an intussusception; signs of mechanical small bowel obstruction and a palpable mass generally allow one to make the proper decision to operate upon these patients.

Hemophilia. Abdominal pain is caused by spontaneous hemorrhage retroperitoneally or into the mesentery or wall of the bowel. There often is a family history or a personal history of previous bleeding episodes or ecchymoses. Cryoprecipitate therapy for 12—18 hours should induce an improvement or remission of the abdominal pain. Remember, hemophiliacs can also develop appendicitis, which needs surgical treatment just as in any other patient.

Appendicitis in the Older Child

Appendicitis is the most common acute abdominal surgical problem of childhood. Its incidence is correlated with age, peaking in frequency from 12—14 years with progressive diminution in frequency in both older and younger ages. Appendicitis is almost unheard of during neonatal life. It is rare during the first two years of life and uncommon before the age of five years. The rarity, coupled with the pre-school youngster's inability to cooperate in history and physical examination, explain why more than 90 % of children under five years of age with appendicitis are already complicated (perforated) by the time laparotomy is undertaken. The complication rate steadily diminishes in the older child as his cooperativeness and ability to render a dependable history improve, and is less than 5 % during adolescence.

Effective antibiotics, coupled with earlier diagnosis, better supportive care, improved anesthesia and better surgery have all served to reduce the mortality rate from appendicitis to less than 1 %. However, the morbidity rate remains significant in terms of wound infections, intra-abdominal abscesses, paralytic ileus, and later bouts of adhesive intestinal obstruction. It is to reduce the morbidity rate by still more careful and early surgical care that our efforts must now be directed.

Pathophysiology

Obstruction of the appendiceal lumen triggers appendicitis, regardless of age (Fig. 12.1). An occasional fecalith is found in the young child, and rarely pinworms and parasites seem to be the offending agent. Since these obstructing agents cannot be identified in children very often, appendiceal submucosal lymphoid hyperplasia in re-

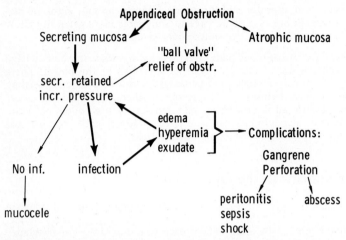

Fig. 12.1.   Pathophysiology of appendicitis (from: R. D. Liechty and R. T. Soper: Synopsis of Surgery. Mosby, St. Louis, Mo., 1972)

sponse to a systemic viremia might be the villain which obstructs the lumen and triggers appendicitis in young children.

The appendiceal obstruction entraps mucus within the distal lumen, excreted by the still-functioning mucosal cells of the appendix. Within a matter of hours, the luminal volume is exceeded, and intraluminal pressure rises as the appendix progressively distends with bacteria-ladened mucus. In the observant older child, one occasionally gets a history that the very first pain of the illness was colicky in nature, reflecting peristaltic efforts to discharge the appendiceal contents into the cecum against the obstruction. However, the colicky pain quickly abates and is replaced at this stage by vague pain of visceral origin difficult to describe or localize, generally referred to the periumbilical area. Anorexia and nausea quickly supervene, followed by vomiting which is far too early to attribute to paralytic ileus, and must be reflex in origin. Ultimately, the intraluminal pressure exceeds capillary pressure to add anoxia to the intestinal wall. The intraluminal bacteria quickly penetrate the now edematous, inflamed and hypoxic wall of the appendix as the hours pass by.

The bacterial element of the inflammation provokes a low-grade temperature elevation (38—39 ° C.) which may be higher in the young child. A moderate leukocytosis (12—18,000) with a shift to the left occurs. Diapedesis of organisms across the edematous, inflamed, and ischemic appendiceal wall produces inflammation of adjacent tissues, to set into motion the mechanisms which localize or wall off the inflammatory reaction. The omentum moves into the area, and adjacent loops of small bowel begin to surround the turgid appendix. Because of anatomic proximity of the appendix to the parietal peritoneum, the latter becomes secondarily inflamed to produce the shift in pain from the vague, difficult to describe central abdominal discomfort of visceral afferent origin to the sharp, easy to describe and localize right lower quadrant pain carried by somatic afferent nerves (T_{11}–L_1). As the somatic nerves become irritated, not only is the pain pattern altered, but also the muscles innervated by these nerves go into spasm to produce the guarding and localized tenderness so necessary for diagnosis. Paralytic ileus ensues to add mild generalized abdominal distention and absent bowel sounds to the picture (Fig. 12.2).

If, by chance, the appendix lies retrocecally or down in the pelvis near the sigmoid colon or bladder, the parietal peritoneum-somatic

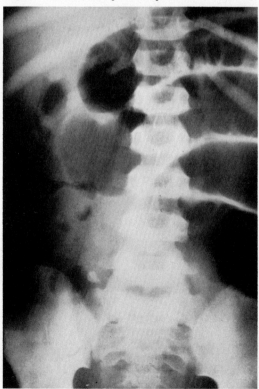

Fig 12.2.
Plain radiograph of abdomen in child with appendicitis showing paralytic ileus and the offending calcified fecalith which triggered the appendicitis

innervation component is absent, and the clinical picture remains vague and difficult to define by both history and physical examination. An inflamed psoas muscle produces a positive psoas sign and obliteration of its shadow on x-ray to suggest retrocecal appendicitis. Dysuria and a few red and white blood cells in the urine suggest a perivesical location, and diarrhea and an exquisitely tender cul-de-sac on rectal examination suggest a so-called "pelvic appendicitis". Constipation characterizes most appendicitis due to the generalized paralytic ileus, but the inflamed pelvic appendix irritates the adjacent sigmoid colon to produce hyperperistalsis and diarrhea.

The final event in the vicious cycle is perforation of the appendix through a now necrotic portion of its wall (Fig. 12.3). This leads to a spreading generalized peritonitis if the tamponading mechanisms

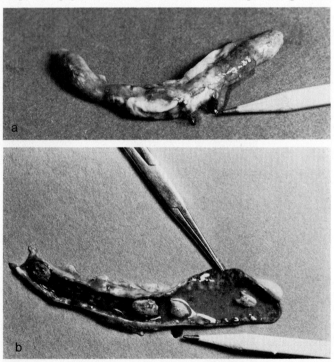

Fig. 12.3.   Upper photograph shows the turgid, gangrenous appendix with perforation at the point of the pencil. The lower photograph of the opened specimen reveals pus and fecaliths; the fecalith at left obstructed the lumen to trigger the appendicitis (from: R. D. Liechty and R. T. Soper: Synopsis of Surgery. Mosby, St. Louis, Mo., 1972)

are inadequate (as they are in the young child) or signs of a localized periappendiceal abscess when the process is successfully contained by omentum or adjacent loops of bowel. In either event, gram-negative septicemia and a remarkable worsening of the general condition of the patient rapidly supervenes to herald these complications of appendicitis.

There is one exception to this chain of events, where the vicious cycle of increasing intraluminal pressure-infection-edema-ischemia is broken when obstruction of the lumen relents, whatever its cause. The fecalith may be expelled into the cecum, or the submucosal lymphoid hyperplasia may abate, allowing the pent-up secretions within the appendiceal lumen to innocuously discharge into the cecum to terminate the attack until and unless luminal obstruction recurs. About 10 % of children with appendicitis have had, upon careful questioning, a previous similar episode which spontaneously resolved. One cannot predict by any clinical yardstick those that will relent in this manner; therefore, every suspected appendicitis should be treated surgically.

Signs and Symptoms

Characteristically, acute appendicitis originates rather blandly with a "stomach ache" which is vague, difficult to describe and localize and is generally epigastric or periumbilical in location. The patient becomes anorexic and then nauseated, and begins to occasionally vomit six to twelve hours after onset of his clinical disease. During the second twelve hours of the illness, the discomfort gradually increases as a mild temperature elevation ensues. The patient begins to feel unwell generally, and ceases normal activity.

During the second 24 hours of the disease, the patient's general condition gradually worsens, and he develops a furred tongue, dry mouth and mild abdominal distention. There is a gradual shift in the pain from vague central abdominal pain to the sharp pain the older child is able to accurately describe and localize to the right lower abdominal quadrant in the area of McBurney's point, located one-third of the distance between the anterior superior iliac spine and the umbilicus. At this stage, the patient notices that cough or motion worsens the discomfort; he prefers to lie down with at least the right hip flexed. Temperature and leukocytosis increase, and the patient becomes obviously more ill.

Further neglect allows perforation to occur, with signs of septicemia and generalized peritoneal irritation with paralytic ileus producing board-like abdominal rigidity and a silent abdomen. Occasionally, the child may come to the physician first after several days of a "flu-like" illness, and on examination be found to harbor a moderately tender mass in the right lower abdominal quadrant or cul-de-sac without signs of generalized peritoneal irritation. This implies a so-called "missed appendicitis" with perforation which is well tamponaded and walled off in an abscess cavity adjacent to the appendix. These patients often are best treated by nasogastric suction, parenteral fluids, and antibiotics. As they improve under this regimen the tender mass gradually diminishes in size, ultimately to disappear completely. The feeding and activity of the patient is gradually restored, and he can be discharged from the hospital safely, but must return in about six weeks for a so-called "interval appendectomy" since subsequent attacks of appendicitis will predictably recur.

Treatment

Supportive Care

Nasogastric suction and intravenous administration of fluids and electrolytes are needed in most patients with acute appendicitis; in those with a complication such as perforation, it is carried out rapidly and coupled with intravenous antibiotics, with restoration of a good urinary output prior to operation. There is no place for non-surgical treatment of appendicitis, except in the patient with a "missed appendicitis" who responds well to supportive and antibiotic care; even these patients require interval appendectomy within six weeks.

If acute suppurative appendicitis cannot be ruled out, the patient should be subjected to immediate laparotomy. If he is not very acutely ill and is obviously in the early stages of whatever the disease is, he may be admitted to the hospital for repeat examinations every two to three hours, simply postponing the decision concerning operation. This kind of leeway avoids unnecessary operations and yet, more importantly, does not delay appendectomy when it is necessary. Even the experienced, conscientious surgeon occasionally explores a patient with the mistaken preoperative diagnosis of appendicitis, only to find another disease at laparotomy. No apologies need be tendered for the occasional unnecessary laparotomy.

Appendicitis in the Very Young

Approximately 10—20 % of acute appendicitis occurs in children under five years of age. The pathophysiology parallels that already outlined for the older child, with one important difference: the speed of progression is markedly accelerated. From obstruction to free appendiceal perforation requires only a few hours, in turn likely due to the tiny appendiceal lumen, abundant lymphoid tissue, vigorous reaction (edema, pus) to infection and ineffective mechanisms to localize inflammation. A thin, short omentum contributes to the latter.

Clinically, appendicitis in the very young child is a short, non-specific and acute illness culminating within hours in generalized peritonitis. In 80—90 %, the appendix has perforated when the patient is first seen, testimony to the speed of progression. Fever, flushed face, irritability and refusal of feedings herald the disease. Copious vomiting ensues quickly, generally bile-stained, with ill-defined abdominal pain and distention, oliguria, dehydration and sometimes diarrhea quickly following. Within 12 to 24 hours a healthy baby becomes acutely and critically ill.

Examination reflects severe dehydration in a crying or apathetic baby who is acutely ill with a high fever (to 40° C) and tachycardia. Attempts at physical examination are generally resisted, although the severely shocked infant may appear to sleep through all but the abdominal exam. The exquisitely tender abdomen typically is distended, tympanitic, silent and board-like, with little evidence of a mass or localization of peritoneal irritation. Rectal exam reveals a full, boggy and tender cul-de-sac. The WBC count is elevated, but may be disarmingly normal in the very ill. Urine is scanty, concentrated and ketotic. Serum electrolytes are elevated (dehydration) and the pH is low.

Vigorous resuscitation with nasogastric suction, intravenous fluids and broad spectrum antibiotics is mandatory. These measures lower the baby's temperature and pulse rate, reverse the signs of dehydration and improve renal function within one to two hours, allowing emergency laparotomy to then be undertaken safely. Through a right lower quadrant muscle-splitting incision, appendectomy is carried out, free pus cultured and the abdominal cavity is lavaged with a saline-antibiotic mixture.

Postoperative recovery is often just as spectacularly rapid as was the course of the illness itself. Often peristalsis returns in 48 hours, paralleling general activity and well being. Few events are more gratifying to the surgeon than the spectacular recovery of a young child from this life-threatening event.

Differential Diagnosis

Mesenteric lymphadenitis. Reactive enlargement of the mesenteric lymph nodes adjacent to the terminal ileum leads to abdominal pain and right lower quadrant tenderness often confused with appendicitis. Mesenteric adenitis is typically preceded by an upper respiratory infection, and indeed may be a response of the lymphoid tissue to such a systemic infection. Abdominal pain is generally vague and centrally located and the right lower quadrant tenderness is not as well localized or acute as in appendicitis. The temperature is apt to be higher with mesenteric adenitis, without the acute shift to the left in the differential count. Observation and reexamination generally show either no progression or gradual improvement; confirmation of diagnosis is more certain if one can palpate multiple tender nodules in the right lower abdominal quadrant (the enlarged, inflamed nodes themselves), best accomplished in the cooperative older patient or the young patient when he is either asleep or sedated. Often mesenteric adenitis is indistinguishable from early acute suppurative appendicitis, except at laparotomy.

Acute gastroenteritis. Children develop acute nonspecific gastroenteritis frequently in childhood, and often come to the physician because their abdominal pain suggests appendicitis. The temperature is apt to be higher than is characteristic of appendicitis. The abdominal tenderness is diffuse rather than localized, the abdomen is slightly distended and hyperactive peristalsis is heard. Diarrhea or vomiting is common, and the white blood cell count is normal.

Acute granulomatous ileitis. Acute transmural granulomatous enterocolitis (Crohn's disease) often cannot be distinguished from appendicitis when it involves the terminal ileum or cecum. In the cooperative or sedated patient one may palpate a tubular, tender mass which then needs to be distinguished from a small periappendiceal perforation or a wad of omentum tamponading an acutely inflamed appendix. The laboratory tests do not help in differentiating the two diseases, and laparotomy is commonly undertaken to rule out appendicitis.

Since most patients with acute ileitis (75 %) have a spontaneous remission, often without further exacerbations, the involved bowel should never be removed at the first attack. The diagnosis is confirmed by a very hyperemic, indurated distal ileum or cecum with enlarged regional lymph nodes. The regional mesenteric lymph nodes should be biopsied and cultured, but no biopsy of the inflamed bowel is taken for fear of postoperative fistula developing through the biopsy site. The important question concerns whether appendectomy should be done so that this confusing differential diagnosis will not recur in the future. We favor appendectomy if the base of the cecum is not involved in the inflammation. If the cecum is inflamed, appendectomy commonly leads to fecal fistulization through the appendiceal stump.

Recurrent Abdominal Pain in Children

Recurrent abdominal pain is a very common problem, especially during the early years of school from age five to ten years, and requires a planned approach to diagnosis. It is easy for the physician to submit a patient with recurrent abdominal pain to innumerable investigations looking for disorders of varying degrees of rarity, when a detailed history, an in-depth interview with the parents and complete physical examination will often provide accurate diagnosis. Only a few patients need submit to anything but quite simple tests.

Too often extensive workups are carried out which discover no organic basis for the pain, and an automatic label of "psychogenic pain" is unfairly pinned on the patient. Significant psychopathy in the patient or family must be found before the pain can be ascribed to psychogenic causes. Further, psychic abnormalities do not confer immunity from organic disease: a very psychogenically disturbed child can develop appendicitis or intussusception to cause one of his recurrent bouts of abdominal pain. Thus, each bout of abdominal pain must be individually evaluated as a separate entity. Cessation of pain after removal of an organic cause does not necessarily mean that all the preceding attacks of pain were due to that cause. The emotional climate may have been changed by the operation with cure of both the organic and psychic pain. On the other hand, children with recurrent pain should not be operated simply on the off-chance of finding an organic cause, and, failing this, that the psychic difficulty might be helped. Seldom is exploratory surgery indicated in patients with recurrent abdominal pain of unknown origin.

The following points help distinguish organic from functional recurrent abdominal pain in children:

Description

Organic pain is fairly constant and is described accurately and precisely, whereas functional pain is more vague and varies from one episode to another.

Localization

There is generally good localization of organic pain, often peripherally or laterally in the abdomen; in contrast, functional pain is poorly localized and is commonly central or periumbilical.

Severity

Organic pain occupies a middle ground between the extremes of bland or excessively severe pain in the child with functional problems.

Time Factor

Organic pain commonly relates to body functions and prevents sleep, whereas functional complaints occur generally during waking hours with stressful situations.

Attacks

Organic abdominal pain attacks tend to last longer than the fleeting attacks of functional pain.

Vomiting

Common in the child with organic complaints, often bile stained; vomiting is rare in the child with functional pain, and consists of ingested food.

Age

No age is exempt from organic pain in childhood; functional complaints begin at the age of four or five, peak at the age of ten, and then gradually taper off into adolescence.

Past history

In the child with organic pain, the past history reflects a fairly pain-free environment and a stable personality; patients with functional pain tend to be worriers, and often were infant spitters.

Family History

Patients with organic pain often have a fairly stable or normal family environment, with little more than the normal parental or sibling pain problems; children with functional complaints often have parents and siblings with painful conditions, with considerable tension and anxiety in the interfamily relationships.

After careful history of the patient and the family and a complete physical examination, the urinary tract is investigated by examining a fresh urine specimen looking for cells, sugar, protein, or acetone. Intravenous pyelogram and voiding cystogram help avoid overlooking a cause for abdominal pain where irrevocable damage can take place before a frank declaration of the problem is made. A complete blood count is always indicated, including examining the red blood cells for sickle cells and spherocytes, anemia, and punctate basophilia of lead intoxication. Contrast studies of the gastrointestinal and gallbladder systems are seldom helpful.

Laparotomy is indicated in those with an organically demonstrable cause for pain, and in only the very rare patient with a negative workup in whom, in the judgment of the surgeon, the risks of not operating are greater than those of laparotomy.

13 Bleeding from the Alimentary Tract

R. T. Soper

General

Gastrointestinal bleeding occurs throughout childhood, from the neonatal period through adolescence. However, it is more common and at times is life-threatening in young babies, partly because of the nature of the lesions that produce hemorrhage in this age group and partly because of infants' low actual circulating blood volume. In general, the older the child the less difficult it is to diagnose and manage gastrointestinal bleeding. Fortunately, the majority of infants and children have a very mild, minor and self-limited bleeding episode which is managed safely and easily.

Important Questions to Answer in GI Bleeding

The first question that demands a prompt answer is whether or not the material being passed actually is blood. This is a most important query in the patient with minor bleeding per rectum. Is the reddish stool color due to ingested dyes or from foods such as raspberries or beets? Is the black, tarry stool from ingested iron? Chemical tests quickly answer this question.

Verified gastrointestinal bleeding prompts this question: is the bleeding simply one manifestation of a generalized bleeding diathesis? Bleeding diatheses in the patient or family and skin purpura or petechiae prompt one to obtain sophisticated blood coagulating studies.

Having ruled out systemic causes, the third question demanding accurate answer relates to the volume and/or speed of gastrointestinal bleeding. Is the bleeding massive as defined by a large volume of gross blood vomited or passed per rectum, signs of shock or the verified loss of 20—25 $^0/_0$ of the total circulating blood volume within a 24-hour period? If so, supportive care is given coincident with diagnostic workup: nasogastric suction, iced saline or bicarbonate gastric lavage with upper gastrointestinal hemorrhage, rapid restoration of blood volume with lactated Ringer's while cross-matching blood, blood transfusions, central venous pressure determinations, and accurate recording of hourly urinary output. The general well-being of the patient is supported during attempts to induce cessation of bleeding or to pinpoint precisely its origin. In contrast, minor, slow or chronic gastrointestinal bleeding can be approached in a much more leisurely and complete manner, without any threat to life or well-being.

The next question to settle is the level of origin of the gastrointestinal bleeding. For this purpose, the gastrointestinal tract is divided into upper and lower compartments. Upper gastrointestinal hemorrhage originates from the esophagus, stomach or duodenum; the blood often presents as hematemesis or is retrieved from the stomach by nasogastric tube; it is also passed per rectum in some altered form. In contrast, lower gastrointestinal bleeding arises distal to the ligament of Treitz and presents only per rectum; blood originating from the anus or lower rectum is bright red in color, blood from the right colon is dark red when passed, and blood of small intestine origin varies from a tarry appearance to a dusky maroon color, dependent on volume and rate of loss.

The final important question to answer concerns the nature of the bleeding lesion itself, epitomizing the ultimate diagnostic goal. This will be discussed later.

Age Correlation

Neonatal Period

In the neonatal period, bleeding is relatively uncommon and is not fully explained in approximately half the cases. Swallowed maternal blood, either aspirated during delivery or ingested by nursing from a fissured nipple, is passed per rectum as black, tarry stool. Blood of maternal origin is quickly distinguished from the baby's blood by detecting adult hemoglobin by the Abt test. Hemorrhagic disease of the newborn produces gastrointestinal bleeding due to a deficiency of serum prothrombin conversion accelerator; 1 mg of vitamin K should stop the bleeding within just a few hours.

Peptic ulceration of the stomach or duodenum is heralded by either perforation or upper gastrointestinal hemorrhage. These neonatal ulcers are likely of "stress" origin because they produce little inflammatory response and are generally discrete, small and punched out, speaking in favor of rapid evolution. Perforation occurs in the ulcers located on the anterior or superior "free" portions of the stomach or (mostly) duodenum. Bleeding characterizes ulcers of the greater or lesser curvatures of the stomach or the medial surface of the duodenum. The bleeding ulcer produces tarry stools and a falling hematocrit, and fresh or slightly altered blood is retrieved from the stomach by tube. Gastric lavage with iced saline or bicarbonate often terminates the bleeding, with blood transfusions restoring diminished blood volume. If bleeding persists or recurs, laparotomy is necessary for suture-ligation of the bleeding point. Since newborns with "stress" ulcers have no true acid-peptic ulcer diathesis, conventional ulcer operations (vagotomy-pyloroplasty, etc.) are rarely justified. Upper gastrointestinal x-rays are, of course, contraindicated in patients with a perforated ulcer. Rarely do they diagnose a bleeding stress ulcer, because the superficial mucosal erosion does not harbor barium in a "niche" which is necessary for the radiographic diagnosis; at best, some element of spasm in the neighborhood of the ulcer is seen at fluoroscopy.

Neonatal Necrotizing Enterocolitis

This condition is a recently-recognized calamity of the first month of life which may be clinically heralded by lower gastrointestinal bleeding. Its pathophysiology (Fig. 13.1) is triggered by ischemia of the ileum or right colon occurring secondary to diversion of portal

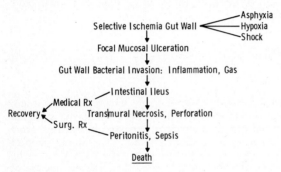

Fig. 13. 1.   Pathophysiology of neonatal necrotizing enterocolitis

blood away from the gastrointestinal tract during a period of shock which, in turn, is generally occasioned by a period of temporary perinatal hypoxemia (hypothermia, fetal distress, traumatic delivery, cardiopulmonary arrest, etc.). The intestinal reaction begins about five days after the original shock-provoking episode, with bloody diarrhea followed by abdominal distention and bilious vomiting. The superior mesenteric artery spasm induces superficial mucosal necrosis with invasion of the bowel wall by intestinal bacteria. Subsequent manifestations include gas within the wall of the afflicted intestine (Figs. 13.2 and 13.3) (as bubbles or linear gas shadows seen on plain radiographs) or later, as gas-forming coliform bacteria metastasize via the portal vein to the liver, by intrahepatic gas (Fig. 13.2). Curiously, the mild cases are the ones who have bloody diarrhea as the main clinical manifestation, whereas the more severely ischemic intestine progresses rapidly to gram-negative sepsis and even bowel wall necrosis with perforation (Fig. 13.4). Supportive

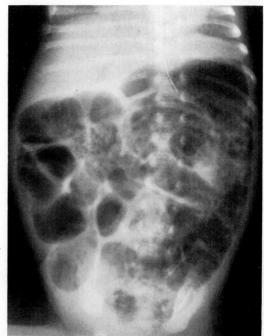

Fig. 13.2.
Plain radiograph of
newborn with necro-
tizing enterocolitis.
Intramural bowel
gas shows as linear
or cystic bubbles,
with portal vein gas
as linear streaks in
the liver shadow

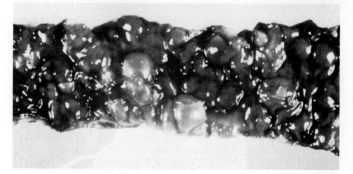

Fig. 13.3.   Intestine from patient in Fig. 13.2.; note the submucosal air cysts which elevate the mucosa

care precedes laparotomy in the severely afflicted patients, where intestinal bypass or resection is carried out. Understandably, the mortality rate is high for this neonatal calamity. Vigorous supportive

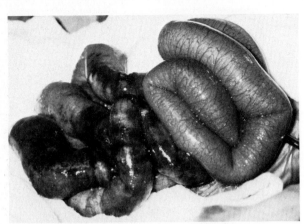

Fig. 13.4.   Operative findings of hemorrhagic, necrotic intestine in new-born with necrotizing enterocolitis

care (nasogastric suction, parenteral fluids and antibiotics, enteral antibiotics, etc.) avoids operation in the mild cases.

One Month to Two Years of Age

In the patient from one month to two years of age, a different set of causes for gastrointestinal bleeding is found. The most common and benign of all is small droplets of bright red blood passed during and just after a painful and hard bowel movement, due to fissuring of the anal mucosa (see Chapters 6 and 9).

Midgut volvulus can produce rectal bleeding in infants, but bilious vomiting and abdominal distention suggest the correct diagnosis (Chapter 5) which leads to urgent laparotomy.

"Stress" Ulcer

"Stress" ulcers of the stomach and duodenum also occur in this age group, generally following operation performed for some other reason or after an acute, febrile illness such as meningitis, sepsis, trauma or severe burns. The same principles apply as outlined previously in the stress ulcer of the newborn: scant diagnostic help from contrast studies of the upper gastrointestinal tract, supportive fluid and blood transfused while the stomach is lavaged with iced saline or bicarbonate, and operation to control bleeding that persists or recurs.

Idiopathic Intussusception

Idiopathic intussusception is the most common serious cause for lower gastrointestinal hemorrhage from 3—18 months of age (see Chapter 5).

Meckel's Diverticulum

This can cause a variety of symptoms, including abdominal pain (diverticulitis) indistinguishable from appendicitis (Chapter 12). It can also cause obstruction (Chapter 5). In addition to these problems, and constituting the most frequent complaint, Meckel's diverticulum can produce lower gastrointestinal bleeding. The bleeding generally is intermittent and recurrent, and has assumed a maroon, deep red color by the time it is passed per rectum. The bleeding episode is generally not accompanied by pain, distention or vomiting. Meckel's

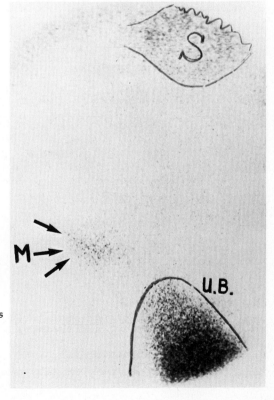

Fig. 13.5.
Scan of abdomen ten minutes after injection of radio-active technetium showing uptake in ectopic gastric mucosa in a Meckel's diverticulum (M), in addition to the normal uptake in stomach (S) and urinary bladder (U.B.)

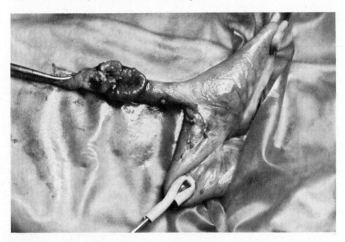

Fig. 13.6. Operative photograph of perforated ulcer in Meckel's diverticulum (from: R. D. Liechty and R. T. Soper: Synopsis of Surgery. Mosby, St. Louis, Mo., 1972)

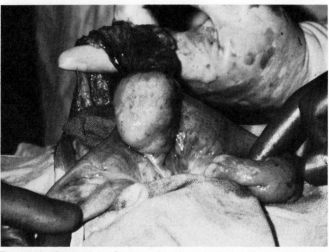

Fig. 13.7. Operative photograph of omentum adherent to apex of a Meckel's diverticulum which contained a bleeding peptic ulcer.

diverticula are rarely demonstrable by radiocontrast studies of the bowel. However, those that bleed generally contain ectopic gastric mucosa so that radioactive technetium (Fig. 13.5), which collects in gastric parietal cells, will show a "hot spot" in the ectopic gastric mucosa of the diverticulum. Most Meckel's diverticula become symptomatic during the second year of life (Figs. 13.6 and 13.7), but many are not discovered until later in childhood. Surgical excision constitutes adequate treatment.

Non-specific gastroenteritis (viral or bacterial in origin) occasionally is so severe as to produce bloody diarrhea. Stool cultures should confirm diagnosis, the bloody diarrhea ceasing as the infection is brought under control by non-surgical measures. The bleeding is never massive and transfusions are rarely required. Ulcerative colitis is extremely rare in the very young.

Duplication of the intestine is discussed in Chapter 5 and is a rare cause of gastrointestinal hemorrhage.

Bleeding From 2—10 Years of Age

The incidence of gastrointestinal hemorrhage gradually diminishes throughout these childhood years. Stress ulcers of the stomach and duodenum sporadically occur in response to acute febrile illnesses, burns, CNS operations or infections, automobile accidents or major surgical operations. Chronic adult-type acid-peptic ulcers begin to occur during late childhood, gradually increasing in frequency through adolescence and into young adulthood; they will be discussed later.

Intestinal Polyps

Various types of intestinal polyps are the most common cause of bleeding during these middle years of childhood.

Juvenile polyps comprise about 80—90 % of all childhood polyps and begin to provoke their most common sign (bright red blood per rectum) in the third year of life, increasing in frequency to peak from four to eight years of age with a rapid fall-off thereafter. Sixty percent involve boys, 85 % of polyps are apparently solitary, and about 90 % are confined to the rectum and sigmoid colon. Almost all produce relatively unaltered blood which coats or follows the bowel movement, often self-amputating or on occasion prolapsing from the rectum.

Grossly, the juvenile polyp is round, smooth, pedunculated and has a shiny or glary appearance (Fig. 13.8). Histologically it consists of numerous cystic dilated glands, abundant stroma with areas of surface ulceration and acute and chronic inflammatory changes. Juvenile polyps are hamartomas, rather than neoplasms, with no malignant potential. Their cause is unknown, but most experts implicate

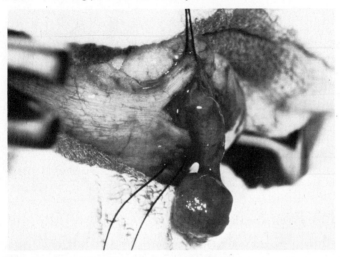

Fig. 13.8.   Juvenile polyp at colotomy removal

mechanical, allergic or inflammatory factors. Rarely, the larger polyps trigger intussusception.

Physical examination typically reveals a healthy child with no signs of chronic anemia who harbors a soft, smooth polyp on rectal digital exam. Proctosigmoidoscopy reveals a polyp with the gross characteristics listed above. Excision of a rectal polyp is safely performed through the sigmoidoscope with cautery of the base. Once the polyp is histologically confirmed as juvenile in type, the treatment is very permissive. These polyps never become malignant, and only rarely develop serious complications such as significant hemorrhage or intussusception. Barium enema air-contrast studies outline the occasional juvenile polyp which is above reach of the sigmoidoscope (Fig. 13.9). Juvenile polyposis is a rare variant of this problem, severe bleeding and protein-losing enteropathy resulting from the hundreds of juvenile polyps these unfortunate patients harbor (Fig. 13.10).

Hyperplasia of submucosal lymphoid tissue in the colon and terminal ileum occasionally aggregate enough to elevate the mucosa and, by definition, produce a rather sessile intestinal polyp. These so-called *lymphoid polyps* occur during the first three to four years of life and are heralded clinically by the passage of unaltered blood per rectum, or perhaps are recognized incidentally at barium enema done for some other purpose. They are generally multiple and are prone to occur in the terminal ileum, the cecum and rectosigmoid. At proctosigmoidoscopy lymphoid polyps are recognized as sessile elevations

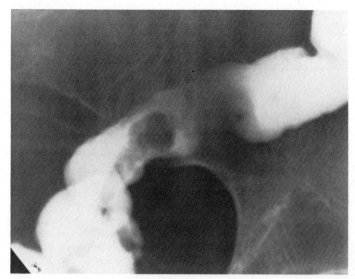

Fig. 13.9.   Barium outlining polyp in Fig. 13.8.

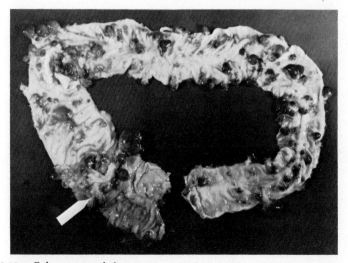

Fig. 13.10.   Colon resected from patient with juvenile polyposis (from:
R. T. Soper and T. H. Kent: Surgery 69: 692—698, 1971)

of normal bowel mucosa; their lymphoid nature is disclosed on histologic examination. Air-contrast barium studies show the small (2—4 mm), uniform, polypoid filling defects involving all or parts of the colon; a fleck of barium in the center of these polyps represents umbilication which is rather unique to lymphoid polyps. Etiology is unclear, but lymphoid hyperplasia in response to infection or allergy is a likely etiologic factor. Their real importance in children is to distinguish them from intestinal lymphoma or from premalignant adenomatous polyps, which require more aggressive surgical or other treatment. The lymphoid polyp of childhood is not premalignant, never causes serious symptoms and disappears with time either spontaneously or in response to low dose steroids or intestinal antibiotic "sterilization".

Peutz-Jeghers Polyps

Peutz-Jeghers polyps become symptomatic during childhood or adolescent years by the passage of altered blood per rectum and/or episodes of colicky pain suggesting intussusception. Melanin pigmentation of the oral and anal mucous membranes are external manifestations of the syndrome (Fig. 13.11). The polyps are generally localized to the small intestine and number from 1 to 10; occasionally they are more numerous and are found within stomach or colon. Malignant degeneration is extremely unusual with this type of

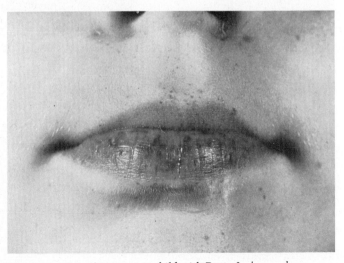

Fig. 13.11.   Buccal pigment in child with Peutz-Jeghers polyps

hamartomatous polyp. Upper gastrointestinal contrast studies generally pinpoint the polyps as filling defects in a youngster with pigmentation of the lips, mouth and anus. Treatment is tailored to symptoms: no treatment is justified for the relatively asymptomatic patient, whereas polypectomy is required if obstruction, intussusception or severe bleeding are produced. The disorder is inherited.

Hereditary (Familial) Polyposis

The only type of adenomatous neoplastic polyps that occurs with any frequency in childhood are those associated with hereditary polyposis or Gardner's syndrome. Both of these conditions are transmitted genetically as autosomal dominant conditions, a few arising sporadically from spontaneous mutation. In addition to colonic polyps, patients with Gardner's syndrome harbor adamantinomas, fibromas, chondromas, and other benign soft and hard tissue neoplasms. Both diseases are characterized by innumerable adenomatous polyps that ultimately involve all the colonic mucosa (Fig. 13.12). Typically, the polyps begin to appear during the second decade of life, producing symptoms (protein-losing enteropathy, melena, intussusception) during the third decade of life and developing into aggressive, invasive neoplasms of the colon during the fourth decade of life. These dangerous, premalignant adenomatous polyps must be histologically differentiated from any other type of benign polyp; it is just as

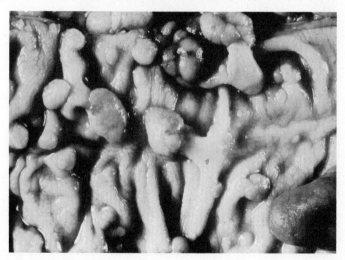

Fig. 13.12.   Fine "raspberry" papillations characterizing the many adenomatous polyps of the colon in this child with familial polyposis

wrong to perform colectomy for benign polyps of the colon as it is to allow the cancer-bearing colonic mucosa to remain in a child with familial polyposis or Gardner's syndrome. Every child in a family with established familial polyposis or Gardner's syndrome should be periodically studied for polyps (Fig. 13.13).

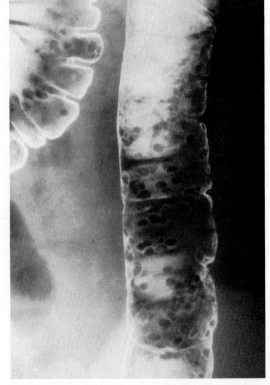

Fig. 13.13.
Air contrast barium enema showing hundreds of polyps in a patient with familial polyposis

Total proctocolectomy removes all the cancer-bearing colonic and rectal mucosa and is the surgical treatment most certain to prevent cancer of the colon from developing later in these unfortunate children. Regrettably, this operation necessitates permanent abdominal wall ileostomy with its own psychological and physiological problems. Abdominal colectomy and ileoproctostomy preserve anal bowel function, but do so at the expense of also retaining premalignant mucosa of the rectum. Recently, an endorectal technique of stripping away the rectal mucosa has been devised. This operation removes all intraabdominal colon and the premalignant rectal mucosa, while retaining normal bowel continence by bringing the ileum through the retained rectal muscle to just above the anal verge. This operation should be undertaken prophylactically once diagnosis has been clearly established and before any neoplastic change has occurred in the mucosa of the colon.

The remaining polyps of childhood are extremely rare: intestinal lymphomas or neurofibromas, ectopic pancreatic tissue within bowel wall or Burkitt's tumors which have a polypoid structure. The majority produce symptoms by melena, intussusception or bowel obstruction. Intestinal contrast studies often show characteristic filling defects. Surgical resection is indicated.

Esophageal Varices

Hemorrhage from esophageal varices constitutes one of the most alarming types of gastrointestinal hemorrhage because it is vomited in a spectacular fashion, thoroughly frightening parents to bring in the patient promptly for evaluation. Portal hypertension is the underlying cause for esophageal varices, occasioned by some obstruction to the flow of venous blood through the portal vein or liver. In adults, portal hypertension is generally due to intrahepatic obstruction from cirrhosis of the liver. In contrast, the majority of childhood portal hypertension is occasioned by thrombosis of the portal vein before it enters the liver. Intrahepatic obstruction occurs from posthepatitis cirrhosis or occasionally from primary hepatic fibrosis or cysts. Major variceal hemorrhage in a patient with a sick liver (cirrhosis) carries a much higher mortality rate from hepatic failure and encephalopathy than if he possesses a normal liver (extrahepatic portal vein obstruction), where prognosis relates solely to the acute blood loss.

Massive hematemesis generally heralds variceal bleeding, often followed by melena. History of neonatal or childhood hepatitis makes primary intrahepatic obstruction the likely cause, especially if the patient has jaundice, spider hemangiomata, palmar erythema or other stigmata of chronic hepatic disease. Lacking these, portal vein thrombosis is the likely cause, and a history of umbilical vein catheterization, umbilical sepsis or ascites should be sought. Often, none of these questions is answered affirmatively.

The first order of business is to assess the volume and speed of hemorrhage. A nasogastric tube is passed with a balloon on its tip (Fig. 13.14); the balloon is inflated and then drawn snugly up against the gastroesophageal junction. Since most of the blood entering esophageal varices comes from the wall of the stomach via collaterals developed as a result of portal hypertension, the proximal gastric

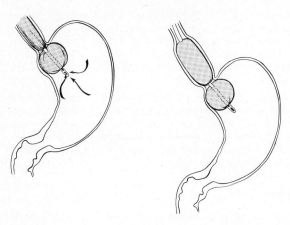

Fig. 13.14.   Left: nasogastric tube with intragastric balloon inflated and drawn up against gastroesophageal junction. Right: esophageal balloon inflated to directly compress esophageal varices

balloon tamponades the blood at this point and often rapidly terminates or diminishes hemorrhage from esophageal varices. If esophageal varices continue to bleed, the blood is constantly regurgitated since it can no longer enter the stomach downstream; the esophageal balloon is then inflated (Fig. 13.14). If no blood is regurgitated, the stomach is then aspirated empty and lavaged with iced saline or iced bicarbonate. If blood continues to return from the stomach tube, then the blood obviously is arising in the stomach or duodenum. If no blood is either regurgitated or retrieved from the stomach after gastric lavage, this is strong presumptive evidence for esophageal variceal hemorrhage temporarily tamponaded by the gastric or esophageal balloons.

If variceal bleeding persists or recurs, emergency ligation of the esophageal varices must be carried out either through the thorax or abdomen, which often prevents further bleeding for one or two years.

If the bleeding is less vigorous, a carefully performed esophagram (Fig. 13.15) often shows indentation and irregularities of the lower esophageal mucosa characteristic of varices. The varicosities are confirmed by esophagoscopy. In patients with chronic liver disease, blood must be purged from the gastrointestinal tract as rapidly as possible to reduce absorption of protein which, in the face of a failing liver, produces hyperammonemia and encephalopathy. This is best

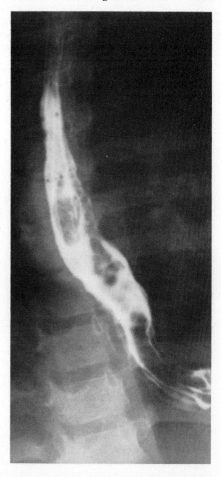

Fig. 13.15. Esophagram showing filling defects characteristic
of esophageal varices

achieved by instilling laxatives and nonabsorbed antibiotics into the
stomach and administering enemas.

Once the bleeding episode has been controlled and the general status
of the patient is improved, more specific diagnostic measures may
be safely undertaken. Under general anesthesia, a needle is placed
into the splenic pulp percutaneously to measure splenic pulp pressure, which faithfully reflects portal vein pressure. Normal portal
vein pressure is 5—15 cm of water; anything above 25 cm of water
pressure is diagnostic of portal venous hypertension. Dye injected

into the splenic pulp fills the portal venous system (Fig. 13.16). From serial films one can detect portal vein thrombosis, the presence of collaterals and often visualize esophageal varices.

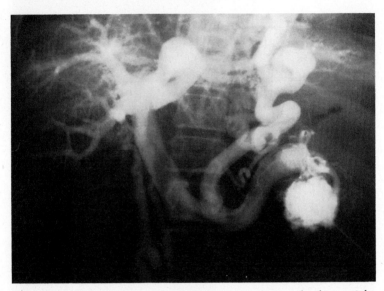

Fig. 13.16. Needle injects radiopaque dye into splenic pulp (lower right pool of dye) which rapidly fills dilated splenic and portal veins; the dilated, tortuous coronary vein (center running cephalad) is the major collateral vessel filling the esophageal varices

Definitive treatment consists of establishing an effective shunt between some part of the portal venous system and the systemic veins, generally the inferior vena cava. The shunt provides easy egress of blood from the obstructed portal system into the systemic veins, lowering portal venous pressure and reducing blood flow through the dangerous, naturally-occuring porta-systemic collaterals (the esophageal varices). Splenectomy sometimes is carried out to immediately improve the thrombopenia and leukopenia of hypersplenism, but if the portal venous pressure is successfully lowered by the shunt, the spleen should diminish in size and the hematologic manifestations of hypersplenism gradually revert to normal. If possible, portasystemic venous shunts are delayed until the child is 8—10 years of age since the larger the veins the better are the chances for a long-term patent anastomosis. Mesenteric-caval shunts can be performed in younger children safely.

Bleeding in Adolescence

Chronic Peptic ulcer

Older children and adolescents develop peptic ulcers which assume more and more the characteristics of chronic peptic ulcer of adulthood. Heralding complaints include repeated episodes of epigastric abdominal pain akin to excessive "hunger pangs" with the fasting-pain-eating-relief cycle as the adult peptic ulcer. The ulcer generally has a deep enough crater to be demonstrated radiographically, as well as other suggestive radiographic signs such as increased peristalsis, excessive secretions and an irritable duodenal bulb.

Chronic peptic ulcer in childhood is almost exclusively a disease of the duodenum, with a slight male sex predisposition. They begin to appear in children five to seven years of age, with a slightly increasing incidence throughout the remainder of childhood. Many of the children have emotional problems in school or in their family situation which are thought to be contributing etiologic factors. The majority respond to measures which improve the emotional environment, antispasmodics, antacids and tranquilizers. Only rarely do complications arise which demand surgical therapy: intractability to medical treatment, cicatricial contracture with obstruction, bleeding or perforation. Vagotomy coupled either with pyloroplasty or gastric antrectomy is very satisfactory surgical treatment.

Zollinger-Ellison Syndrome

Reportably rare is the child with the Zollinger-Ellison syndrome, by definition consisting of gastric hypersecretion produced by functioning non-beta islet cell tumors of the pancreas leading to intractable, atypically-located peptic ulcers which persist or recur despite vigorous conventional medical and surgical treatment. Diarrhea may accompany the peptic ulcer symptoms. Markedly elevated serum gastrin, and high gastric acid secretions which are not augmented by histamine stimulation suggest the diagnosis, along with contrast studies showing large or multiple ulcers with prominent gastric rugae. Operation generally reveals multiple pancreatic tumors which may have already metastasized to liver. Total gastrectomy is the surgical treatment of choice, to completely remove the target organ responsible for the symptoms.

Chronic Ulcerative Colitis

Approximately 10—15 % of chronic ulcerative colitis originates during childhood, carrying a more serious prognosis than when it begins later in life because of retardation of body growth and sexual development; also the younger the age of onset the more likely malignant transformation may ultimately occur. It can usually be distinguished easily from the other types of childhood colitis which cause bloody diarrhea by its chronicity and consistently negative stool examinations for ova, parasites and pathogenic organisms. The differential diagnosis includes intestinal infections from Shigella and Salmonella, Endamoeba histolytica, actinomycosis and histoplasmosis.

Mucous and later bloody diarrhea of a chronic and recurrent nature clinically herald chronic ulcerative colitis. Crampy abdominal discomfort and gradual weight loss supervene with ultimate personality changes of irritability and dependency. Joint pains, clubbing of the fingernails and growth failure with retardation of sexual development are the major systemic manifestations of the disease in children.

During the early stages of ulcerative colitis, proctoscopy reveals edematous, friable mucosa which bleeds readily upon contact with the scope. Later, the rectal valves become foreshortened and blunted and superficial mucosal ulcerations appear which, as they enlarge and coalesce in a longitudinal fashion, leave behind edematous, intact mucosa referred to as "pseudopolyps". In its late stages, inflammation and fibrosis produce rigidity of the bowel detected on sigmoidoscopy and barium enema. In this stage, barium enema

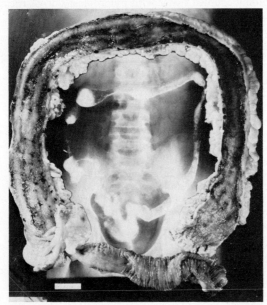

Fig. 13.17.
Barium enema and resection specimen of adolescent male with far advanced chronic ulcerative colitis

shows a smooth, narrowed colonic lumen with loss of haustrations, the so-called "lead pipe" colon of advanced ulcerative colitis (Fig. 13.17).

The prognosis in chronic ulcerative colitis of childhood is serious, but variable. Medical treatment includes a low residue diet, bedrest, and administration of vitamins, iron and a nonabsorbable sulfa like Azulfidine. Withdrawal from the home or school environment to a hospital with a sympathetic physician often helps induce a remission. Systemic steroids help control the disease, but have significant side effects that must be appreciated: occult perforations of the gastrointestinal tract plus growth and sexual retardation. Local steroids in the form of enemas produce fewer systemic side effects, and may induce remission.

Somewhere between 20 and 40 % of children with chronic ulcerative colitis ultimately come to surgical treatment for complications of the disease or its treatment. Of those treated surgically, about a quarter require emergency operations for an acute complication such as toxic megacolon (paralytic ileus of the colon with enormous dilatation and imminent perforation), massive hemorrhage or frank bowel perforation. The remainder have chronic indications: colonic obstruction, intractability to medical management, growth or sexual retardation and suspected carcinoma of the colon. Only about 5 % of patients with chronic ulcerative colitis actually develop carcinoma of the colon, but the percentage is higher in those contracting the disease in childhood (10—15 %). The incidence of cancer increases dramatically after ten years of chronic inflammatory activity.

Proctocolectomy with ileostomy, either staged or undertaken at one operation, is the surgical treatment of choice. Getting rid of the involved bowel produces dramatic improvement in these youngsters, and should not be withheld until the patient is moribund or profoundly retarded in terms of growth and sexual development. The etiology of ulcerative colitis is unknown: viral, psychological and autoimmune theories of origin all lack verification.

Granulomatous (Transmural) Enterocolitis

(Regional enteritis, regional ileitis, regional ileocolitis and Crohn's disease.) Granulomatous enterocolitis is an uncommon disorder, which generally begins in adulthood. However, about 15 % of cases originate in children ten years of age or older. The cause of the disease is unknown, although allergic, infectious and autoimmune factors have been suggested as contributing factors.

In the majority, granulomatous enterocolitis originates in, or is totally confined to, the distal ileum. Spread commonly occurs proximally and occasionally distally to the colon, often leading to multiple sites of involvement with uninvolved "skip areas" intervening. Early in the disease, the involved mucosa ulcerates and the wall of the intestine becomes grossly thickened, erythematous and edematous with thickening of the adjacent mesentery and rubbery enlargement of the regional mesenteric lymph nodes. Ultimately, all layers of the bowel become involved to justify the descriptive term *transmural*. When this disease attacks primarily the colon, the transmural inflammation serves to distinguish it from the primarily mucosal inflammation of chronic ulcerative colitis.

Approximately 75 % of patients with acute terminal ileitis have spontaneous resolution of their disease, often with no recurrence. Repeat bouts of enteritis or enterocolitis is the rule, however, and in the later stages of the disease fibrous tissue develops in the involved bowel wall producing rigidity, contracture and narrowing of the bowel lumen. A moderately tender mass can usually be palpated at this stage, clinically associated with periodic bouts of crampy abdominal discomfort, diarrhea, weight loss and anemia. Fever and leukocytosis parallel the disease activity, and for unknown reasons perianal abscesses, fissures and fistula-in-ano are common (Chapter 6).

Late stages of transmural enterocolitis are characterized by deep ulcerations which penetrate through the bowel wall to produce abscesses and inflammation of adjacent viscera leading to both external and internal fistulas. Signs and symptoms of chronic low grade intestinal obstruction induced by the luminal narrowing are often superimposed.

Diagnosis

The diagnosis of transmural enterocolitis is generally made by contrast (barium) x-ray studies. During early stages the radiographic signs include a modest narrowing of the lumen associated with edema and raggedness of the mucosal pattern with puddling of barium. Later, extreme narrowing of the lumen may occur with scarring, producing a "string sign" with dilatation of proximal loops proportionate to the degree of mechanical intestinal obstruction (Fig. 13.18). Occasionally the barium fills deep ulcerations, peri-intestinal abscesses or fistulas into adjacent viscera.

Treatment

The treatment of granulomatous enterocolitis is medical until and unless complications occur. A nutritious and low residue diet, supplements of vitamins and iron, ingestion of nonabsorbed sulfon-

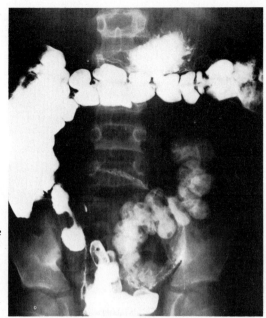

Fig. 13.18.
Late radiograph in barium upper GI series with small bowel follow-through; most of the barium is already in the colon, but a long, narrow "string sign" of terminal ileitis is pictured in a curvilinear pattern centrally.

amides (Azulfidine), physical and psychological rest and symptomatic treatment for diarrhea are all used in various combinations. Systemic steroids and antimetabolites occasionally help. Total parenteral nutrition for a few weeks places the entire gastrointestinal tract at rest, and may induce a dramatic remission.

Surgical treatment (Fig. 13.19) of transmural enterocolitis is carried out for complications of the disease: intestinal obstruction, fistula, intra-abdominal abscess, hemorrhage, or if the patient's general well being is compromised by chronic malnutrition, anemia, pain and debility. Ultimately, over one-half of patients with chronic granulomatous enterocolitis require surgical intervention.

Surgical treatment is tailored to the particular complications which are found, and includes resection or bypass of the involved intestine. Recurrence in previously uninvolved bowel occurs in fully one-third of the patients who are followed up for many years after primary surgical treatment. Repeated resections and bypassing procedures are themselves fraught with nutritional and metabolic disturbances, warranting intensification of medical treatment and, when possible, avoidance of surgical treatment.

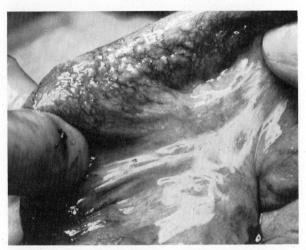

Fig. 13.19.   Subacute granulomatous ileitis at operation; small bowel loop is firm, thickened and injected

Intestinal Hemangioma

Intestinal hemangioma may involve any part of the gastrointestinal tract and may be the cause of repeated bleeding episodes. Cutaneous hemangiomas occasionally are an external manifestation. Plain radiographs (showing calcification of the lesions) and arteriography

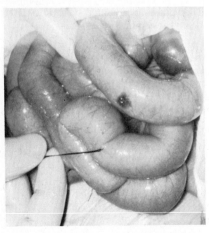

Fig. 13.20.   Dark spot on the bowel wall is an intestinal hemangioma responsible for many bouts of melena.

(which fill the lesion's vascular channels with dye) occasionally help make the diagnosis preoperatively. Generally, intestinal hemangiomas (Fig. 13.20) are discovered only at laparotomy undertaken because of repeated bouts of mild GI hemorrhage. Simple resection suffices as treatment.

14 Abdominal Masses

R. T. SOPER

General

Discovery of an abdominal mass in an infant or child is understandably alarming to the parents and physician. The history often does not help unravel the mystery, because most abdominal masses of childhood evolve slowly enough so that symptoms are subtle and late in developing. Most of the masses are noticed by the parents from changes in the normal contour of the abdomen (Fig. 14.1) or by accidental palpation of the mass while dressing or bathing the child. Masses arise from virtually any of the intra-abdominal or retroperitoneal viscera, both hollow and solid, and range in prognostic significance from very minor and unimportant entities (retention of stool in the constipated child) to problems which threaten the very life of the patient (inflammatory masses, neoplastic masses).

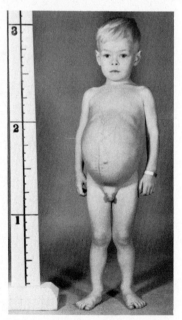 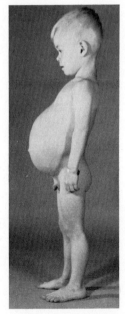

Fig. 14.1. Gross change in abdominal contour imposed by a large liver tumor (from: D. L. Silber, R. T. Soper and T. H. Kent: J. pediat. Surg., Vol. V. 4: 1970)

Enlargement of the liver and/or spleen accounts for approximately half of all childhood abdominal masses. Splenomegaly may be secondary to portal hypertension from either postnecrotic cirrhosis or portal vein thrombosis (Chapter 13). It also occurs from granulomatous or parasitic infestations, lymphomatous involvement and malaria: spleens softened and enlarged by disease are more vulnerable to rupture by minor trauma, justifying early treatment of the primary disease.

Hypersplenism

The term hypersplenism is nonspecific and implies an increased splenic destruction of one or more of the formed elements of the blood (red blood cells, white blood cells or platelets). It is usually associated with splenomegaly, peripheral blood depression of the blood elements destroyed in the spleen and increased production within the bone marrow of the elements which are diminished in the peripheral blood.

Idiopathic Thrombocytopenic Purpura

Diminished circulating platelets associated with a bleeding diathesis characterize this condition. It must be clinically distinguished from thrombopenia and purpura secondary to bone marrow depression seen with a variety of disorders such as tuberculosis, excessive irradiation, leukemia, widespread bony metastases and bone marrow sensitivity to drugs such as sulfonamides, Chloramphenicol, benzol and arsenicals. Secondary thrombocytopenic purpura is not helped by splenectomy.

Idiopathic thrombocytopenic purpura is more common in female than male children; its basic cause is unknown. Clinically the disease is manifested by periodic abnormal bleeding episodes (petechiae, ecchymoses and hematomas following minor trauma). Occasionally, urinary or gastrointestinal bleeding occurs, or menometrorrhagia in adolescent females. Hematomas may develop in the intestinal wall which can obstruct the lumen or act as the lead point of an intussusception. The most potentially dangerous bleeding occurs intracranially, although this catastrophe is most unusual in children. Idiopathic thrombocytopenic purpura is the only hypersplenic state not commonly associated with splenomegaly (80 %).

Diagnosis of idiopathic thrombocytopenic purpura is suggested by a peripheral blood platelet count of 40,000/cu mm or below. Understandably, the bone marrow smear contains increased numbers of platelet precursors (megakaryocytes). The bleeding time is prolonged and the clot retraction is poor, although coagulation time is normal. Petechiae are regularly produced distal to a sphygmomanometer cuff inflated above venous pressure (Rumpel-Leede test). Spontaneous remissions often occur, and may be permanent. Steroid therapy may induce a remission or at least temporarily elevate peripheral platelet counts.

Splenectomy is indicated for idiopathic thrombocytopenic purpura if a remission is not obtained by steroids or if the disease exacerbates while under steroid maintenance. From 60 to 70 % of patients have permanent elevation of platelet counts following splenectomy; the bleeding tendency improves in others even though the platelet count is unchanged.

Idiopathic Splenic Neutropenia and Pancytopenia

These are rare primary types of hypersplenism with a deficiency in one or all of the formed blood elements associated with an increase in marrow activity in those blood elements which are deficient peripherally. Splenectomy is curative.

Much more commonly, these varieties of hypersplenism are *secondary* to other primary disorders producing splenomegaly, including infections (malaria, sarcoidosis), neoplasms (leukemia, lymphoma, Hodgkin's disease), metabolic storage diseases (Gaucher's disease, Niemann-Pick disease, Hand-Schuller-Christian disease, Letterer-Siwe disease), and portal hypertension. Of course, treatment should be directed at the primary disease, rather than the enlarged spleen itself in secondary splenic pancytopenia. Splenectomy occasionally is performed for massive splenomegaly (especially vulnerable to traumatic injury) or to temporarily improve severe hematologic changes.

Congenital Spherocytosis

Congenital spherocytosis is a hemolytic anemia caused by a congenital disturbance of hemoglobin which results in a morphologic alteration of the red blood cell to a spheroid shape, rather than a biconcave disc. About 20 % of cases arise as a spontaneous mutation, the remainder showing a strong family history of anemia and jaundice suggesting a Mendelian dominant trait transmitted by either parent. The mechanical and osmotic fragility of the spherocytes is increased, making them more susceptible to entrapment and hemolysis within the spleen.

Clinically, mild anemia and jaundice with a slightly enlarged spleen develop during the first decade of life. Patients with mild forms of the disease may have a perfectly normal life span, although about 25 % ultimately develop gallstones due to chronic hyperbilirubinemia.

Children with more severe forms of congenital spherocytosis develop periodic crises of abdominal pain, fever, nausea and vomiting, progressive anemia, acholuric jaundice and splenomegaly, sometimes precipitated by systemic infections. Blood smear reveals the spherical erythrocytes characteristic of the disease. The reticulocyte count and red blood cell counts are low during a crisis, but rise during the recovery period.

Short of morphology, the most diagnostic test for congenital spherocytosis is increased red blood cell fragility. The indirect serum bilirubin level is elevated, although there is no biliuria because of the conjugated nature of the bilirubin. Coombs' test for immune globulin is negative, and bone marrow commonly reveals erythroid hyperplasia.

Treatment of the crisis is directed at tiding the patient over the acute episode by means of cautious blood transfusions if necessary. Later, splenectomy can be carried out with less risk to the patient. Splenectomy cures the serious hemolysis of this disorder, but does not alter red blood cell shape or fragility. Since spontaneous remissions do not occur, all symptomatic patients with congenital spherocytosis should have elective splenectomy. The gallbladder is carefully inspected for bilirubin stones or gravel to which hemolysis predisposes the patient.

Hepatomegaly

The liver edge is commonly palpable in the newborn 1—2 cm below the right costal margin; it is generally easily distinguished from pathological hepatomegaly. Most hepatomegaly of older infants and children is "medical" in origin, in which the help of the surgeon is occasionally enlisted for diagnostic biopsy or laparotomy: infection (hepatitis, chronic granulomatous disease, viremia), benign tumors (Fig. 14.2) (hemangioma, hemangioendothelioma, hamartoma), primary malignant tumors (hepatoblastoma), secondary malignant disease (metastasis from abdominal neuroblastoma, leukemic infiltrate, involvement with Hodgkin's disease, lymphoma), storage diseases, congestive heart failure, malnutrition, etc.

The other half of abdominal masses in infancy and childhood involve enlargement of organs other than the liver and spleen, and are much more clearly "surgical" in origin. Here the surgeon is called in early both for diagnosis as well as therapy. This "surgical" half of ab-

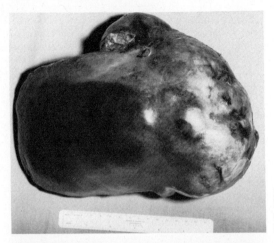

Fig. 14.2.
Hamartoma of liver
resected from boy
pictured in 14.1.

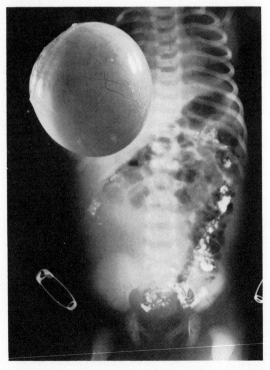

Fig. 14.3.
Right ovarian cyst in
newborn producing
an asymptomatic
abdominal mass
which displaced
intestine

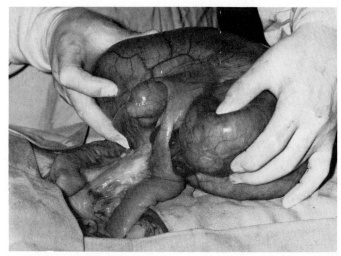

Fig. 14.4. Large mesenteric (lymphatic) cyst of jejunum producing soft, nontender abdominal mass

dominal masses is conveniently subdivided into approximately one-half which involve masses in and of the urinary tract (cystic disease, hydronephrosis, Wilms' tumor) and half consisting of nonurinary masses of either intraperitoneal or retroperitoneal origin. The intraperitoneal masses are generally due to congenital problems involving the hollow viscera or other intraperitoneal structures (Fig. 14.3 and 14.4), whereas the retroperitoneal masses are generally neoplasm (neuroblastoma, rhabdomyosarcoma) arising retroperitoneally.

Physical Examination

One must first exclude ascites and nonpathological abdominal masses (retained material within stomach, colon and urinary bladder). Repeat examination after the stomach and colon have been emptied excludes gastric dilatation and retained stool. Reexamination after the patient voids clarifies the normal bladder full of urine; however, a suprapubic mass which remains after voiding requires bladder catheterization to exclude residual urine from bladder neck obstruction (Chapter 18). Free ascitic fluid should not be confused with an abdominal mass: flank bulging and percussion dullness and central tympany while the patient is supine, dullness shifting with position change and diagnostic needle paracentesis.

Liver and spleen are the most common upper abdominal masses in children. An enlarged liver presents as a right upper quadrant or epigastric mass with a fairly sharp leading edge which moves freely with respiration and is generally non-tender. The spleen enlarges downward and medially as a left upper quadrant mass which also moves with respiration but has a rounded edge and a notch on its upper medial border. It is more superficial than a renal mass, which enlarges downward and does not move with respiration.

Lower abdominal masses generally consist of residual stool within the colon or urine within the bladder, appropriate evacuation clarifying their true nature. Ovarian masses are palpated best on bimanual rectal-abdominal examination; they are unilateral cystic or solid masses which are tender only if twisted or associated with an ectopic pregnancy. Hydrocolopos or hydrometrocolpos presents a midline lower abdominal mass which extends into the pelvis; the mass does not disappear with bladder catheterization.

Lateral abdominal masses are the most important masses of infancy and childhood. Excluding liver and spleen they also are the most

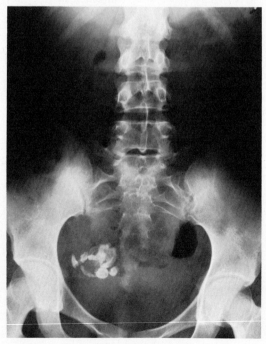

Fig. 14.5.
Coarse calcification in a benign pelvic teratoma arising from the right ovary

numerous. Cystic kidneys, congenital hydronephrosis, Wilms' tumor and neuroblastoma are the four most common causes of lateral abdominal masses, pointing up the importance of careful intravenous pyelography in their evaluation. None of these masses moves particularly with respiration and it is only rarely that one can distinguish cystic from solid tumors on physical examination alone. Transillumination and sonography clearly separate solid from cystic masses. They are typically nontender, and only the neuroblastoma crosses the midline with any frequency.

Workup

Workup of the infant or child with an abdominal mass may be extremely simple, but at times taxes the ingenuity and resources of experienced surgeons and large institutions. Plain radiographs of the chest (for metastases) and abdomen is the first step in laboratory

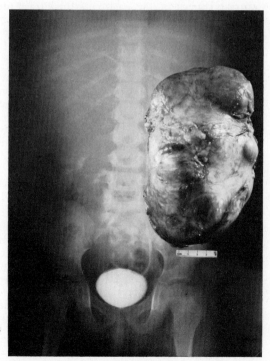

Fig. 14.6.
Finely stippled calcification in a huge right suprarenal neuroblastoma which displaced kidney inferiorly

diagnosis. Displacement of hollow or solid viscera by the mass is noted. Calcification within the mass is important to determine, teratomas having a coarse calcification (Fig. 14.5) with occasionally recognizable teeth or bones in contrast to the finely stippled calcification found in about half the neuroblastomas (Fig. 14.6).

Intravenous pyelography is clearly the most important single study in evaluating abdominal masses of childhood. Delayed films and a longer intravenous infusion of more dye are refinements of this basic study that increase detail and clarity of the film and better evaluate renal function.

Transillumination often helps distinguish solid masses from water-filled cysts. The study needs to be carried out in a totally dark room with an intense light source. Transillumination is especially helpful in newborns, clearly distinguishing hydronephrosis from solid renal or perirenal masses. Understandably, the older the child, the thicker the abdominal wall and the more deeply seated the mass, the less satisfactory is transillumination.

Contrast studies of the gastrointestinal tract often help diagnose masses primary within the gastrointestinal tract. Radioactive scanning is a valuable method of examining masses arising in or secondarily involving the liver, spleen and kidney. Lesions larger than 2–3 cm in size show up as punched out areas within these organs.

Sonography, or diagnostic ultrasound, is a recently developed non-invasive method of detecting consistency, location and size of body organs and masses. Two-dimensional "pictures" of body cavities can be mapped out by sonographic scanning. Abdominal masses produce changes from the normal or expected sonographic recording. Sonography distinguishes masses containing air or fluid from solid masses, and accurately pinpoints their location and dimensions. Since it is a noninvasive study with little risk and can be done quickly, it is being used with increasing frequency in evaluating children with abdominal masses.

Angiography is of considerable help in the diagnosis of abdominal masses. Inferior vena cavograms (Fig. 14.7) often show displacement or compression by retroperitoneal masses. Abdominal aortography (Fig. 14.8) or specific infusions of dye into the celiac axis or renal arteries (Fig. 14.9) via catheters inserted percutaneously into the femoral artery, are more useful than venography. Neoplasms have a characteristic blood supply which allow their identification. Further, the major vessels supplying the mass often are demonstrated, which is of importance to the surgeon at the time he surgically approaches the mass.

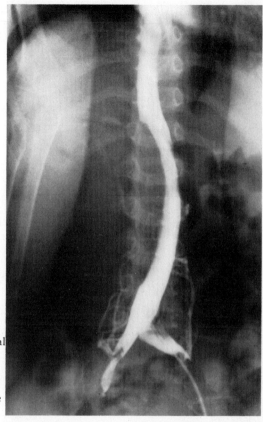

Fig. 14.7.
Inferior vena cavogram showing medial displacement (but not invasion) of the vein by a huge right neuroblastoma arising inferior to the right kidney

Abdominal Neuroblastoma

Cancer ranks second to trauma as a cause of death among children. Neuroblastoma, the most common abdominal malignancy of childhood, accounts for about 9 % of all the malignancies of childhood, ranking behind leukemia (40 %), central nervous system tumors (15 %) and malignant lymphomas (10 %). Since abdominal neuroblastomas generally arise above or around the kidney, they must be preoperatively distinguished from primary malignancies of the kidney (Wilms' tumors) which are almost as common as neuroblastoma, as well as from the more common benign kidney masses of childhood (cystic disease of the kidneys, congenital hydronephrosis). Part

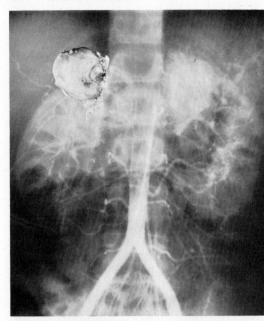

Fig. 14.8.
Abdominal aorto-gram causes a left pheochromocytoma to "light up" in a child being investi-gated for hyper-tension

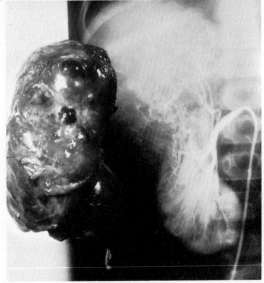

Fig. 14.9.
Right renal arterio-graphy in adolescent female with a Wilms' tumor arising from the upper pole of the right kidney

of the fascination of neuroblastoma revolves around its variability in natural history and clinical course, which may proceed in an anticipated direction or pursue a totally bizarre course. It may spontaneously change from an aggressive malignant neoplasm with metastases to a benign lesion permitting survival of the patient, or may disappear altogether.

Neuroblastoma is truly of embryonic origin, arising from primitive sympathetic system cells (sympathogonia) which originate from primitive dorsal neural crest tissue. Age at diagnosis varies from the neonatal period to about 10 years of age, averaging between 18 months and 2 years at diagnosis. There is a male:female preponderance of approximately 3:2.

Because of its cell type of origin, neuroblastomas can develop wherever sympathetic tissue is found. Approximately 75 % arise intraabdominally, about two-thirds of these originating in and around the adrenal gland. The remainder are scattered retroperitoneally to one side or the other of the vertebral column. Twelve percent occur in the posterior mediastinum and two percent in the neck.

The abdominal neuroblastoma is histologically and clinically more aggressive than the same tumor arising in the posterior mediastinum or neck. Histologically they are composed of very primitive sympathicoblast cells, with no or little tendency to ganglion cell production. About three-fourths of the patients with abdominal neuroblastoma regrettably have metastases at diagnosis. Forty percent have metastases to the long bones or skull, demonstrable either on x-ray, bone scan or microscopic bone marrow examination. About 20 % have metastases to the liver (with hepatomegaly and punched out areas on the liver scan) and about 15 % have spread to regional tissues or distant soft tissue.

The most common reason for a child with abdominal neuroblastoma to come to hospital is discovery of an abdominal mass (Fig. 14.10). Symptoms related to the metastases include bone pain, weight loss, anorexia and anemia. Because the tumor is occasionally hormonally active, humoral symptoms dominate the clinical picture in approximately 10 %: diarrhea, fever, flushing and hypertension. Abdominal discomfort and enlargement herald the abdominal mass. The most outstanding feature on physical examination is a solid abdominal mass which often crosses the midline, although originating with equal frequency on both sides of the abdomen. The mass does not transilluminate, gives a solid echo on sonography and generally is smooth and nontender. It does not move with position change or inspiration.

Plain radiographs of the abdomen show the ground-glass appearance of the mass displacing hollow viscera; 50 % have finely stippled

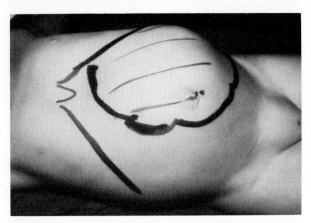

Fig. 14.10.   Child with abdominal mass due to left neuroblastoma

calcification within the mass. Chest and bone x-rays should be obtained, looking for metastases. Intravenous pyelography shows that the neuroblastoma displaces, but does not distort, the renal

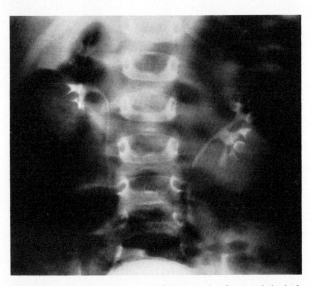

Fig. 14.11.   Suprarenal neuroblastoma displacing left kidney downward but not distorting its collecting system

collecting system (Fig. 14.11). The bone marrow is studied histologically for metastases which are too small to show up on radiographs.

Conventional urinalysis is usually normal. An 24-hour collection of urine for catecholamines should be obtained. The neuroblastoma cells produce excessive quantities of dopa, dopamine and norepinephrine, which are converted to two major terminal urinary metabolites, homovanillic acid (HVA) and vanilmandelic acid (VMA). If both these urinary metabolites are tested for, more than 90 % of patients with neuroblastoma will show abnormally high excretions. No matter how careful and extensive the workup, diagnosis should always be histologically confirmed before treatment is undertaken.

In the 25—30 % of patients without metastases, neuroblastomas may be completely extirpated surgically with relative safety. This demands removal of the adrenal on the involved side and sometimes requires nephrectomy because of the inextricable physical association of the neuroblastoma with the kidney. Even with the complete gross removal of the primary tumor, some Centers would deliver relatively low dosage x-ray therapy (1,500—3,000 R) to the tumor bed postoperatively.

If the primary tumor cannot be completely removed safely, the neuroblastoma is one of the few neoplasms where partial removal of the primary seems to improve prognosis. Postoperative x-ray therapy to the tumor bed of 2,000—3,000 R may be delivered, although some Centers rely entirely on chemotherapy.

The recommended chemotherapy at present includes alternating weekly intravenous infusions of Vincristine, 1.5 mg/m^2 with Cyclophosphamide, 300 mg/m^2, for six weeks. The dosage is then reduced to every other week alternating drugs, continuing until either progressive lesions recur or for at least one or two years.

Prognosis in children with abdominal neuroblastoma is dictinctly related to the age at diagnosis. In patients under one year of age, fully two-thirds survive two years without disease. In patients between 1—2 years of age at diagnosis, only about 20 % survive two years without evidence of disease. If the tumor is first diagnosed above the age of 2 years, only about 5 % survive two years without disease. Those without metastases at diagnosis survive four times as long as those patients who already have metastases.

Wilms' Tumor (Nephroblastoma)

The so-called Wilms' tumor is the only malignant neoplasm of the kidney seen in children. It ranks in frequency just behind the neuroblastoma in malignancies of childhood. Histologically, Wilms' tumors embrace a variety of tissue types in which glandular and muscular elements often predominate although histologically recognizable myxomatous tissue, fat and cartilage have also been described. Approximately 5 % of Wilms' tumors are bilateral. The diagnosis of Wilms' tumor is made before the age of three-and-one-half years in about half the cases, at least 90 % of patients presenting under eight years of age. Similar to abdominal neuroblastoma, patients with Wilms' tumors come to diagnosis after incidental discovery of a loin mass by the mother or physician.

Although Wilms' tumor remains encapsulated for a lengthy period of time, local invasion into renal substance and perinephric tissue has occurred in about 80 % of children at the time of diagnosis. Regional lymph nodes are involved in approximately 30 % and hematogenous metastases to lungs in about 50 %. Wilms' tumor rarely metastasizes to bone, in clear distinction to neuroblastoma.

Physical examination reveals a loin mass in well over 90 % of children with Wilms' tumor. The mass generally does not extend across the midline, in distinction to neuroblastoma. It is firm and non-tender and does not move with respiration or position change.

Plain and GI contrast radiographs often show displacement of bowel away from the tumor. Intravenous pyelogram shows distortion of the internal architecture of the kidney (Fig. 14.12). Rarely the kidney does not visualize even with infusion pyelography, signifying that the tumor has completely filled the renal pelvis and proximal ureter. In the newborn, the most common enlargement of the kidney which

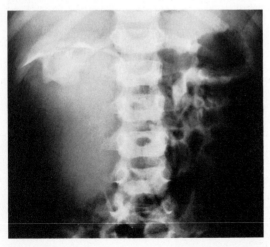

Fig. 14.12.
Upward displacement and distortion of the collecting system produced by a large Wilms' tumor arising in the lower pole of the right kidney

shows no excretory function is a multicystic kidney. One of the great values of the intravenous pyelogram is to document a normal kidney on the opposite side. It is imperative to know that the opposite kidney is normal before the involved kidney is removed.

Inferior vena cavography may show blockage of the inferior vena cava due to extension of the tumor into the renal vein and thence into the cava. Aortography and especially infusion of dye into the renal artery (Fig. 14.9) precisely outlines the tumor and its blood supply but generally is not required for a correct preoperative diagnosis. Chest x-ray should always be obtained looking for metastases. Transabdominal nephrectomy is carried out as the primary treatment of Wilms' tumor. This approach allows evaluation of the other kidney and provides exposure for early ligation of the renal veins to reduce the chances of tumor embolization. The periaortic lymph nodes on the side of the tumor are removed in addition to the kidney and its surrounding fat and adrenal gland.

Actinomycin-D and Vincristine are the best chemotherapeutic agents to use postoperatively, starting on the day of surgery. Radiation therapy is generally begun one or two weeks postoperatively to a tumor dose of 3,000–4,000 R. Bilateral Wilms' tumors are treated. with a combination of partial nephrectomy and irradiation plus chemotherapy. Repeat courses of chemotherapy are administered for two years after operation.

As with neuroblastoma, prognosis relates to age at diagnosis. In patients diagnosed under the age of two years, 70–80 % survival is expected, compared to survival of considerably less than half of that in children older than two years. A poor prognosis is generally seen in tumors larger than 300 g in weight as well as those with capsular and renal vein invasion. Recent reports indicate that with early diagnosis and combination surgery, radiotherapy and chemotherapy, overall survival rates of 70–80 % might be expected, regardless of age. Two years survival without recurrent tumor is tantamount to cure, in distinction to the five-year cure rate quoted for adult cancers. Late recurrence of Wilms' tumor does occur, but not often.

X-ray therapy and chemotherapy are used to treat recurrent Wilms' tumor or late metastases, surgical excision occasionally being employed for a solitary metastasis. Pulmonary metastases is the usual cause of death in children with incurable Wilms' tumors.

To be distinguished from a truly malignant Wilms' tumor is the peculiar and benign fibromyomatoid tumor of the neonatal kidney. The distinction is important because this latter tumor is benign and nephrectomy alone is curative without the need for postoperative radiation or chemotherapy. The benign fibromyomatoid tumor is highly cellular with fibromyoblastic stroma in which are imbedded foci of cartilage, hematopoietic tissue and angiomatoid tissue plus dysplastic tubules and glomeruli. Although rare, the fibromyomatoid tumor is the most common neonatal renal neoplasm.

The retroperitoneal space may also harbor masses other than Wilms' tumors or neuroblastomas, including rhabdomyosarcomas, teratomas and retroperitoneal sarcomas. A firm and non-tender lateral abdominal mass incidentally discovered usually brings in the infant or young child for diagnosis. Workup procedure is similar to that for Wilms' tumor or neuroblastoma, the intravenous pyelogram showing displacement of the kidney to distinguish these retroperitoneal masses from a Wilms' tumor, normal urinary catecholamines ruling out neuroblastoma. Diagnosis is made at laparotomy and the treatment hinges on complete surgical removal. Postoperative x-ray therapy and chemotherapy generally are administered for those tumors that histologically prove malignant.

15 Biliary and Pancreatic Disease

R. T. SOPER

Jaundice

Jaundice is a common problem only during the first few days or weeks of life, when distinction between cases which are amenable to surgical correction as opposed to those of "medical" origin is both difficult and critical. Surgically amenable jaundice should be corrected before three months of age and preferably by two months of age, to obviate the otherwise inevitable subsequent problems of cirrhosis, portal hypertension and liver failure.

Over 50 % of term infants and 80 % of premature infants become clinically jaundiced during the first week of life. The jaundice is detected on the second day of life, peaks on the third or fourth day and rapidly disappears thereafter. This "physiologic" neonatal jaundice is largely composed of unconjugated bilirubin which poses no threat of kernicterus and therefore requires little active therapy. It is partially related to the high red blood cell count at the time of delivery; as these excessively fragile red cells hemolyze, the immature liver cannot produce enough glucuronide enzyme to deconjugate the bilirubin from globin. Jaundice disappears as the number of red cells diminish to normal, their fragility improves and the liver enzymes become adequate to handle normal amounts of bilirubin breakdown. Newborns who are icteric at birth generally have a nonphysiologic type of hemolytic disorder, the most common of which is Rh incompatibility: a sensitized Rh negative mother carries and delivers an Rh positive baby. In utero hemolysis of the fetus' red cells occurs, and at delivery the baby is anemic and jaundiced. Kernicterus is a serious threat. ABO incompatibility is a much less common cause of hemolytic disease of the newborn.

Jaundice appearing in the second or third week of life has a host of possible causes, most of them non-surgical:

1) Non-hemolytic familial inborn errors of enzyme deficiency: Gilbert's disease and Crigler-Najjar disease.

2) Infections: septicemia, congenital syphilis, cytomegalic disease, toxoplasmosis, herpes.

3) Drugs: vitamin K, sulfa drugs.

4) Breast feeding.

5) Absorption of hematoma.

6) Thrombocytopenic purpura.

7) Congenital spherocytosis.

8) Infant of a diabetic mother.

9) Galactosemia.

10) Storage diseases: Gaucher's, Niemann-Picks.

11) The **inspissated bile syndrome** (Fig. 15.1):

This last-named entity generally develops in a severely dehydrated newborn, or one who recovers from one of the aforementioned hemolytic diseases of the newborn. The jaundice is associated with acholic stools and a rising direct bilirubin fraction and is therefore clearly obstructive in nature. Operative findings (Fig. 15.1) include thickened, inspissated plugs of bilirubin blocking the common bile duct. Treatment (Fig. 15.2) is limited to saline irrigation of the biliary ducts system through a tube introduced into the fundus of the gallbladder.

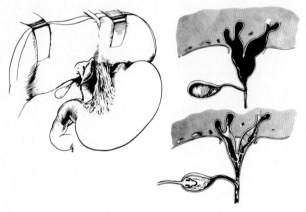

Fig. 15.1.   Inspissated bile syndrome

Jaundice which becomes apparent during the second month of life can be caused by late onset of the diseases mentioned above. Occasionally it is associated with hypertrophic pyloric stenosis, the malnutrition associated with this disorder diminishing the glucuronidase liver enzyme which deconjugates bilirubin. The elevated bilirubin is indirect in type and the jaundice rapidly disappears after surgical correction of the hypertrophic pyloric stenosis.

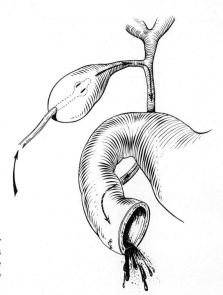

Fig. 15.2. Saline irrigation through fundus of gallbladder washes the obstructing plugs of inspissated bile from the common bile duct down into the duodenum

Obstructive Jaundice

Neonatal Hepatitis and Biliary Atresia

When all the above causes for late neonatal jaundice have been excluded by appropriate blood and urine studies, we are left a residue of jaundiced newborns now six to eight weeks of age with "obstructive" jaundice in whom the differential diagnosis of *neonatal hepatitis* versus *biliary atresia* becomes paramount. These infants are clinically well, have bilirubins ranging from 8–15 mg⁰/₀, acholic stools, dark-colored urine and moderately enlarged livers. Since significant hepatic cirrhosis occurs by three months of age in both of these conditions, identification of the surgically correctable ones must be made before that time.

Laboratory tests which favor biliary atresia include an increase in the unconjugated fraction of bilirubin, absent bilirubin in the stool, increase in urinary bilirubin, decreased urine urobilinogen and indirect tests reflecting hepatic obstruction such as elevated alkaline phosphatase, thymol turbidity and the various flocculation tests. However, intrahepatic obstruction of bile caused by neonatal hepatitis cannot be distinguished from bile obstruction due to atresia by these laboratory data. Serum transaminase activity is modestly elevated in both disorders. I—131 labeled rose bengal theoretically should all be retained within the liver in patients with biliary atresia, with free passage of the dye into the intestine for excretion per rectum in patients with hepatitis. However, overlap exists in even this test so that clear distinction often cannot be made. Exploratory laparotomy is then necessary to precisely distinguish between biliary atresia and neonatal hepatitis.

Preoperatively, the patient must be prepared by vitamin K if the prothrombin time and PTT are elevated. Through a short right upper quadrant transverse incision open biopsies of the liver are taken and the gallbladder is identified; if present, a small catheter is sutured into the fundus of the gallbladder for saline irrigation of the biliary duct and operative cholangiography. If the gallbladder is not seen, or if the cholangiograms are abnormal or if the liver biopsies suggest biliary atresia on frozen section examination, then the incision is extended so that the entire extrahepatic biliary system can be meticulously explored.

Regrettably, only about 10 % of babies with biliary atresia have an anatomically correctable type of lesion (Fig. 15.3). Anatomic correctability implies a bile-distended proximal segment of bile ducts, which is anastomosed with intestine to allow the bile to drain into the intestinal tract (Fig. 15.4). About 90 % of biliary atresia cases have no such dilated bile-filled proximal ducts detectable at laparotomy (Fig. 15.5); these patients have a grim prognosis, the majority dying from six months to two years of age from progressive cirrhosis and hypersplenism. Recently, pediatric surgeons from Japan have anastomosed the hilum of the liver where the atretic bile ducts emerge to a Roux loop of jejunum in hopes that undrained intrahepatic lakes of bile converging toward the hilum will now have

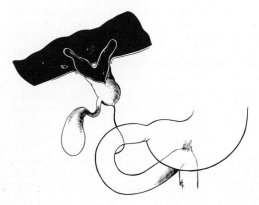

Fig. 15.3.
"Correctable" type of biliary atresia

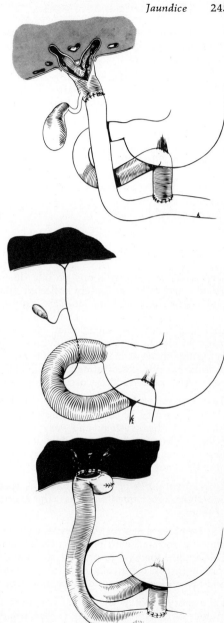

Fig. 15.4.
Surgical correction of condition shown in Fig. 15.3.
by anastomosis of dilated
common bile duct to a
Roux-en-Y loop of jejunum

Fig. 15.5.
"Uncorrectable" type of
biliary atresia

Fig. 15.6.
Surgical correction of condition shown in Fig. 15.5. by
hepatic portojejunostomy

access to the intestine (Fig. 15.6). The cure rate with this operation (hepatic portojejunostomy) is only about 20 %, but this is far better than doing nothing.

The cause of biliary atresia is unknown. There are many who feel that in the final analysis biliary atresia and neonatal hepatitis will turn out to represent simply different stages of inutero hepatitis.

In view of the poor results of surgical treatment of biliary atresia, it is understandable that liver transplantation has emerged as a viable method of treatment when liver failure ultimately develops in the somewhat older child with biliary atresia and/or severe neonatal hepatitis. As transplantation immunology becomes more specific and effective, liver transplantation may indeed prove worthy of serious consideration in every patient with incorrectable biliary atresia or severe neonatal hepatitis.

Choledochal Cyst

Congenital cystic dilatations of bile ducts occasionally develop in infants and children, loosely collected under the term "choledochal cyst". Recurrent bouts of jaundice, right upper quadrant abdominal pain and a palpable mass constitute the classic triad on which the clinical diagnosis of choledochal cyst rests. Diagnosis is generally made within the first or second decade of life, but has been reported in young adults. Children of oriental extraction seem predisposed to choledochal cyst, constituting approximately one-third of the reported cases. About three-fourths occur in females.

There are many different anatomic varieties of choledochal cyst (Fig. 15.7). They may be solitary or multiple, may involve any portion of the biliary duct system, and vary in size from 1 cm to enormous cysts holding several liters of bile. The cyst wall varies from a few mm to 1 cm in thickness, and the composition of the wall and lining mucosa is not uniform. The cause of choledochal cyst is unknown.

Only about 20 % of patients have the classic triad of jaundice, pain and right upper quadrant mass, the majority harboring one or two of them.

The jaundice is obstructive in type, with acholic stools and dark urine and is associated with pruritus. Occasionally, bacterial infection occurs within the cyst to produce the characteristic chills and fever of cholangitis. In older children, firm and cirrhotic livers, splenomegaly and hematologic changes of hypersplenism are found.

Laboratory workup should include liver function studies, chemical studies of the stool and urine to detect bile, and plain radiographs to

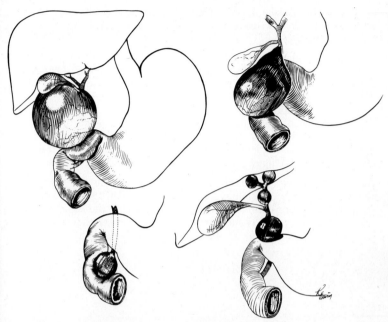

Fig. 15.7.   Different anatomic types of choledochal cysts

show the "ground glass" appearance of the right upper quadrant mass. Oral cholecystography is of no help in the presence of jaundice, but between episodes of jaundice may show a collection of dye within the cyst which must then be differentiated from gallbladder. Intravenous cholangiograms may help confirm diagnosis. Upper gastrointestinal contrast series often reveal medial and downward displacement of the duodenal loop by extrinsic pressure from the cyst.

Treatment of choledochal cyst is entirely surgical. A side-to-side anastomosis of the cyst into the duodenum or a Roux-en-Y anastomosis of cyst to jejunum should be carried out. Cyst excision with choledochojejunostomy also is effective treatment.

Gallbladder Disease in Children

Gallbladder disease in children is unusual, less than 1,000 cases being recorded to date. Eighty to ninety percent of the children are female, with a mean age of about nine years. More than 50 % have a history of gallbladder disease in other family members, some of whom have inherited a causally associated hemolytic state (spherocytosis or sickle cell anemia).

Hemolysis appears to be an important etiologic factor in only 10—15 % of children with gallbladder disease, the chronic hemolytic disease (spherocytosis, sickle cell anemia) producing increased bilirubin concentrations in bile which favors its precipitation into stones. Cystic duct compression from adjacent vessels or lymph nodes is reported, as well as congenital abnormalities which kink or produce valves within the cystic duct. Acute cholecystitis is sometimes triggered by dehydration from some other cause, such as severe trauma, infection, enteritis, upper respiratory infection, scarlet fever, etc.

As in adults, cystic duct obstruction appears to be the triggering event in the pathophysiology of cholecystitis (Fig. 15.8). If the obstruction is intermittent or partial, as is usually the case, chronic recurrent cholecystitis ensues. In the unlikely event that the cystic duct obstruction is complete, acute unrelenting cholecystitis ensues.

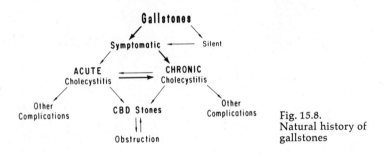

Fig. 15.8.
Natural history of gallstones

About 70 % of childhood cholecystitis is chronic in type. A smaller percentage of children with cholecystitis have associated stones within the gallbladder (50 %) than the 85—95 % of adults with cholecystitis. Common duct stones are rare in children, occurring in only about 5 %.

Cholecystitis typically occurs in overweight adolescent girls with episodes of abdominal discomfort which is often periumbilical and difficult to describe or localize, rarely radiating to the back or scapular tip. Nausea and vomiting is common, and right upper quadrant tenderness is found in about half of the children during an acute episode. Fatty food intolerance is experienced by about one-third of the children, and few give a history of jaundice either currently or in the past.

The diagnosis of cholecystitis is difficult to establish in children because of its rarity and the atypical and nonspecific nature of the pain. Acute appendicitis is the most common preoperative diagnosis in children with acute cholecystitis; the reverse side of this coin is the fact that 15—20 % of children with chronic cholecystitis will have had a previous (negative) exploration for appendicitis. Oral or intravenous cholecystography (Fig. 15.9) often helps confirm diagnosis. Prior to undertaking surgical treatment of gallbladder disease in children, a chronic hemolytic disorder (spherocytosis, sickle cell anemia) should be ruled out by appropriate hematologic studies.

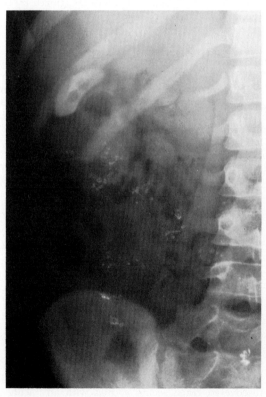

Fig. 15.9.
Oral cholecysto-
graphy revealing
two stones (as filling
defects) in gall-
bladder

The surgical treatment of gallbladder disease in childhood is cholecystectomy. Common bile duct exploration is rarely necessary, and is somewhat dangerous because of the small size of the common bile duct. Splenectomy can be done at the same time as cholecystectomy should the patient have congenital spherocytosis. Cholecystostomy is resorted to only rarely in the youngster who is acutely ill with empyema of the gallbladder.

Pancreatic Disorders in Children

Introduction

Diseases of the pancreas are rare in children. The most common time-honored pancreatic disorder recognized by the pediatric surgeon is annular pancreas (Chapter 5).

Pancreatitis

Pancreatitis can occur in many different clinical forms which include acute pancreatitis, chronic relapsing or recurrent pancreatitis and pancreatitis secondary to trauma, often associated with pseudocysts. The etiology of childhood pancreatitis is obscure, as many as two-thirds having no clear etiologic agent.

Some of its recognized causes are:

1) Drugs: steroids (Cortisone, ACTH), hydrochlorothiazide.

2) Trauma: pancreatic fracture generally overlying L_2 vertebral body, followed later by pseudocyst.

3) Hereditary, familial: generally associated with hyperlipidemia or amino-aciduria.

4) Congenital anomalies: annular pancreas, duplication cysts.

5) Parasitic: Ascaris lumbricoides.

6) Viral (mumps): rare, even in children.

7) Miscellaneous: polyarteritis nodosa, hyperparathyroidism, post-operative, cystic fibrosis.

Acute Pancreatitis

The majority of pancreatitis in children is of the acute variety with hemorrhage and often infarction with septicemia. They are often discovered when seeing a child with an "acute surgical abdomen" (Chapter 12). Often acute pancreatitis appears to be either secondary to, or at least associated with, other major acute problems such as severe dehydration, acidosis, severe vomiting or diarrhea, septicemia, thermal burns and diabetic acidosis. In these situations, it is often impossible to tell which is the cart and which the horse. In pancreatitis associated with sepsis, coliform organisms appear to predominate (E. coli, Enterococcus, A. aerogenes, Proteus, Pseudomonas).

The clinical manifestations of acute pancreatitis include abdominal pain with tenderness and guarding superimposed upon a youngster who is already severely ill with one of the aforementioned clinical problems. Late manifestations include tachycardia, jaundice and shock with coma. Physical examination is non-specific in the sense that the child has a somewhat distended and silent abdomen with generalized tenderness and guarding, with shock out of proportion to his primary illness. Elevated serum or urine amylase confirms the pancreatitis part of the diagnosis. Paracentesis sometimes yields rusty ascitic fluid which contains an enormously high amylase level.

The medical treatment of acute pancreatitis includes pain relief with an analgesic that does not have the smooth sphincter contracting effect that morphine has (Demerol), large amounts of intravenous fluids, electrolytes (particularly calcium), vitamins and calories while putting the pancreas at rest via nasogastric suction and anticholinergic drugs. If severe shock is present, central venous pressure must be monitored and blood and/or plasma administered. Antibiotics control secondary infections.

Laparotomy is rarely indicated during the acute phase if the diagnosis is clear and if trauma is ruled out. If the disease is discovered at exploratory laparotomy, the lesser sac should be drained and a gastrostomy performed for decompression; no biliary drainage is instituted (as in adults) because of the low association of biliary disease and pancreatitis in children. The disparate group of etiologic factors previously mentioned needs to be looked for and treated or withdrawn.

Chronic Pancreatitis

Only a handful of children with chronic relapsing or recurrent pancratitis have been reported. As in adults, it is characterized by recurrent attacks of abdominal pain difficult for children to describe, sometimes radiating or boring directly through into the lumbar spine. Sometimes calcification of the pancreas is seen on plain radiographs. The gland has a firm, fibrosed appearance; the pancreatic duct exhibits ectasia and a "chain of lakes" appearance on pancreatography. Steatorrhea, weight loss and diabetes occur late.

The diagnosis is generally confirmed only at laparotomy, where operative pancreatic ductogram is performed (Fig. 15.10). Since ductal obstruction is almost always associated with chronic pancreatitis, the operation should improve drainage of the pancreatic duct: trans-

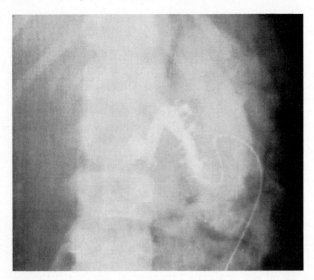

Fig. 15.10. Terminal pancreatic duct filled with radiopaque material during operation shows dilated, tortuous duct which is completely obstructed near the head of the pancreas

duodenal division of the sphincter of Oddi, removal of stones and gravel from the pancreatic duct, intestinal drainage into a Roux-Y jejunal loop via lateral or terminal pancreaticojejunostomy. Total or near-total pancreatectomy is resorted to when the drainage procedures fail or are impossible to perform.

Pseudocysts of the Pancreas

Most cysts of the pancreas are really pseudocysts (lacking an epithelial lining) occurring secondary to trauma. A handful of truly congenital cysts of the pancreas (with an epithelial lining) have been reported which are unilocular and should either be removed or internally drained into the intestine.

Rarely pseudocysts of the pancreas follow mumps and other infections, but a history of upper abdominal trauma several days or weeks earlier is obtained in well over 50 % of children with pancreatic pseudocysts. Falls across bars or onto bicycle handles or posts are the most common inciting trauma. There is a male:female ratio of 2:1, in keeping with the pronicity to trauma of young boys. About one-third of the cases follow acute idiopathic hemorrhagic pancreatitis. Pseudocysts are generally unilocular and may communicate with the main pancreatic duct, in which case the cloudy fluid contains high levels of amylase.

A pseudocyst of the pancreas is suggested by a history of upper abdominal trauma or pancreatitis followed by a symptom-free interval of several weeks or a few months, when the youngster begins to complain of epigastric abdominal pain with anorexia and later vomiting and weight loss. A nontender spherical epigastric mass is often palpated at this stage, and radiocontrast studies of the gastrointestinal tract reveal upward and anterior displacement of the stomach, widening of the duodenal "C" loop and inferior displacement of the transverse colon.

Treatment of pancreatic pseudocyst consists of internal drainage of the cyst into the gastrointestinal tract.

Pancreatic Neoplasms

Pancreatic neoplasms are rare in infants and children. There are a handful of children reported with adenocarcinoma of the pancreas, their complaints centering around chronic abdominal pain associated with an epigastric abdominal mass, icterus, anorexia and vomiting. Radiocontrast studies of the gastrointestinal tract reveal findings similar to a pseudocyst. Diagnosis is confirmed by biopsy at laparotomy. Pancreatectomy or pancreaticoduodenectomy should be undertaken in those few patients without metastases.

More common than adenocarcinoma are nonbeta islet cell tumors producing the Zollinger-Ellison syndrome (See Chapter 13).

A handful of children have been reported with functioning islet cell adenomas of the pancreas; excessive amounts of insulin produce hypoglycemia. The adenoma generally is benign but often is buried within the pancreatic substance so as to make its discovery at operation difficult indeed. To be excluded in these children are the many nonsurgical causes of hypoglycemia: abnormalities of the endocrine system and liver, metabolic errors, prediabetes, and patients with idiopathic spontaneous hypoglycemia. Islet cell adenoma is seen at all childhood ages, but predominates early in life. The tumor is multicentric in about 15 % of cases. About 75 % are found either in the body or tail of the pancreas, 25 % in the head of the pancreas and 2 % are located in ectopic pancreatic tissue. Severe recurrent hypoglycemic attacks with convulsions bring these children in for diagnosis. After exclusion of nonsurgical causes, laparotomy is required for diagnosis. If an adenoma is found and can be safely resected, all is well. However, if no adenoma is detectable, subtotal pancreatectomy (removing 80 % of the tail and body of the gland) is generally recommended as a safe and effective procedure. If the tumor is completely removed, prognosis is excellent; if not, recurrent hypoglycemia is the rule.

16 The Inguinoscrotal Region

R. T. Soper

Introduction

Inguinoscrotal masses vary in severity from the very common and innocent hydrocele to the life-threatening strangulated inguinal hernia or the malignant testicular neoplasm. Indirect inguinal hernia is one of the more common inguinoscrotal masses, its repair constituting the most frequent elective abdominal operation in children.

Since many surgical problems of the inguinal area are in some way related to testicular descent, it is understandable that the majority occur in males. Further, there is an inverse relationship to age, almost all inguinoscrotal abnormalities being more common during the first year of life and gradually declining in incidence in a progressive manner thereafter. Exceptions to this age relationship will be pointed out.

Embryology-Anatomy

In the male, the *gubernaculum testis* is a slender band which attaches the lower pole of the retroperitoneal testis to the bottom of the scrotum. Near the end of the second trimester of gestation, there is a diverticulum of primitive peritoneum (*processus vaginalis*) which elongates into a sac extending downward through the inguinal canal adjacent to the gubernaculum. During the last trimester of gestation, the testicle migrates caudad passing through the inguinal canal from internal (or deep) to external (or superficial) ring, carrying with it thinned out contributions from the three muscle layers of the abdominal wall. The left testicle descends earlier than the right and ends up lower in the scrotum; this later and lesser descent of the right testis perhaps explains its higher incidence of both hernia and maldescent. Descent of the testes into the scrotum is complete in more than 95 % of term newborns, but in about 30 % of immature newborns testicular descent is completed only during the first few weeks of extra-uterine life.

The processus vaginalis (Fig. 16.1) retains a connection to the peritoneal cavity until soon after birth; normally, this lumen then obliterates from the internal inguinal ring down to the testicle (Fig. 16.2), retaining patency only in the portion that surrounds the testicle known as the *tunica vaginalis*. Obliteration of the processus vaginalis is incomplete at birth, but continues throughout infancy and on into young childhood; in some patients it never does close

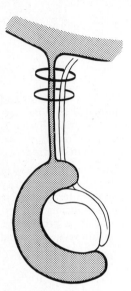

Fig. 16.1

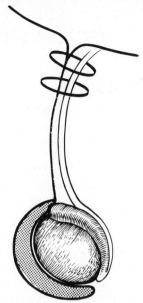

Fig. 16.2

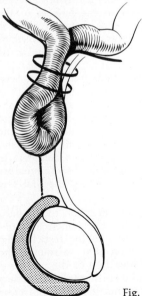

Fig. 16.5

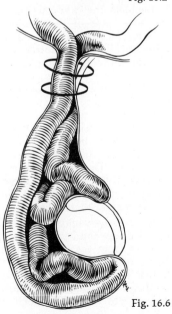

Fig. 16.6

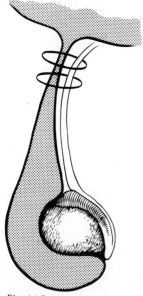

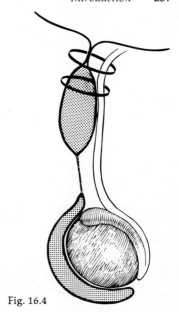

Fig. 16.3   Fig. 16.4

properly. Imperfect closure of a processus vaginalis, or reopening of one that has been partially or imperfectly closed, is the basis for the development of both hydrocele (peritoneal fluid dissecting down a patent processus vaginalis) (Fig. 16.3 and 16.4) and indirect inguinal hernia (Fig. 16.5 and 16.6) (when the processus enlarges sufficiently to accept intestine). An arrest or misdirection in the descent of the testicle results in the various forms of cryptorchidism. The precise causes for the maldescent of the testicle or imperfect obliteration of the processus vaginalis are unknown.

An analogous situation exists in the female fetus, with the exception that the gonad does not penetrate the abdominal wall. The peritoneal

---

Fig. 16.1.   Stippled areas indicate peritoneal fluid traveling through a patent *processus vaginalis* to fill the *tunica vaginalis* surrounding the testis. The rings mark the internal (deep) and external (superficial) inguinal rings
Fig. 16.2.   After closure of the *processus vaginalis*
Fig. 16.3.   Complete (communicating) hydrocele
Fig. 16.4.   Hydrocele of cord
Fig. 16.5.   Indirect inguinal hernia, ordinary type
Fig. 16.6.   Indirect inguinal hernia, large (scrotal) type

eventrations into the canal of Nuck adjacent to the round ligament are small, and the developing uterus discourages visceral descent into the inguinal canal. This accounts for the much lower incidence of inguinal hernia in the female.

Surgical Diseases of the Inguinoscrotal Region

Hydrocele

Hydroceles are almost exclusively limited to the male, and consist of collections of fluid within different portions of a still-patent or imperfectly closed processus vaginalis (Fig. 16.3 and 16.4). In virtually all cases, the fluid originates in the peritoneal cavity and dissects down through an imperfectly closed processus vaginalis to gravitate to the lowest level that is not obliterated.

The majority of hydroceles disappear before the first birthday, likely from obliteration of the connection with the peritoneal cavity. Hydroceles that persist beyond, or arise after, the first two years of life tend to persist. Those that enlarge the peritoneal connection to ultimately allow bowel to enter constitute the 15 % of hernias pre-

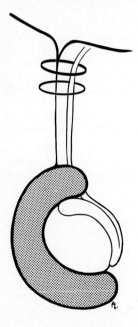

Fig. 16.7.   Hydrocele of the testicle

ceded by hydroceles. If the hydrocele is limited to the tunica vaginalis surrounding the testicle, it is termed a "hydrocele of the testicle" (Fig. 16.7); if it is limited to the processus vaginalis cephalad to the testicle it is referred to as a "hydrocele of the cord" (Fig. 16.4). The connections of hydroceles to the peritoneal cavity vary in size. In those with large connections (the so-called "communicating hydrocele" (Fig. 16.3), the fluid can be squeezed out of the hydrocele back into the peritoneal cavity freely, only to refill during the next few minutes or hours as the youngster strains or assumes an upright posture. Hydroceles with tiny connections to the peritoneal cavity cannot be emptied manually in this manner; small droplets of peritoneal fluid are forced down the tiny connection as the patient strains or forcefully increases intra-abdominal pressure, no similar reversal of pressure relationships existing to force the hydrocele fluid back into the peritoneal cavity.

A typical history of hydrocele is a scrotal or inguinal canal mass which varies in size directly with activity and is not associated with local or intestinal complaints. Physical examination reveals a nontender and nonerythematous mass; local pressure reduces the size of the mass only in those few with large connections to the peritoneal cavity. Ordinarily, the cephalic end of the hydrocele does not extend to the external inguinal ring nor is the mass easily reduced with local pressure. Brilliant transillumination of the hydrocele clearly distinguishes it from inguinal hernia, testicular tumor or other inguinoscrotal masses.

Treatment

During the first two years of life, no treatment of hydrocele is indicated. The majority spontaneously disappear during this time without sequellae. Those that persist beyond, or originate after, the second birthday persist as hydroceles or develop into hernias when the proximal peritoneal connection enlarges. These should be treated surgically.

Inguinal Hernias

Approximately 1 % of boys develop inguinal hernias. Virtually all inguinal hernias of childhood are indirect in type, the sac originating at the internal inguinal ring and traversing the inguinal canal, to suggest their embryologic origin from the processus vaginalis (Fig. 16.5 and 16.6). The direct inguinal hernia and the femoral hernia are extremely rare in childhood, and will not be further considered here.

Because of its relationship to testicular descent, indirect inguinal hernia is 10 to 20 times more likely to develop in males than in females. Understandably, inguinal hernia is more common in children with chronic elevations of intra-abdominal pressure, i. e. ascites, abdominal tumors, intestinal obstruction, etc. Three inguinal hernias occur on the right side for every two on the left side. Somewhere between 15 and 20 % of children with one inguinal hernia later develop a hernia on the other side. This propensity to bilateral hernia bears an inverse relationship to the age at which the first hernia occurs; those who develop the first hernia at a young age are more apt to develop a hernia on the other side than if the first hernia occurs late in childhood.

The diagnosis of inguinal hernia is easy if one finds a groin mass that is readily reducible and does not transilluminate (Fig. 16.8). However, often the inguinal mass has disappeared by the time the child is brought in for examination and cannot be reproduced even as the youngster strains or cries. In these cases, palpation of the cord structures against the pubic bone after they emerge from the external inguinal ring commonly reveals a thickening and a slippery sensation to the index finger as it passes from lateral to medial across the cord structures. This is reliable indirect evidence of the presence

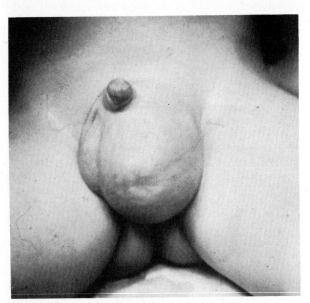

Fig. 16.8.   Left scrotal hernia

of a hernia sac, and is referred to in the American literature as the "silk glove sign". This sign is dependent upon the presence of a hernia sac lubricated with a small amount of peritoneal fluid which produces both the thickening and the slippery sensation to palpation, even when intestine is not resident in the hernia sac. Since the inguinal canal is small in infants and young children, inversion of scrotal skin by the examining finger in an attempt to evaluate the inguinal canal is useless; furthermore, it is painful and destroys whatever rapport one might have established with the patient. In the male, the hernia sac may descend anywhere from the internal ring down to the base of the scrotum surrounding the testicle. In the female, the mass presents in the inguinal canal and the upper part of the labia majora lateral to the mons veneris. Presence of a bean-sized, movable and sometimes irreducible nodule in the inguinal canal of a female indicates a sliding inguinal hernia containing a gonad.

The lesion most frequently confused with inguinal hernia is a hydrocele, which we have already discussed. Enlarged inguinal lymph nodes occasionally prompt a visit to the physician; their multiplicity, firmness, irreducibility, rubbery consistency and lateral location all should clearly distinguish them from inguinal hernia. Examination for hernia is not complete without careful documentation of the size and position of the testes.

Incarceration and strangulation are the two most serious complications of inguinal hernias. The reported incidence of incarcerated inguinal hernias in children varies from 2 % to 18 % in different series. Regardless of actual incidence, it is clear that incarceration and strangulation are inversely related to age; the younger the child the more likely it is that his hernia will incarcerate. In infants, incarceration often heralds the inguinal hernia.

Treatment

Acutely incarcerated hernias are more benign in the infant and child than in the adult. Most of them can be safely and completely reduced by sedating the youngster while he is positioned in a head-down, feet-up position; should this fail in 15 to 20 minutes, a combination of gentle taxis and pressure exerted from below toward the inguinal canal safely reduces the majority. Bowel gangrene, the most serious complication of strangulated hernia, occurs in less than 5 % of incarcerated hernias of children. If the hernia is safely reduced, repair should be delayed for three to four days while the patient remains under observation, to diminish sac edema and friability and make hernia repair technically easier.

If gentle efforts at hernia reduction fail, or if there are signs of impending or actual strangulation, immediate surgical exploration is mandatory. Local erythema and redness, difficult reduction, signs and symptoms of intestinal obstruction, melena, fever, leukocytosis and shock are all signs of strangulated inguinal hernia which demand immediate surgical exploration. Neglected and tightly incarcerated inguinal hernias may infarct the testicle from compression of the vascular components of the cord; prompt surgical reduction avoids this misadventure.

In general, inguinal hernias are surgically repaired whenever they are diagnosed, unless a specific contraindication exists: intercurrent unrelated disease, prematurity or other anomalies that are more serious than the hernia itself. Commonly, hernioplasty is safely deferred in the newborn for a few weeks providing the neck of the sac is large, reduction is easy and frequent examinations can be performed. Control of an inguinal hernia by a truss is discouraged because it is difficult to fit, messy, requires frequent reapplication and is dangerous if applied when bowel is herniated into the sac.

Inguinal hernia repair can be carried out on an outpatient basis when the hernia, the patient and his home environment are all ideal. Physical activity is not restricted after this operation, which then becomes a rather minor incident in the life of an otherwise healthy child.

Since the incidence of bilateral inguinal hernias is only 15 to 20 %, routine exploration of the contralateral groin is not recommended. However, if the history (a bulge or mass) or physical examination (thickened cord, silk glove sign) suggests a possible hernia on the other side, or if the first hernia occurs on the left side or in a female (with a higher incidence of contralateral hernia) or at a relatively young age (less than 2 years old), simultaneous contralateral groin exploration is often advised. Under these circumstances, ligation of a sac or patent processus vaginalis on the other side might obviate a subsequent hernia from developing.

The female commonly herniates ovary into the hernia rather than the more malleable intestine found routinely in the male hernia sac. Thus, the incidence of incarceration is doubled or trebled in the female. About 25 % of female inguinal hernias are sliding hernias of the broad ligament, demanding careful opening of the sac on its anterior surface to avoid injuring the fallopian tube or ovary. The absence of cord structures in the female groin allows sacrifice of the round ligament, analogous to the cord, with complete closure of the internal inguinal ring. Contralateral groin exploration is routinely carried out, because females have bilateral hernias more often than males. About 1 % of inguinal hernias in apparent females (to external examination) actually represent some kind of intersex problem (see Chapter 17) with gonadal and/or genital abnormalities. Testes or ovotestis may reside within the hernia sacs in these intersex patients, requiring biopsy of the gonad for more precise identification of the problem. This possibility makes it advisable to obtain buccal chromatin smears preoperatively on all female children with inguinal hernias, as well as to critically inspect the external genitalia and carefully palpate for the uterus on rectal examination. If the buccal smear is chromatin-negative, the patient should have more sophisticated studies of sexual status before the hernia is repaired.

Cryptorchidism

There are few things more alarming to the parents of a baby boy than to find one or both sides of his scrotum empty. The real tragedy lies in the patient whose empty scrotum is neglected until irreparable damage has occurred to spermatogenesis, or some other complication of cryptorchidism has occurred. Basically there are five explanations for an empty scrotum: (1) A retractile or retractable testicle, (2) anorchia, (3) failure of normal descent of the testicle, (4) maldescent of the testicle (ectopia) and (5) remote infarction of the testicle (torsion).

A retractile testicle is simply one that is pulled cephalad out of the scrotum by the cremaster muscle; gentle examination by warm hands can bring down such a testis into the scrotum. Retractile testes are very common up to the age of puberty and are not abnormal in composition, function or descent; they should never be confused with truly cryptorchid testes. Anorchia refers to agenesis of the testicle; it occurs rarely, comprising less than 5 % of cryptorchidism. An ectopic testicle is one that has descended through the inguinal canal in a normal fashion, and then has become lodged in the perineum, the pubopenile area or in the femoral area. The remainder, comprising the bulk of cryptorchidism, are testes that have descended only part of the way from their point of origin in the urogenital ridge to the scrotum. They may be found in a retroperitoneal intra-abdominal location, within the inguinal canal or lying just outside the external ring in a suprascrotal position.

At least half of the testes which are incompletely descended at birth descend into the scrotum in a normal fashion during the first year of life. Therefore, correction of cryptorchidism should be withheld until during or after the second year of life. Somewhere between 15 to 20 % of cryptorchidism is bilateral.

There are five good reasons for considering early repair of cryptorchidism. First and foremost is the physiologic damage that an inguinal or abdominal position exerts on the developing testis, probably because of higher environmental temperature than when the testis resides in the scrotum. Impaired spermatogenesis and characteristic histologic changes predictably develop in cryptorchid testes, beginning around the third year of life. Secondly, there is good statistical evidence suggesting that testicular carcinoma is ten times more common in cryptorchid than in normally descended testes; malignant degeneration generally occurs after puberty. Thirdly, an empty scrotum exerts a severe psychological and cosmetic handicap to the patient, particularly during young school years. Fourthly, abnormally positioned testes are more subject to trauma and torsion. Finally, fully 90 % of undescended testes are associated with indirect inguinal hernias which themselves justify surgical correction. Taken together, particularly in view of the unpredictable and meager success rate when gonadotrophins are administered to patients with undescended testes, orchidopexy should be undertaken somewhere after the second and definitely before the fifth year of life.

Orchidopexy is performed through a groin crease incision similar to that employed in the repair of inguinal hernia. The testicle may be biopsied to assess the histologic nature of the gonad. A degenerated gonad is excised; in these patients, as well as when no testis is found, a silastic prosthesis is implanted in the scrotal sac for cosmetic reasons.

Masses of the Testicle

Inflammatory testicular masses are fairly common in infants and children secondary to trauma, torsion or more rarely epididymo-orchitis. Differentiation of these three causes for tender, inflamed testicular masses is not easy, at times requiring surgical exploration for precise distinction.

Epididymo-Orchitis

The condition is unusual during childhood unless the lower urinary tract has been instrumented. It is generally unilateral. Bilateral orchitis from a viral agent, such as mumps, is extremely rare before puberty. Tenderness, erythema and enlargement of a painful testis associated with temperature elevation and leukocytosis are the usual clinical findings. If the testicle rides low in the scrotum the diagnosis of epididymo-orchitis can be safely made; cold compresses and antibiotics are the usual treatment. If the inflamed testicle rides high in the scrotum, it cannot be distinguished from testicular torsion short of surgical exploration.

Testicular Trauma

This generally occurs in active, athletically-inclined older boys, and is unusual in the young child. A testicle ectopically entrapped in the abdominal wall or suprascrotal position is particularly vulnerable to crushing trauma than the normally descended testicle which swings freely in the scrotum. Generally there is no leukocytosis or temperature elevation, but considerable ecchymosis and hemorrhage. Cold packs and bed rest suffice for treatment. Permanent damage to the traumatized testis is unusual.

Torsion of the Testicle   (Fig. 16.9)

The term implies an axial twist of the cord structures. The twist first interferes with lymphatic and venous return from the testicle and later with its arterial inflow, to produce swelling, infarction and

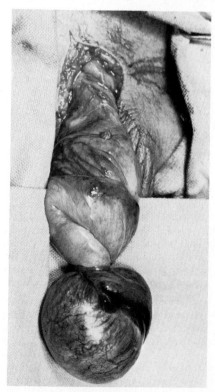

Fig. 16.9.
Torsion of the testicle

gangrene. The twist is possible because of increased mobility of the cord when it is suspended freely within the tunica vaginalis; the precise instigating cause (activity, trauma, etc.) is unknown. Often clinically indistinguishable from torsion of the spermatic cord is torsion of the *appendix testis* or *appendix epididymis* (Fig. 16.10).

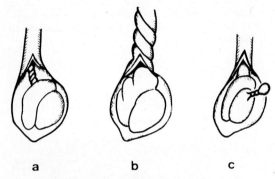

a   b   c

Fig. 16.10.   The various types of testicular torsion:
a) torsion above tunica vaginalis;
b) torsion inside tunica vaginalis;
c) torsion of appendage of testis

Testicular torsion can develop throughout childhood, but the majority involve children less than two years of age. In the infant, it presents as an apparently painless reddish or purplish, hard, nontender mass in the upper portion of the scrotum which does not transilluminate. There are few systemic reactions and no temperature elevation. In older children, torsion usually is heralded by a sudden attack of severe testicular pain associated with nausea and vomiting; examination reveals a high-riding testis which is enlarged, tender and reddish in color. Understandably, this may be confused with acute epididymo-orchitis or testicular trauma, often requiring surgical differentiation. Rarely, torsions occur bilaterally simultaneously. Because of a similar anatomic predisposition on the contralateral side, the opposite testicle should always be fixed to the scrotum.

Because of the threat to testicular integrity, surgical correction is indicated whenever the diagnosis of torsion of the spermatic cord is suspected. At operation the testicle is delivered into the wound and the tunica vaginalis is incised. Only then can one clearly separate torsion of the spermatic cord from torsion of the appendix or epididymis of the testis, or from inflammation or trauma to the testis. The twisted appendices are removed and the twist in the spermatic cord is relieved. The *tunica albuginea* of the testis is anchored to the inner layers of the scrotum with a few interrupted sutures to prevent recurrence. The tunica albuginea of a traumatized or inflamed testis is incised to relieve intratesticular pressure. A grossly necrotic testis undergoing liquefaction is excised and replaced by a silastic prosthesis. A testicle of questionable viability is never removed. Sometimes the torsion episode goes unrecognized, to result later in an "empty scrotum".

Time is of the essence in treating testicular torsion. Testicular survival is virtually 100 % if surgical correction is undertaken within ten hours, but falls to 50 % survival in those operated from ten to twenty-four hours after torsion has occurred; no testicular salvage is likely if torsion has been present over twenty-four hours. Clearly, the sooner the patient is operated upon, the better.

Testicular Neoplasms

Neoplasms of the testicle and paratesticular tissues within the scrotum are rare. The noninflammatory nature of the mass on clinical examination clearly distinguishes them from testicular trauma, torsion or inflammation; their irreducibility and failure to transilluminate separate them from hydroceles and hernias.

Testicular neoplasms generally present as painless solid masses. Seventy-five percent develop during the first three years of life, many being present at birth. Neoplasms are more apt to develop in testes that have failed to descend properly, and of course in this situation are extrascrotal in location. They are asymptomatic in the very young, often discovered on routine examination by the mother or physician. Older children describe a vague discomfort or heaviness or dragging sensation in the scrotum.

About 70 % of the primary testicular neoplasms in children arise from germinal cells of the testis, presenting as hard, solid and encapsulated tumors. Embryonal carcinoma, teratocarcinoma, and the well differentiated teratoma are the common tumors. Treatment consists of radical orchiectomy.

The nongerminal neoplasms of the testicle comprise about 30 % of testicular tumors. They arise from Sertoli cells, interstitial cells and supporting stroma. They are usually benign and certain ones tend to virilize the patient, inducing macrogenitosomia. Radical orchiectomy suffices for treatment of the benign tumors.

Rarely, distant tumors metastasize to the testis, particularly leukemia, lymphoma, reticulum cell sarcoma and adrenal malignancies. Biopsy and orchiectomy confirm diagnosis to direct appropriate definitive therapy.

Rarely, tumors arise in the epididymis, cord and supporting stroma as well as other paratesticular tissue. About one-third of them are malignant rhabdomyosarcomas which require radical excision. The remainder are benign tumors, including lipoma, fibroma, myxoma, mesothelioma, hemangioma and lymphangioma, for which simple excision suffices.

17 The External Genitalia and Intersexuality

P. P. RICKHAM and M. ZACHMANN

Malformations of the external genitalia are frequent in boys and rare in girls. Although many of the malformations are relatively minor, they nevertheless cause great parental anxiety. Undue importance is often attached to these relatively minor abnormalities because of an astonishing ignorance about external genitalia. The parents need assurance by the attending doctor that their child will function sexually in a normal fashion with these minor abnormalities, and that in most instances something can be done surgically to restore him or her to near normalcy.

The Female

Adherent Labia Minor

This is the most common abnormality of the external genitalia in girls. The labia minora are glued together by flimsy adhesions leaving only a small opening anteriorly for the external urethral meatus. It appears as if the girl had no vagina (Fig. 17.1).

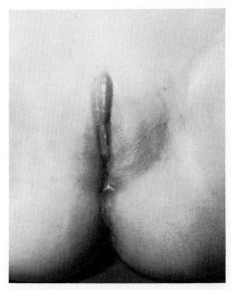

Fig. 17.1.
Adherent labia minora

Treatment

The condition is very easily cured by separating the labia with the aid of a probe. In babies no anesthetic is required.

Vaginal Obstruction

The vagina may be obstructed by an atresia in its lower end, or more commonly by an imperforate hymen. Whatever the cause, obstruction of the vagina may give rise to two different conditions: hydrocolpos or hematocolpos.

Hydrocolpos
(Hydrometrocolpos)

In the embryo, maternal estrogens cause excessive uterine and vaginal excretions; if the vagina is blocked it distends with a whitish, mucoid fluid proximal to the obstruction (Fig. 17.2). These infants are born with a midline suprapubic swelling and on examination of the vulva an atresia or more commonly a bulging hymen will be noticed (Fig. 17.3).

Treatment

The hymen is opened to drain the fluid away. Since ascending infections of the dilated genital passages are common, these patients should be treated with antibiotics for at least two weeks after operation. Since many of these children have associated malformations of the urinary tract, urologic investigation is in order.

Hematocolpos

Many infants with imperforate hymen never develop hydrocolpos. The condition is therefore not discovered until the children reach puberty and start to menstruate. They will then complain of typical periodic menstraul-like pains without any vaginal bleeding. Slowly over a period of months a progressively enlarging suprapubic midline tumor becomes apparent. It consists of the vagina and uterus distended with blood.

Treatment

Treatment consists in incising the hymen and draining the old blood away. There is a considerable risk of infection which may be prevented by antibiotics.

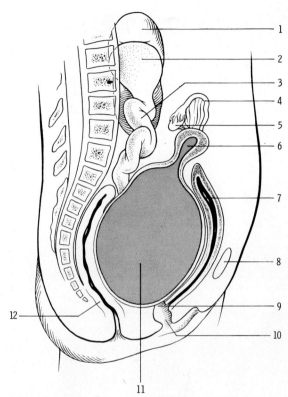

Fig. 17.2. Sagittal section through child with hydrocolpos:

1 Left kidney	7 Bladder
2 Dilated renal pelvis	8 Pubic symphysis
3 Tortuous ureter	9 Vaginal septum
4 Uterine tube	10 Lower vagina
5 Ovary	11 Hydrocolpos
6 Dilated uterus	12 Rectum

(After H. W. Jones. In: Handbuch der Urologie, ed. by C. E. Alken, V. W. Dix, W. E. Goodwin, H. M. Weyrauch, E. Wildbolz. Vol. VII/1, Springer Verlag 1968)

Vaginal Discharge

Vaginal discharge is not uncommon in small girls before puberty. Since the most common demonstrable cause is a foreign body pushed up into the vagina by the patient, the discharge tends to be foul

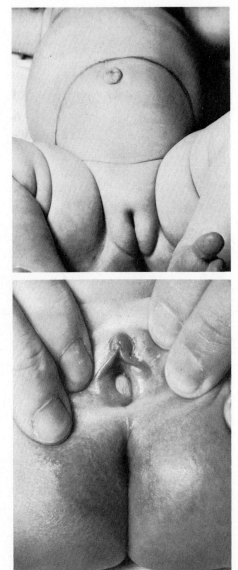

Fig. 17.3.   A. Abdominal mass in infant with hydrocolpos; B. Bulging vaginal septum in the same infant

smelling. Vaginitis is another recognized cause of discharge, generally induced by the patient scratching the perineum. Predisposing conditions such as threadworms and urinary infections should be looked for and treated. In older girls, specific infections such as gonorrhea and trichomonas do occur and the causative organisms should be searched for.

In many children, however, none of the above predisposing causes is found. Prepubertal girls lack the defense mechanisms that discourage vaginitis in the adult: the glycogen-containing cells have not yet developed in the vaginal wall, the vaginal secretions are not yet acid and Döderlein's bacillus is absent. Poor personal hygiene is said to be a common cause of vaginal discharge in girls. More frequently, one finds overanxious mothers constantly cleaning their child's vulva thus causing irritation and infection.

Treatment

Firstly an attempt is made to eliminate the specific cause (see above). This entails vaginoscopy for foreign bodies, cellophane swabs for threadworms, urine cultures and bacterial swabs of the vagina. If no specific cause is found and if the vaginitis persists even after rectifying management errors, a two week course of stilbestrol 0.1 mg daily usually clears up the discharge by altering the vaginal mucosa. It is doubtful if antiseptic Sitz baths and pessaries, which are usually prescribed, are very effective.

The Male

Phimosis, Paraphimosis, Ammoniacal Dermatitis

Phimosis is a condition where the foreskin cannot be retracted fully beyond the corona of the glans penis.

"Physiological" Phimosis

The foreskin separates only relatively late during embryonic life from the epithelium of the glans. In many newborn infants flimsy adhesions bind the undersurface of the foreskin to the glans, preventing full retraction of the foreskin (Fig. 17.4). Forcible retraction of the foreskin at this age causes splitting and bleeding of the skin and may lead to later scarring and phimosis. These adhesions disappear spontaneously in the majority of cases during the first two to three years of life. Therefore, in newborn infants inability to retract the foreskin fully is the normal state of affairs and should not

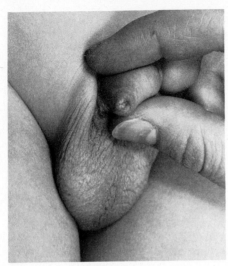

Fig. 17.4.
Infantile phimosis
impossible to retract

give rise to undue anxiety. During the first few years no smegma forms beneath the foreskin. Smegma has a mildly irritative action and infection of retained smegma causing balanitis is common in older boys.

True Phimosis

Inability to fully retract the foreskin after the child has reached his third birthday is definitely abnormal and should be treated by circumcision. In the untreated patient recurrent infection beneath the foreskin (balanitis) is likely to occur for the reasons aforementioned. In addition, recurrent irritation by retained smegma is one of the predisposing factors of penile carcinoma of adulthood.

Balanitis

This is infection of the glans nearly always occurring in the uncircumcised patient due to retained smegma becoming infected. The foreskin becomes red, edematous and very tender and the child may develop a temperature elevation.

Treatment

Treatment consists of Sitz bath and if necessary local and/or systemic antibiotics. If the foreskin is too tight the pus beneath it may be unable to drain and in these cases a dorsal slit of the foreskin is necessary. The patient should be circumcised later on when infection and edema have subsided.

Paraphimosis

In these cases a tight foreskin has been forcibly retracted and cannot now be brought forward again because of foreskin edema and engorgement with blood. Gangrene of the foreskin may develop.

Treatment

The paraphimosis must be reduced under anesthesia, grasping it with the index and middle fingers of both hands and pushing the glans back with the thumb. If this maneuver is unsuccessful, the dorsum of the foreskin may need to be split before it can be reduced.

Circumcision

Ritual and Social Circumcision

Ritual circumcision is practiced by Jews, Mohammedans and many other religious sects. It is basically a hygienic measure as in hot climates balanitis is common and severe. Circumcision is also performed for social and hygienic reasons on most North American babies and on a considerable percentage of British infants. On the European Continent it is uncommonly performed except for medical reasons.

Medical Indications for Circumcision

Medical indications for circumcision are few: inability to retract the foreskin fully after the third birthday, paraphimosis and recurrent balanitis. A relative medical indication is a very tight foreskin in a young infant which prevents exposure of the external urethral meatus. However, even the tightest foreskin may loosen up in time.

Operation of Circumcision

In the newborn this is a very minor procedure and does not necessitate hospitalization. In older children hospitalization for at least one night is advisable as reactive hemorrhage following an erection is not uncommon. The operation, carried out under general anesthesia, consists of removing excess foreskin and stitching the skin of the penile shaft to the cuff of skin left behind the corona.

Contraindications for Circumcision

Today the risks from anesthesia and operation are minimal but accidents may still occur. Circumcision should never be carried out in the presence of infection, especially ammoniacal dermatitis (see below), since meatal ulcer frequently develops later on. Circumcision is also strongly contraindicated in every degree of hypospadias.

Ammoniacal Dermatitis (Diaper Rash)

This is a common complaint of infants in cold climates and affects boys more than girls. The urea in decomposing urine is split by bacteria into ammonia and water and the strongly alkaline ammonia irritates the baby's skin. The foreskin, scrotum and less frequently the whole perineum and lower part of the trunk are bright red, blistered and painful.

Treatment

The infant's diapers should be changed frequently, leaving his perineum and genitalia exposed to the air whenever possible and applying slightly acid or buffered creams or ointments to the affected skin.

Meatal Ulcer

This is a shallow, bright red and very painful ulcer around the external urethral meatus produced by ammoniacal dermatitis. It may induce slight hematuria. The ulcer heals by cicatrization, frequently producing meatal stenosis which may later on necessitate its operative enlargement (meatotomy). Meatal ulcer does not occur in the uncircumcised, and is one of the main arguments against routine circumcision. It is especially common in those children who were circumcised during or shortly after an attack of ammoniacal dermatitis.

Treatment

The treatment of meatal ulcer is essentially the same as for ammoniacal dermatitis plus the local application of protective ointments to the meatus several times per day.

Hypospadias

This relatively common malformation is caused by the failure of the urethral groove to close during embryonic life. The urethra thus opens on the ventral aspect of the penis. Since embryonic closure of the urethral groove occurs from behind forwards, hypospadius is classified according to the position of the abnormal meatal opening: perineal, scrotal, penile (Fig. 17.5) (undersurface of the shaft of the

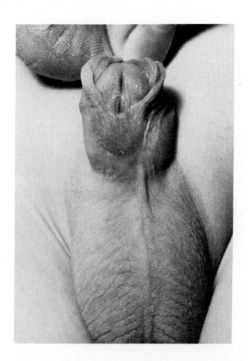

Fig. 17.5. Penoglandular hypospadias

penis) and glandular hypospadias. The more severe types (perineal, scrotal) are uncommon and are associated with a bifid scrotum (Fig. 17.6).

In all types of hypospadias the foreskin is deficient ventrally and has a characteristic "hooded" appearance (Fig. 17.7). In all but the mildest cases there is a ventral curvature of the penis (chordee) caused by fibrosis of the corpus spongiosum distal to the abnormal urethral opening (Fig. 17.8). Urinary incontinence is never associated with hypospadias, as the bladder neck and sphincter muscle are normal.

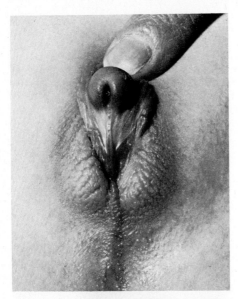

Fig. 17.6.
Penoscrotal hypospadias

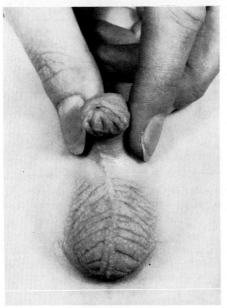

Fig. 17.7.   Hooded foreskir
in child with hypospadias

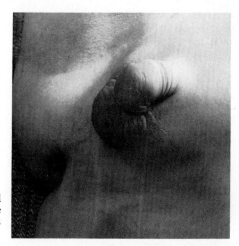

Fig. 17.8. Chordee in child with hypospadias. The penis is bent through a right angle

Treatment

These children must never be circumcised since the foreskin is needed for repair of the defect. Treatment can be divided into three stages:

1) Meatotomy done early in life if the external urethral meatus is too small.

2) Relieving the chordee and stretching the penis, usually performed during the second year of life. This relatively small operation can be combined with meatotomy, if necessary.

3) Bringing the meatal opening forward as near as possible to the tip of the glans. This operation should be carried out well before the patient reaches school age, since by then he should be able to urinate forwards when standing up. The operation is often combined with temporary diversion of the urinary stream by means of a perineal urethrostomy.

Epispadias

Epispadias is the reverse of hypospadias, the abnormal urethral opening being situated along the dorsum of the penis. It is much rarer than hypospadias. The penis distal to the opening is flattened; instead of a urethral tube there is a shallow urethral groove lying dorsal to and between the two corpora cavernosa (Fig. 17.9 a, b). Except in the mildest cases there is usually an accompanying defect of the bladder sphincter mechanism and the patient is incontinent. There is usually also a dorsal chordee and often a grossly shortened penis.

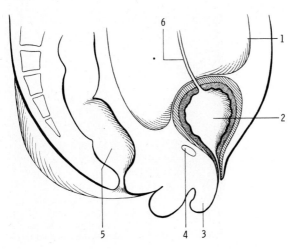

Fig. 17.9 a). Diagram of epispadias; sagittal section:

1 Peritoneum 4 Pubic symphysis
2 Bladder 5 Rectum
3 Penis 6 Ureter

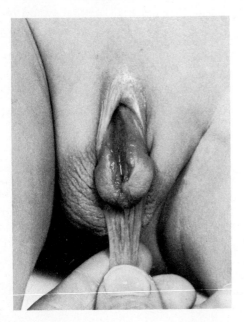

Fig. 17.9 b).
Total epispadias

Treatment

Operation to form a new urethral tube is similar to that performed for hypospadias, but straightening of the penis may be much more difficult. Operations on the bladder neck to cure incontinence are only occasionally successful. Some patients may therefore need urinary diversion into the bowel later on (see below).

Exstrophy of the Bladder

This severe and fortunately rare malformation occurs once in 10,000 births and affects boys more than girls. There is failure of ventral fusion of the lower abdominal wall, leaving a wide gap at the site of the symphysis pubis and a circular or oval suprapubic midline defect. The bladder occupies this gap in the abdominal wall as a flat plaque. The bladder mucosa is exposed as a bright red velvety area above the pubis, and on careful inspection the trigone can be identified, as well as the ureteric openings ejecting urine from time to time. There is complete epispadias and a grossly shortened and dorsally bent penis (Fig. 17.10 a, b). In girls the urethral groove is only a few millimeters long and the clitoris is split. Understandably, there is complete urinary incontinence (Fig. 17.11 a, b).

Treatment

This is at best unsatisfactory. Plastic reconstruction of the bladder in infancy only occasionally restores urinary continence. Many of the children need urinary diversion later on, generally by transplanting the ureters into the sigmoid colon. Although these patients frequently become continent of both stool and urine following this operation, unfortunately long term follow up often shows deterioration of renal function secondary to recurrent urinary infections with hydroureter and hydronephrosis (Fig. 17.12). Cutaneous ureterostomy may then be necessary, or the ureters may be anastomosed into an isolated loop of ileum which opens onto the abdominal wall. A closely fitting bag can be applied around the ileal stoma, rendering the patient dry.

Intersexuality

M. Zachmann

The term intersexuality originally referred to the patient with external genitalia which were neither clearly female nor clearly male. In a broader sense, however, this term concerns all *disorders of sexual differentiation*. Since the conditions leading to intersexuality vary considerably, a certain classification or schematization is required.

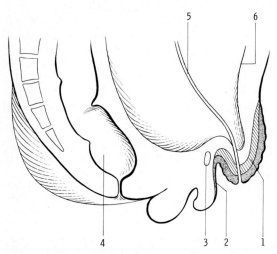

Fig. 17.10 a).   Diagram of male exstrophy, sagittal section:

1 Muscle layer of exstrophic bladder
2 Open urethra and epispadias
3 Pubic symphysis
4 Rectum
5 Ureter
6 Peritoneum

(After V. F. Marshall and E. C. Muecke. In: Handbuch der Urologie, ed. by C. E. Alken, V. W. Dix, W. E. Goodwin, H. M. Weyrauch, E. Wildbolz. Vol. VII/1, Springer Verlag 1968)

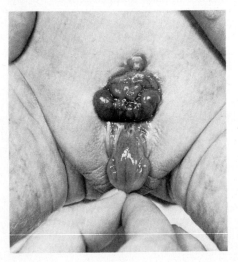

Fig. 17.10 b).   Male exstrophy and epispadias

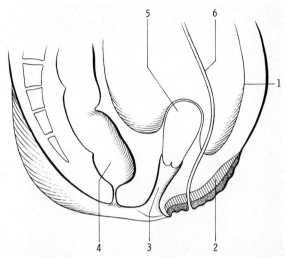

Fig. 17.11 a). Diagram of female epispadias:

1 Peritoneum
2 Muscle layer of exstrophic
   bladder
3 Vagina

4 Rectum
5 Uterus
6 Ureter

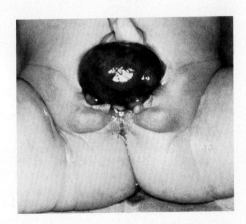

Fig. 17.11 b). Female
exstrophic bladder with
bifid clitoris

The conditions leading to *congenital intersexuality* may be divided
into 3 main groups:

1) **Abnormal gonadal development** (frequently associated with disorders of the sex chromosomes).

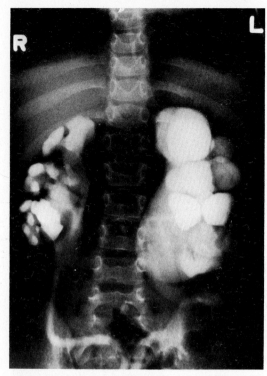

Fig. 17.12.
Pyelogram showing gross bilateral hydronephrosis after implantation of the ureters into the sigmoid colon

2) **Abnormal genital development in the presence of normal testes** (male pseudohermaphroditism) and
3) **Abnormal genital development in the presence of normal ovaries** (female pseudohermaphroditism).

In a still broader sense the acquired types of intersexuality should be mentioned, including hirsutism and virilization in the female and gynecomastia and feminization in the male sex.

This classification is based on the propositions by Prader. Traditional classification which differentiates only between true hermaphroditism and male and female pseudohermaphroditism is at present not sufficiently extensive.

Before discussing individual disturbances, some *embryological comments* are required: the *sex chromosomes* (XX in the female, XY in the male) determine whether the gonadal *anlage* differentiates in the female or the male direction. This takes place in the first weeks of fetal life. Normally, a *testis* develops in the 6th to 8th fetal week if there is a Y-chromosome, an *ovary* somewhat later when 2 X-chromosomes are present and a Y-chromosome is missing. After the differentiation of the gonads has taken place, they themselves influence the *prenatal genital differentiation*.

In the 3rd fetal month, ductus deferens, epididymis and seminal vesicles develop as internal genitalia in the *male sex* from the Wolffian duct. The penis develops from the genital tubercles, the penile urethra from a fusion of the genital folds.

In the female sex uterus, Fallopian tubes and the superior part of the vagina develop as internal genitalia from the *Muellerian duct*. The labia minora and majora develop from the genital folds.

Genital differentiation in the male sex is basically different from that in the female. In the *male,* differentiation is an *actively induced process*: testosterone from the fetal testes masculinizes the external genitalia and a peptide which has not yet been characterized suppresses the development of the uterus and Fallopian tubes from the Muellerian duct (Muellerian inhibiting substance). In contrast, *female* genital differentiation is a *passive autonomous process:* the Muellerian structures develop and the external genitalia become female in the absence of testes, even if no ovary and no estrogens are present.

In view of the heterogeneity of the conditions leading to intersexuality, numerous and sometimes highly specialized *methods of examination* are required to reach a correct diagnosis. The external genitalia are accessible to direct examination. However, the findings are confusing for the inexperienced examiner. The continuum of changes between purely female and purely male external genitalia were divided by Prader into five stages (Fig. 17.13). These are practically useful and may be described as follows:

Type I: Enlargement of clitoris, otherwise female genitalia.

Type II: Enlargement of clitoris and funnel-like urogenital sinus, where vagina and urethra are visible.

Type III: Narrower urogenital sinus, still funnel-shaped.

Type IV: Only small urogenital opening on the base of the phallus.

Type V: Normal male pattern.

It should be stressed that the findings on examination of the external genitalia never allow one to make a diagnosis, since disorders with identical external appearance may have entirely different causes.

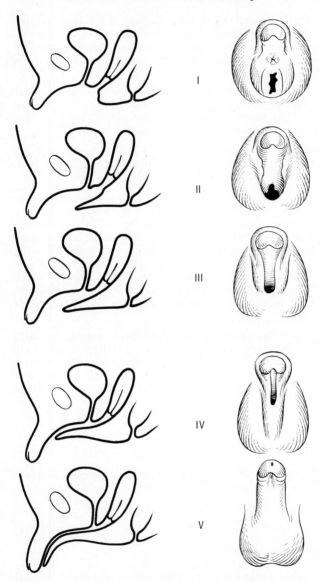

Fig. 17.13.   Intersexual external genitalia, type I to V. For detailed explanation see text

In addition to the external, the *internal genitalia* should also be evaluated, which is considerably more difficult. Some years ago, only examinations by catheters, radiographic studies and laparotomy were available. More recent technical innovations, especially *laparoscopy*, have greatly enhanced diagnosis, allowing biopsies of the gonads.

Chromosome Studies

These are frequently mandatory, although they are complicated and possible only in special laboratories. Frequently, however, determination of *sex chromatin* from the buccal smear and the hair root is sufficient. However, one should realize that this examination does not supply the same information as the analysis of the sex chromosomes. It rather only indicates the number of X-chromosomes. The buccal smear is positive when at least two X-chromosomes are present and negative if there is only one. Recently, fluorescent staining of the Y-chromosome has been developed. These two examinations allow precise differential evaluation of the sex chromosome structure.

Steroid hormone studies further differentiate intersexuality. However, the simple group determinations (17-ketosteroids, 17-hydroxy-corticoids) are of limited value, especially in children. Specific steroid analyses are required in the various types of congenital adrenogenital syndromes and the types of intersexuality due to defects of the testosterone biosynthesis (see below). Recent development of specific gas chromatographic, radio-immunological and other methods allow one to determine specifically almost every steroid hormone which is of biological significance.

Clear conclusions are frequently possible only after stimulation with chorionic gonadotropin or ACTH (especially in infants and children).

Abnormal Gonadal Development

"False" sex chromosomes lead to abnormal development of the gonads in *Turner's syndrome* (XO) and in *Klinefelter's syndrome* (XXY). Since in these disturbances the external genitalia are normally female or male respectively, they are mentioned here only for the sake of completeness, and are not discussed in detail. The same is true for the so-called *pure gonadal dysgenesis*, where the genitalia are unequivocally female. In contrast, patients with so-called *asymmetrical mixed gonadal dysgenesis* have intersexual genitalia. Here, there is a testis on one side and a rudimentary gonad (streak) on the other side. This condition is generally caused by a sex chromosome mosaicism XO/XY.

True Hermaphroditism

This condition also belongs in the group of abnormal gonadal development. It is diagnosed when the gonads contain testicular as well as ovarian tissue. Little is known of the cause; generally no disorder of the sex chromosomes can be demonstrated. Most cases are chromatin positive and about half the cases have a female XX-chromosomal structure. Most frequently external genitalia of type III and IV are found. The gonads may be located intra-abdominally, but also inguinally, scrotally or labially. There may be bilateral ovotestes, a testis on one and an ovary on the other side, or a unilateral ovotestis with testis or ovary on the other side. The diagnosis of true hermaphroditism should be especially considered in chromatin positive cases where an adrenogenital syndrome (see below) can be excluded.

Male Pseudohermaphroditism

If the testis is developed normally and is also able to produce testosterone normally, but not the peptide which suppresses the Muellerian structures, the syndrome of *persistent oviducts* develops. In this syndrome which is also called *internal* male pseudohermaphroditism or hernia uteri inguinalis syndrome, the patients are externally completely normally developed males with normal pubertal development and are usually fertile. However, these patients frequently have uni- or bilateral cryptorchidism and inguinal hernias. The syndrome is of surgical importance because at operations of such hernias, uterus and Fallopian tubes are unexpectedly found and lead to diagnostic confusion. In several of the reported cases, a testicular tumor (seminoma, carcinoma or teratoma) has developed.

In male pseudohermaphroditism with intersexual external genitalia, or *external* male pseudohermaphroditism, congenital defects of testosterone biosynthesis should be considered. Recently, a number of congenital defects of steroid biosynthesis have been discovered, most of which concern the adrenals. If the early stages of steroid biosynthesis are concerned and if the cortisol synthesis is also affected, an *adrenal hyperplasia* develops because of the increased pituitary ACTH secretion; this produces a *salt-wasting syndrome* due to impaired aldosterone biosynthesis. In this way *lipoid-hyperplasia* of the adrenals (where the enzyme deficiency is so complete that no testosterone is formed and the external genitalia are female even in XY-individuals) and *3β-hydroxysteroid dehydrogenase deficiency* (a special and rare type of congenital adrenal hyperplasia) manifest themselves. A special defect is *17-hydroxylase deficiency*. Cortisol cannot be formed here either, but there is no increased ACTH secretion and no adrenal hyperplasia because corticosterone is formed, which replaces cortisol to some extent.

Defects of biosynthesis in the later steps lead only to male pseudo-hermaphroditism, without adrenal hyperplasia and the salt-wasting syndrome, since cortisol and aldosterone are formed normally.

17,20-desmolase deficiency and 17-ketosteroid-reductase deficiency belong to this group. With the exception of the genital abnormality, these cases are completely healthy.

The syndrome of *testicular feminization* also has to be classified as male pseudohermaphroditism. This is a well-known clinical syndrome, where externally female individuals with breast development have normal testes (mostly inguinal), absent pubic and axillary hair ("hairless women") and male sex chromosomes. Uterus and fallopian tubes are absent and the patient therefore exhibits primary amenorrhea. Testosterone in blood and urine show adult male values in spite of the clinical absence of any testosterone effect.

This condition is considered as an *end-organ-resistance* to normally formed testosterone. The mechanism of this resistance is not yet clear, but there are many possibilities: most probable is an increased binding of testosterone in plasma to globulin, reducing the free testosterone which is necessary for the androgenic action.

Besides this classical type, there are also cases of so-called *incomplete* or *partial testicular feminization*. Here, the external genitalia are not entirely female but a genital type I—III clitoral hypertrophy as well as some degree of development of pubic hair are present. Some rare syndromes, such as Gilbert-Dreyfus and Reifenstein's syndrome as well as hereditary vulviform pernineal hypospadia, which will not be discussed in detail here, also belong in this group.

Female Pseudohermaphroditism

Female pseudohermaphroditism is a condition where male or intersexual genital development is found in individuals with XX-karyotype and normal ovaries.

The most frequent cause of these disorders is one of the forms of congenital adrenal hyperplasia where excessive testosterone is formed; in the majority of cases this is the adrenogenital syndrome with *21-hydroxylase deficiency* which is relatively frequent (about 1 in 5000 newborns). It may occur with or without salt-wasting and is characterized biochemically by an increase of the 17-ketosteroids and of pregnaentriol as well as by the presence of pregnaentriolone in urine. In a minority of the cases, there is an *adrenogenital syndrome with 11β-hydroxylase deficiency*. In this type there is no salt-wasting syndrome, but hypertension develops frequently. Adequate treatment with gluco- and mineralocorticoids, respectively, normalizes the biochemical findings in all these types as well as in the above mentioned lipoid-hyperplasia and the 3B-hydroxysteroid-dehydrogenase deficiency. Of course, steroid replacement does not influence the genital malformation which developed prenatally.

If female pseudohermaphroditism is found, *transplacental virilization* must always be considered. In this condition, a normal female fetus is masculinized by androgens from the mother through the placenta. This is possible when the mother has received androgens, anabolic steroids or some gestagens, which are testosterone derivatives, during pregnancy. Many of these compounds are no longer on the market. It is, however, possible that even progesterone in high doses may be metabolized to testosterone and may virilize the fetus. Also androgens produced by the mother herself, as from maternal *ovarian or adrenal tumors,* can virilize a fetus. However, this occurs rarely since the majority of females with such tumors are amenorrheic and sterile.

Therapeutic possibilities

In the cases of a clear enzyme defect, the *biochemical disturbance* cannot be corrected, but the imbalance can be normalized by administering appropriate exogenous hormones. In the various types of adrenogenital syndrome, cortisol normalizes growth and skeletal maturation and inhibits the precocious development of secondary sex characteristics (with normal pubertal development at the expected time) and mineralocorticoids correct the salt-wasting syndrome. In defects of testosterone biosynthesis, exogenous testosterone induces a male puberty, if one decides to raise these patients as males.

Besides the treatment of the biochemical disturbance, as optimal a correction of the *genital malformation* is also of utmost importance. This immediately raises the question as to which sex the child with intersexual genitalia should be assigned. The *responsibility* for this decision is immense and leads to very important consequences with respect to the psychosocial development of the patient. The decision has to be made *individually* in each patient and as early as possible (during the 1st year of life), considering the points of view of the pediatric endocrinologist, the pediatric surgeon and the child's psychiatrist.

The following points may be used as *guidelines:*

The opinion that the chromosomal sex is the "true" sex is obsolete, and no effort should be made to assign a patient to his chromosomal sex. More importance is given to the cause of the disorder, the external aspect of the genitalia and the psychosexuality (in older children).

In the presence of entirely female external genitalia (e. g. Turner's syndrome, testicular feminization, pure gonadal dysgenesis) the child should be raised as a girl. This is most frequently done automatically since, at birth, there are no doubts concerning the "sex" of the child.

In cases with intersexual external genitalia or in female patients with male external genitalia, one should insist on elucidating the cause, if possible, during the 1st year of life. If the patient is *a girl with female pseudohermaphroditism*, she should be raised as a girl, the surgical correction of the external genitalia being carried out later on. Subsequently normal female pubertal development and fertility may be expected. In the case of *boys with male pseudohermaphroditism*, they should be assigned to the sex which best suits the external genitalia.

Changes of sex should not be carried out after the 3rd year of life because of the deleterious psychological consequences, even if the child has been assigned the wrong sex.

One should avoid early operation before diagnosis is clear. Especially the gonads should not be removed, since this precludes a possibly normal later pubertal development, and the diagnostic possibilities (e. g. stimulation tests with gonadotropins) are considerably reduced. In summary, one can say that the problems of intersexuality are often difficult diagnostically and therapeutically, that premature decisions with respect to sex assignment should be avoided and that competent colleagues should be consulted before serious interventions, such as gonadectomy or surgical correction of the external genitalia, are carried out.

18 Urinary Disorders

P. P. RICKHAM

Urinary disturbances are common in childhood. In surgical practice, the most frequent cause for such problems is congenital malformations of the urinary tract. For the most part, symptoms of urinary disease in childhood are the same as those found in adults, but certain differences are worth mentioning.

Urinary Infections

Urinary infections are common in childhood, affecting girls more than boys. Even after painstaking investigations it is frequently impossible to find a cause for many of the infections, but in the majority of cases two causes may be identified: stasis and foreign bodies.

Stasis

Stasis of urine may be caused either by anatomical lesions (strictures in the ureter, valves in the posterior urethra, etc.) or functional disturbances (vesico-ureteric reflux, hydronephrosis without obstruction at the pelvi-ureteric junction, neurogenic bladder disturbances, etc.).

Foreign Bodies

A foreign body may be introduced into the urinary system from without (Fig. 18.1), i. e. pushed through the urethra into the child's bladder or left inside the urinary tract at operation (a non-absorbable suture) or it may develop within the urinary tract (a urinary calculus or a blood fibrin clot). All of these may act as a foreign body, providing a nidus which triggers infection.

Signs and Symptoms

In older children, the signs and symptoms of urinary infection are similar to those encountered in adults, although the reaction in children is on the whole more violent. In young children and babies the temperature may often be very high, associated with rigors and convulsions. Frequency and burning pain on micturition are symptoms which are difficult to elucidate in a small child. However,

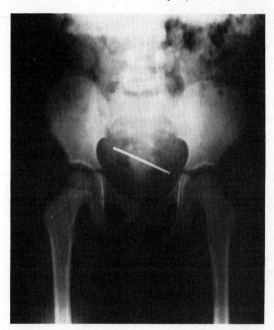

Fig. 18.1.
Foreign body
(hairpin) in the
bladder

vomiting and diarrhea are common. In babies, poor feeding, failure to gain weight and unexplained anemia may be the only symptoms of urinary infection.

Diagnosis

The diagnosis of urinary infection rests upon finding significant bacteriuria or pyuria. More than 10 leukocytes per field and more than 10^5 bacteria per ml of urine are generally regarded as significant. The urine specimen must always be cultured. Sterile pyuria may occur with tuberculosis or walled off abscesses in the urinary tract, but is more frequently found in patients who are already under antibiotic therapy.

Obtaining a Urinary Specimen

In older children, a midstream specimen taken after cleaning the glans or vulva is usually satisfactory. In infants a sterile bag must be applied after cleaning the external genitalia, but it must be admitted that urinary specimens thus obtained are occasionally contaminated. Catheter specimens should only very rarely be resorted to, especially in little boys, as considerable trauma to the delicate urethral mucosa with subsequent edema and difficulties in urination may result. Suprapubic vesical puncture with a sterile needle to obtain a sterile specimen of urine is increasingly popular with pediatricians.

Other Investigations

Urinary infection is so common in children that many pediatricians will not submit the child to any investigation other than urine examination and culture until the second attack. Most pediatric surgeons advise that even after the first infection at least an intravenous pyelogram should be performed, and if possible a micturating cystourethrogram. This precaution is taken because it is not at all uncommon to find a foreign body or an underlying abnormality of the urinary tract. Size of the kidneys and thickness and scarring of the renal cortex can also be evaluated.

Other studies (cystoscopy, urethroscopy and retrograde pyelography) are carried out if the above-described investigations are insufficient to make a definite diagnosis.

Chronic Urinary Infection

Many of the chronic or recurrent urinary infections, especially in girls, result from an underlying anatomical abnormality in the urinary tract (see below). There are, however, a considerable number of girls with chronic or recurrent infections where even an extensive workup discloses no cause for urinary stasis. In these cases antibiotic treatment is carried out for many months or even years. Periodically the antibiotics are changed if justified by urine culture and sensitivity studies. A high fluid intake and alkalinization of the urine is achieved since the organisms often prove to be E. coli living in a strongly acid urine. Since every attack of urinary infection destroys some renal substance, treatment is aimed at prevention of further attacks (Fig. 18.2).

Enuresis

From the surgeon's point of view, enuresis is not a disease but a symptom. It is very commonly encountered in childhood, especially in boys. Enuresis is common in normal children under the age of

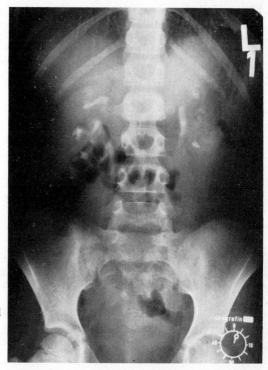

Fig. 18.2.
Bilateral scarred and
deformed kidneys
and pelvis as a
result of chronic
urinary infection

five years. Once school age approaches, treatment becomes more important. In the majority of bedwetters there is no organic cause demonstrable; the enuresis must either have a functional basis or more frequently is due to faulty training of the child. For diagnosis and management of this type of enuresis the reader is referred to textbooks of pediatrics. Should simple conservative treatment fail, or should there be infection or other signs of an underlying urinary abnormality, a thorough urological investigation is indicated: urinalysis, intravenous pyelogram and micturating cystourethrogram.

Malformations of the Urinary Tract

Cystic Kidneys

There are a number of renal cystic diseases which occur in childhood; only the more common ones will be briefly discussed here.

Infantile Polycystic Disease

This is a recessive inherited disease. The children are born with enormous kidneys filled with hundreds of cysts of variable size derived from the collecting tubules. The children die of renal failure soon after birth. It must be distinguished from adult polycystic disease.

Adult Polycystic Disease

This is inherited as a Mendelian dominant. The patients usually die during the third or fourth decade because the kidneys are destroyed by hundreds of slowly distending cysts within the renal substance. During childhood these cysts are very small in size and do not give rise to any symptoms. Symptoms of hypertension and/or renal failure only start during adult life.

Multicystic Kidneys

These are usually unilateral and only occasionally bilateral. They are commonly discovered in newborns with a lumbar mass, one kidney being replaced by a mass of large grape-like cysts. The renal pelvis is never fully patent and the ureter is either absent or hypoplastic (Fig. 18.3). These multicystic kidneys give rise to symptoms because their bulk compresses neighboring abdominal organs. Treatment consists of removing the cystic mass.

Hydronephrosis

Pathology

Hydronephrosis, or distention of the renal pelvis and caliceal system, occurs when the pressure in the renal pelvis is raised above 20 cm of water. It is a progressive disease, the distending calices encroaching upon and finally destroying adjacent renal parenchyma. Hydronephrosis is caused by some obstruction to the urinary flow at or below the pelviureteric junction. We shall first concentrate on obstructions at the pelviureteric junction, for which there are three common causes:

Obstruction in the Lumen of the Pelviureteric Junction. These are relatively uncommon, usually a renal calculus (see below) or a blood clot impacting at the junction of pelvis and ureter to cause obstruction and urinary stasis (Fig. 18.4 a, b).

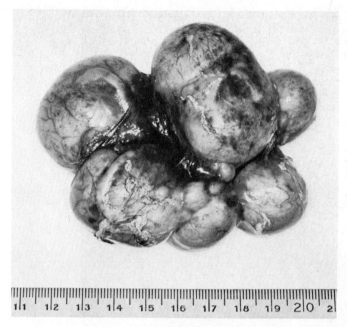

Fig. 18.3.   Multicystic kidney from a newborn infant

Obstruction in the Wall of the Junction. Congenital or acquired strictures of the upper ureter, mucosal diaphragms or valves may all cause urinary obstruction. At times no obvious obstruction can be found and we then speak of an idiopathic hydronephrosis. The most likely cause here is a disturbance of ureteric peristalsis which prevents the urine being propelled down the ureter (Fig. 18.5).

Obstruction outside the Pelviureteric Junction. It is rare for large tumors from other organs to obstruct the upper ureter; more commonly perinephric bands and adhesions kink the ureter or bind it to the wall of the renal pelvis to cause obstruction. An aberrant renal artery running to the lower renal pole has often been blamed for obstructing the ureter. It is doubtful if the artery alone can cause this; careful dissection usually reveals that the ureter is compressed or kinked by adhesions between the artery, the ureter and the renal pelvis.

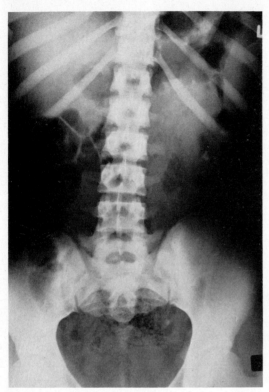

Fig. 18.4 a).
Radiograph showing small stone at the lower end of the left ureter in the pelvis and a small renal stone in the region of the lower pole of the left kidney

Diagnosis

The most common presenting symptom of hydronephrosis in childhood is urinary infection. Pain in the costovertebral angle due to sudden distention of the renal pelvis is only rarely observed, but frequency (or enuresis) is common even without infection. Hematuria may occur after only minimal trauma.

In children even a slightly enlarged kidney can often be palpated on physical examination and the diagnosis is confirmed by intravenous pyelography.

Treatment

Nephrectomy should only be resorted to in hopeless cases with gross pyonephrosis or complete destruction of renal parenchyma. In child-

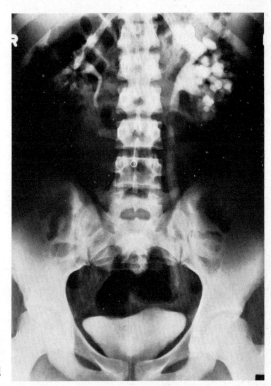

Fig. 18.4 b).
Intravenous pyelo-
gram in same
patient as in 'a),
showing left-sided
hydronephrosis and
hydroureter

hood, preservation of the kidney is all important. Pyeloplasty is performed, eliminating the obstruction. If necessary, the grossly enlarged renal pelvis is partially resected to allow better drainage. The results of this operation are quite good.

Hydroureter

Pathology

Dilatation of the ureter (and subsequent hydronephrosis) occurs whenever there is obstruction of the urinary flow lower down in the ureter. In the majority of cases the obstruction occurs at the distal end of the ureter, on occasion due to a stricture or valve. More commonly, no anatomical obstruction can be found; the last 1 or 2 cm

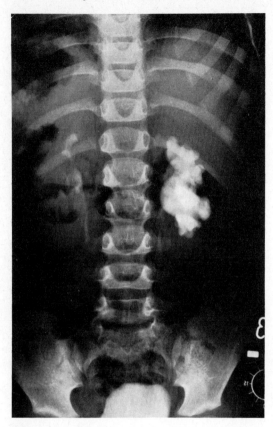

Fig. 18.5.
Left-sided hydrone-
phrosis due to
obstruction at the
pelviureteric
junction. Note
normal left ureter

of ureter is perfectly normal in diameter while the proximal ureter is
markedly dilated, elongated and tortuous (megaureter) (Fig. 18.6).
This so-called "functional" obstruction is likely due to a disorder in
peristalsis in this distal short segment of ureter, but the exact mechanism is not yet understood.

Diagnosis

As every hydroureter ultimately causes hydronephrosis, the signs
and symptoms are those of hydronephrosis. In thin children it is
occasionally possible to feel the grossly dilated ureter on abdominal
palpation or rectal examination. The exact diagnosis is finally made
by pyelography.

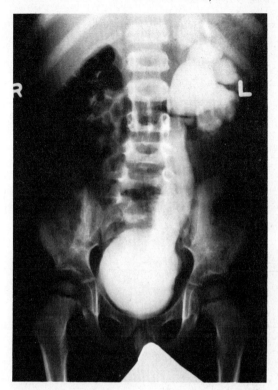

Fig. 18.6.
Massive left
megaureter and
hydronephrosis

Treatment

Treatment consists of excising the distal narrow ureteric segment and reimplanting the remaining ureter in a valvular fashion into the bladder, attempting to prevent any urinary reflux (see below). Tortuous ureters have to be dissected free and stretched, and very large ureters may be thinned by longitudinal excision of part of their wall. The results of this operation are on the whole satisfactory, but in general the larger the megaureter the more doubtful is the prognosis.

Vesicoureteric Reflux

When we talk about reflux in the urinary system we usually mean vesicoureteral reflux. The normal ureter enters the bladder obliquely where its terminal opening is surrounded by strong muscle bundles. This arrangement enables the ureter to eject urine into the bladder without hindrance. During the act of micturition, the bladder contracts with considerable force to expel the urine. The valvular mechanism at the ureteric opening prevents reflux of urine up this opening. If the valvular mechanism is disturbed (congenital or acquired) or if the intravesical pressure becomes abnormally high during micturition (urethral or bladder neck obstruction) reflux will occur. Persistant reflux distends the affected ureter and slowly produces hydroureter and later hydronephrosis. As urine is pushed up into the ureter and renal pelvis at each act of micturition, the residual urine in the affected pelvis will develop stasis and infection.

Diagnosis

The child nearly always presents with signs and symptoms of recurrent urinary infection. It must be pointed out that if a micturating

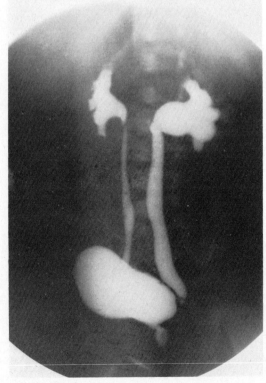

Fig. 18.7. Micturition cystourethrogram showing massive reflux of dye into both ureters and renal pelvis during micturition. Hydronephrosis and hydroureter more marked on the left

cystourethrogram is performed in a child currently suffering from urinary infection, a small amount of reflux nearly always occurs; it is of no practical importance and will disappear when the infection has been cured. However, persistent reflux or reflux of dye as far as the renal pelvis cannot be ignored (Fig. 18.7), especially if dilatation of ureter and pelvis is already present. In boys, reflux is often associated with an obstruction at or below the bladder neck; in girls, where it is more common than boys, it is not usually associated with any definite obstruction.

Treatment

Obstruction at or below the level of the bladder neck has to be removed (see later). However, more commonly no obstruction can be discovered and treatment is at first medical, the appropriate antibiotics being given for at least 6 and perhaps 12 months. The urine should be examined and cultured at frequent intervals. In milder cases, the reflux may thus be cured and the attacks of urinary infection case. Some pediatric surgeons in addition advise that the child should micturate two or three times in succession once every two hours. The rationale behind this treatment is that with the first act of micturition some urine will reflux into the affected ureter and renal pelvis, and later slowly trickle back into the bladder; the child can often expel urine a second or even third time a few minutes after the first micturition. Double or triple micturition thus gets rid of the functional residual urine. Operation is indicated if the upper urinary tract is already markedly dilated when the child is first seen, or if with conservative treatment infections recur or progressive worsening of the hydronephrosis develops. At the operation of ureteroneocystostomy the ureter is divided as it enters the bladder and is reimplanted into the bladder in such a way that further reflux is prevented. Prognosis following this operation is good unless marked hydroureter is already present.

Duplicated and Ectopic Ureters

Incomplete Duplication

Duplication of the ureter is common. In the incomplete variety the two ureters join somewhere above the ureterovesical junction. Many children with incomplete duplication are asymptomatic and are discovered accidentally on pyelography (Fig. 18.8). Occasionally patients complain of pain and suffer from urinary infection produced by urinary stasis secondary to disordered ureteric peristalsis.

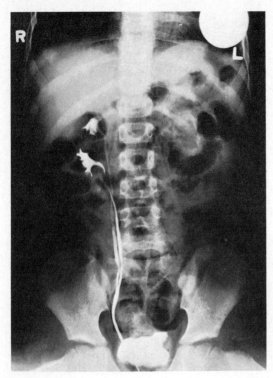

Fig. 18.8.
Incomplete duplica-
tion of right ureter
shown on retrograde
pyelography

Complete Duplication

Here the two ureters open separately in the bladder. The ureter
coming from the upper renal pelvis crosses the other and opens
below it in the trigone (Fig. 18.9). There may be no symptoms, but
symptoms secondary to reflux up one or both duplicated ureters are
frequently encountered (Fig. 18.10). Hydronephrosis may occur; if so,
partial nephrectomy with excision of the ureter associated with the
hydronephrotic and at times functionless kidney is carried out.

Ectopic Ureters

An ectopic ureter does not open in the normal place at the lateral
angle of the vesical trigone; instead, it opens lower down in the
trigone, the bladder neck, the urethra, the cervix, vagina or vulva.
Frequently the ectopic ureter is one of a pair of duplicated ureters,

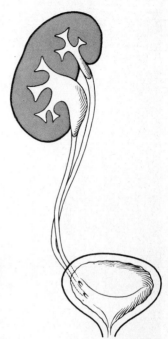

Fig. 18.9. Schematic drawing showing complete duplication of right ureter (After A. D. Amar and J. A. Hutch. In: Handbuch der Urologie, ed. by C. E. Alken, V. W. Dix, W. E. Goodwin, H. M. Weyrauch, E. Wildbolz. Vol. VII/1, Springer Verlag, 1968)

the other one (from the lower pelvis) opening in the normal position in the trigone. Ectopic ureters are frequently associated with urinary stasis and infection. Furthermore, an ectopic ureter opening below the level of the bladder neck produces urinary incontinence, the urine dribbling away as it is ejected from the ureteric opening. Ectopic ureters are also frequently associated with ureteroceles (see below). If an ectopic ureter causes symptoms it should be excised together with the renal pelvis and kidney belonging to it (partial nephrectomy and ureterectomy).

Ureteroceles

If the ureteric orifice of the bladder is narrow and stenotic the ureter just proximal to the opening will tend to dilate, forming an ever-enlarging submucous intravesical swelling. These cystic swellings are called *ureteroceles* (Fig. 18.11). They are diagnosed by observing a spherical filling defect on cystography (Fig. 18.12). In time, the stenotic ureteric meatus produces obstruction of urinary flow and

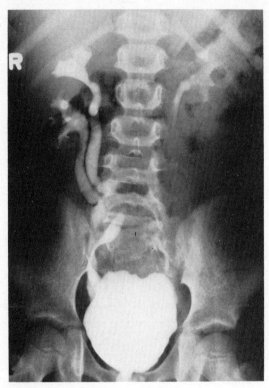

Fig. 18.10.
Micturating cysto-
gram showing reflux
into both dilated
ureters on the right.
There is also some
reflux into the left
renal pelvis

leads to hydroureter and hydronephrosis. Treatment consists in excising the ureteric swelling and reimplanting the ureter into the
bladder.

Ectopic ureters are commonly associated with ureteroceles. If the
ectopic ureter opens into the urethra, the ureterocele may obstruct
the urinary flow from the bladder; in girls it may prolapse through
the external urethral meatus as a dark-red, cystic swelling at the
vulva.

Obstruction at or below the Bladder Neck

The main causes for bladder neck obstructions will be described
below. First, let us review the deleterious effects of obstruction:

1) The obstructed bladder empties slowly, with difficulty and never

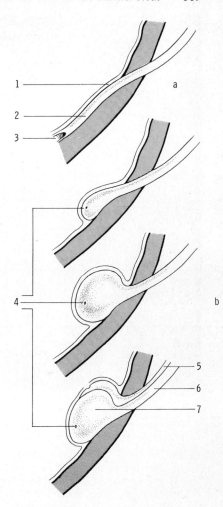

Fig. 18.11. Formation of ureterocele. Schematic cross section of bladder wall.

a) Normal vesicoureteric junction;
b) Development of ureterocele;
1 Bladder mucosa
2 Ureter
3 Normal ureteric meatus
4 Stenosed ureteric meatus
5 Upper ureter
6 Lower ureter
7 Ureterocele
(After A. D. Amar and J. A. Hutch. In: Handbuch der Urologie, ed. by C. E. Alken, V. W. Dix, W. E. Goodwin, H. M. Weyrauch, E. Wildbolz. Vol. VII/1, Springer Verlag, 1968)

completely. It slowly dilates and even after micturition is completed an increasing amount of residual urine is left in the bladder. Urinary stasis ultimately leads to infection and stone formation (see below).

2) Because of the increased work necessary to empty against an obstruction, the muscle in the bladder wall becomes hyper-

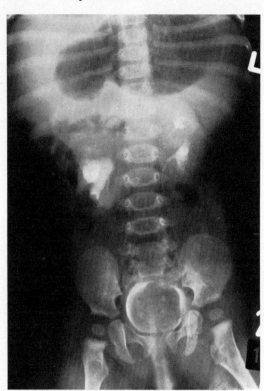

Fig. 18.12.
Pyelogram showing
large round vesical
filling defect of dye
due to ureterocele.
There is a double
pylon on the left,
but the ureterocele
belonged to a non-
secreting superior
segment of the left
kidney.

trophied. This is reflected on cystoscopy by the interlacing, thickened muscle bundles referred to as trabeculation.

3) In the areas between these hypertrophied interlacing muscle
bundles the bladder wall becomes thinned by the increased intravesical pressure. These thinned areas start to bulge outwards
forming little pockets called diverticula. Urine tends to stagnate
in diverticula, since their walls are formed of mucosa and fibrous
tissue only and cannot contract on micturition. The residual
urine in each diverticulum thus becomes a nidus for infection and
stone formation.

4) The increased intravesical pressure ultimately causes vesicoureteric reflux (see above) which may be unilateral at first, but
ultimately becomes bilateral.

Bladder Neck Obstruction

Pathology

Many girls with recurrent urinary infections develop a large bladder and vesicoureteral reflux associated with muscular hypertrophy of the bladder neck. In the past it was presumed that the hypertrophy of the bladder neck sphincter muscle was the primary cause for this condition, and treatment was therefore directed towards weakening the sphincter. Many pediatric surgeons are convinced, however, that the primary pathology is the vesicoureteric reflux, and that dilatation of the bladder and hypertrophy of the bladder neck are secondary phenomena, which will disappear once the reflux is corrected.

Valves in the Posterior Urethra

The most common cause of subvesical urinary obstruction is urethral valves which occur almost exclusively in the posterior urethra of boys. They are small mucosal folds rather similar to the endothelial valves found in veins situated just distal to, or running down from, the *veru montanum* (Fig. 18.13). In spite of their flimsy nature they obstruct the urinary stream, but allow unhindered passage of a catheter from the external urethral meatus into the bladder. The bladder becomes secondarily dilated and hypertrophied, and ultimately vesicoureteric reflux follows.

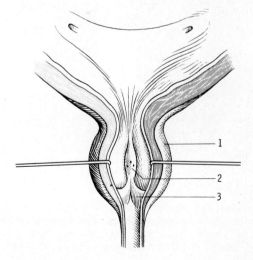

Fig. 18.13.
Schematic drawing of anatomy of posterior urethra after opening the prostate anteriorly in the midline

1 Prostate;
2 Colliculus seminali;
3 Posterior urethral valves

Signs and Symptoms

In girls with bladder neck obstruction and in small boys with posterior urethral valves, the presenting symptoms are usually urinary infection. In small infants the condition may be so advanced when first seen that renal failure secondary to gross bilateral hydroureters and hydronephrosis dominates the clinical picture. Older boys with urethral valves may complain of difficulty in starting micturition and having to forcibly express their bladder; however, the force of the urinary stream is poor and at times urine is passed in dribbles.

Diagnosis

The diagnosis is confirmed by micturating cystourethrogram to evaluate the shape of the bladder, bladder neck and urethra and to demonstrate vesicoureteric reflux. Bladder neck obstruction from urethral valves produces a grossly dilated and elongated posterior urethra obstructed by a minute filling defect, the mucosal valves (Fig. 18.14).

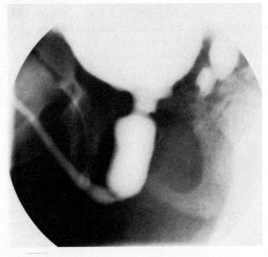

Fig. 18.14. Micturating cystourethrogram showing widened, elongated prostatic urethra with a thin filling defect at its lower end (the urethral valve). Distal to the valve the urethra narrows down to a normal caliber

Treatment

The treatment of bladder neck obstruction has already been referred to above. If the surgeon is convinced that the bladder neck actually obstructs the urinary flow, a wedge shaped resection of the bladder neck is performed with a resectoscope. Urethral valves are destroyed by diathermic cautery. Treatment results are good unless the upper urinary tract is already permanently damaged.

The Neurogenic Bladder

Neurological disturbances of the bladder are relatively common in childhood. Rarely the cause is traumatic in origin, i. e. paraplegia following a spinal injury. More commonly neurogenic bladders are associated with congenital malformations of the spine: lumbosacral myelomeningocele (Chapter 7) and congenital absence of the last three sacral vertebrae. The latter may occur alone or in association with anorectal atresia.

Symptomatology

Traumatic paraplegia from transection of the spinal cord frequently produces an automatically emptying bladder, where the patient may empty his bladder by suitable manipulations such as stroking the inner side of the thigh, percussion of the bladder, etc. These children are at first incontinent, which can often be overcome by suitable training.

In contrast, the neurogenic bladder secondary to myelomeningocele or absent sacral vertebrae is often associated with incontinence. The incontinence is rarely of the flaccid type with complete paralysis of the internal vesical sphincter, the urine dribbling from the urethra after it has been ejected from the ureteric orifices into the bladder. More commonly, one observes so-called "overflow incontinence": the bladder sphincter is spastically contracted, and the bladder distends with urine which is expressed in driblets with difficulty. The bladder wall is usually grossly hypertrophied and trabeculated, and vesical diverticula (see above) are common. The bladder never expels all the urine, and there is an ever-increasing amount of residual urine with the threat of infection secondary to stasis. Sooner or later vesicoureteric reflux develops because of the grossly increased intra-vesical pressure, which in turn leads to hydroureter and hydronephrosis (Fig. 18.15). Overflow incontinence is therefore a dangerous and ultimately fatal condition.

Treatment

In neurogenic bladder secondary to traumatic paraplegia, simple training of the bladder (see above) keeps the patient dry. Occasionally, these same techniques are successful in patients with neuro-

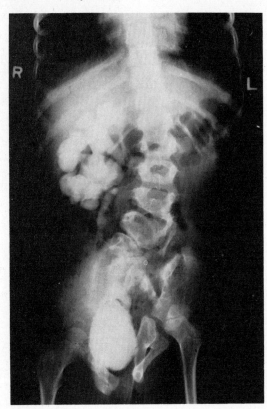

Fig. 18.15.
Neurogenic bladder
with functionless
left kidney and
hydronephrotic
right kidney. Note
gross spinal
deformity

genic bladders secondary to congenital lesions of the spine, provided there is not too much spasm of the urethral sphincter. Recently, some success has been reported by a training method involving filling the bladder repeatedly via a catheter. Whatever training method is attempted, care must be taken that the urine does not get infected and prophylactic chemotherapy is always used. The majority of boys with total flaccid incontinence can be kept dry by a closely fitting penile bag with a suprapubic pressure pad. In boys who cannot manage this bag, and in all girls with flaccid incontinence, the urinary stream ultimately must be diverted to the abdominal wall; urine is then collected in a close fitting urinary bag which is glued to the abdomen. This is achieved either by cutaneous ureterostomy or by transplanting the ureters into an isolated segment of intestine which opens onto the abdominal wall.

In patients with overflow incontinence it is usually possible to destroy the urethral sphincter by forcible dilatation or wedge resection, thus rendering the patient totally incontinent. However, most of these patients later require diversion of the urinary stream as a permanent measure.

Urinary Lithiasis

Urinary stones in children are uncommon in Europe and North America, but are common in many Asiatic and African countries. The reason for this regional variation is obscure, but diet and vitamin intake may play a part. In many cases the etiology of urinary stones is not known and we speak of idiopathic urinary calculi. In a number of instances a cause for calculus formation can be found. The more common causes are:

Inborn Errors of Metabolism

Excessive amounts of certain organic substances excreted in the urine because of an error in metabolism produce urinary stones. Common examples of metabolic stones are cysteine stones in patients with cystinuria and oxalate stones secondary to oxalosis. Both of these are familial metabolic disorders. The oxalates are deposited in the parenchyma of the kidney (nephrocalcinosis) as well as excreted in the urine. Other metabolic calculi are rare.

Foreign Bodies

When a foreign body comes into contact with urine, a stone forms around it. Children occasionally push foreign bodies up the urethra. Unabsorbable suture material used in urinary operations is another well-known cause.

Stasis Calculi

Calculi occur whenever there is stasis in the urinary flow, also predisposing to infection. This is nearly always due to an anatomical abnormality (see above).

Immobilization Calculi

Patients who lie immobilized in bed for prolonged periods, (children with fractures) are predisposed to renal calculi. This is partly due

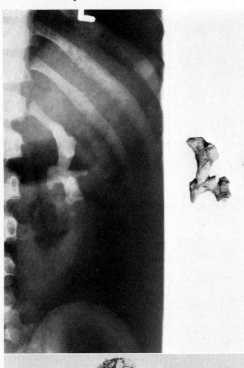

a

Fig. 18.16.
"Staghorn" calculus

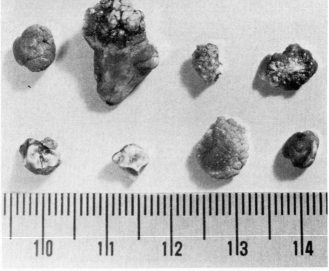

b

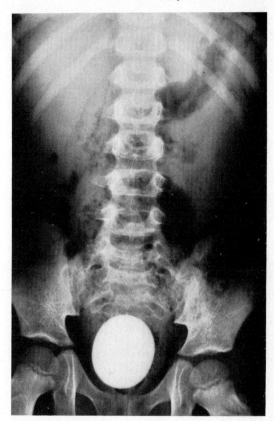

Fig. 18.17.
Large radioopaque
calculus in the
bladder

to urinary stasis induced by prolonged immobilization and partly because the skeleton is decalcified: with disuse of the limbs excessive amounts of calcium and phosphorus are mobilized and excreted in the urine.

Signs and Symptoms

Renal calculi may be symptomless for long periods of time, especially when they lie in one of the calices. They may slowly enlarge and finally form a complete cast of the caliceal system and renal pelvis, a so-called "staghorn" calculus (Fig. 18.16). On the other hand, a small stone may be washed into the pelvis with the urinary stream and impact at the pelviureteric junction or further down the ureter, giving rise to renal colic. Renal colic presents with shock and severe, colicky pain originating in the loin and traveling downwards and inwards towards the genitals, usually accompanied by hematuria. Vesical calculi produce dull suprapubic pain; severe pain, urgency and hematuria on micturition occur when the calculus impacts in the trigone (Fig. 18.17). Regardless of location, urinary calculi ultimately produce urinary infection with characteristic signs and symptoms superadded (see above).

Treatment

Treatment consists of surgical removal of the stone or stones, correcting any predisposing anatomical abnormality, if present. Superadded infections are treated by the appropriate antibiotic.

19 Malformations and Diseases of the Abdominal Wall

U. G. STAUFFER

Umbilical Malformations

Umbilical Hernia

Every fifth newborn has an umbilical hernia; in Negrids umbilical hernias are even more common than in Europids. The umbilical hernia is caused by defective cicatrization of the umbilical ring. The peritoneum of the hernial sac adheres closely to the cutaneous scar of the umbilicus. The hole is usually easily palpable as a ring. It varies in size from only a few millimeters to 3 cm in diameter. When the patient cries or strains the hernial sac protrudes. Depending on the size of the hernial sac, small intestine or omentum may prolapse. Reduction is always easy. Usually, a gurgling noise can be heard when intestinal loops glide back into the abdomen.

An umbilical hernia is not a dangerous condition. It rarely disturbs the patient. Incarceration hardly ever occurs. Most umbilical hernias disappear spontaneously during the first 12 months, and others only during later years of childhood. Operative repair is safely deferred until the child has reached the fourth year of life. Adhesive trusses may soothe anxious parents, but do not influence the likelihood or speed of spontaneous disappearance of umbilical hernias. Since the adhesives may be harmful to the skin, the patient is better off without them.

Paraumbilical Hernias

The hole in the abdominal wall is situated in immediate proximity to the umbilicus, generally above it. The hernial sac does not adhere to the skin, thus differing from umbilical hernia. The hernial opening is usually palpable as a transversely oriented sharp-edged hole. A paraumbilical hernia may coexist with an umbilical hernia, in which case the hernial openings are separated by an easily palpable fibrous cord. In contrast to umbilical hernia, the paraumbilical hernia does not spontaneously disappear. Since the hernial sac is not adherent to the skin, only the fascial gap has to be closed during operation.

Epigastric Hernia

These are situated somewhere between the xiphoid process and the umbilicus. Although generally single, they are sometimes multiple, and are easily palpable as ellipsoid, sharp-edged defects in the linea alba. They hardly ever disappear spontaneously. Epigastric hernias may cause abdominal pain, probably due to a pull on the peritoneum. At operation there is usually a small, pedunculated extraperitoneal lipoma which has prolapsed through the gap; it is removed and the fascial gap closed.

The Discharging Umbilicus

When the umbilical cord is shed during the first week of life, there remains an area covered by granulation tissue. Normally, this becomes covered with ingrowing epithelium within a few days. Because of the threat of infection in this area, good umbilical nursing care is most important during this period of time. Infection is generally prevented by applying sterile compresses and dabbing the umbilical stump with an antiseptic solution (i. e. mercurochrome). Within a few days the umbilicus generally becomes dry. If the discharge continues for several days, an umbilical granuloma or an umbilical polyp are usually found at the base of the umbilicus. Silver nitrate cautery of the granuloma, or tying off the polyp cause both conditions to disappear in a few days. If a discharge persists it is advisable to look for fetal remnants or connections between the umbilicus and the intestinal tract (persistent omphalomesenteric duct) or the urogenital system (patent urachus). The congenital causes for persistent umbilical discharge are discussed later on.

Omphalitis and Umbilical Sepsis

In the pre-antibiotic era, neonatal omphalitis and umbilical sepsis were among the most dreaded of all infections. Since the umbilical vessels are still patent during the first few weeks of life, spreading of the infection and invasion of the bacteria into the blood stream often occurred. The inflammatory process then spread from the umbilical to the portal vein and via the ductus venosus to the inferior vena cava. One of the causes of thrombosis of the portal vein in childhood is portal phlebitis from omphalitis (Chapter 14). Even today, omphalitis is occasionally seen, especially if umbilical hygiene is poor. The umbilicus is bright red and swollen, and there is a persistent discharge which is blood stained and purulent. Bacteriological examination of the exudate reveals staphylococci or E. coli. In most cases, sepsis can be prevented if local disinfectants and antibiotics are given immediately.

Umbilical Granuloma

The umbilical scar heals more slowly than normal and red granulation tissue appears at the base of the umbilical depression. The granulation tissue grows exuberantly and cannot be covered by skin. Histological examination sometimes reveals ectopic intestinal mucous membrane (pseudopolyp of the umbilicus), representing small remnants of the fetal connection of the intestinal tract to the umbilicus (see below). Treatment is simple. Pedunculated granulation tissue is easily removed. If the base is broad, silver nitrate cautery is sufficient. In a few days, epithelization of the area occurs.

Persistence of the Omphalomesenteric Duct

In the early embryonic period the omphalomesenteric duct connects the fetal intestine with the vitelline sac. During the sixth or seventh fetal week the connection obliterates, together with its accompanying vessels, and then disappears completely. If this involution is incomplete, several characteristic malformations occur (Fig. 19.1). If the proximal part of the omphalomesenteric duct persists a Meckel's diverticulum is formed (see Chapter 13). If the distal end fails to close a sinus develops which opens at the umbilicus, secretes mucus and is lined with intestinal mucosa. On inspection a bright red, slightly hemorrhagic polypoid structure with a small central opening is observed at the umbilicus (Fig. 19.2). If both ends are closed, but the middle segment is open, mucus filled cysts of different size develop (so-called vitelline duct cysts). The omphalomesenteric duct or vessels may persist as a fibrous cord between the lower ileum and the posterior aspect of the umbilicus, around which a loop of intestine may become ensnared to produce intestinal obstruction.

Rarely does the entire duct persist (persistent omphalomesenteric duct), with a patent connection between the ileum and the umbilicus. After the umbilical cord separates, a round, bright red mucosal ring surrounds a central opening (Fig. 19.3) from which there is intermittent discharge of mucus, gas bubbles or even feces. Occasionally an intussusception through the duct may occur (Figs. 19.1 f, 19.4).

Injection of the duct with radiocontrast material documents its connection with the intestine, and is diagnostic in obscure cases. Frequently, the proximal ileum prolapses through the patent duct wall. Excision of the fistula is the treatment of choice (Fig. 19.5).

Urachal Fistula

During early fetal life the urachus connects the apex of the bladder with the umbilicus. It normally obliterates to a fibrous cord lying

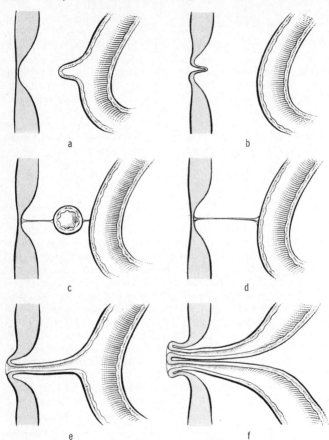

Fig. 19.1.   Remnants of the omphalomesenteric duct:

a) Meckel's diverticulum,
b) Umbilical sinus,
c) Omphalomesenteric cyst,
d) Fibrous band between ileum and umbilicus,
e) Persistent omphalomesenteric duct,
f) Intussusception through the omphalomesenteric duct (see Fig. 19.4)

between the fascia and peritoneum of the lower anterior abdominal wall, forming the median vesicoumbilical ligament. Persistence of its proximal part results in a urachal diverticulum, which is a finger-like pouch situated at the apex of the bladder. If both ends obliterate and only the intermediate segment remains open, a urachal cyst

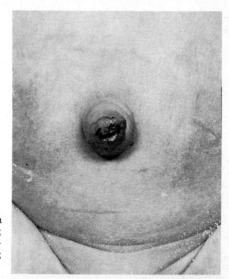

Fig. 19.2. Umbilical sinus. In the center of the discharging umbilicus a polyp-like swelling with a central opening is observed

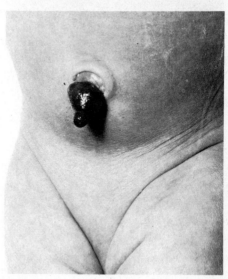

Fig. 19.3.
Persistent omphalomesenteric duct in 3-week-old infant. The duct is everted and flatus and a little stool are discharged from it

develops. Urachal cysts present as spherical tumors somewhere between the umbilicus and the pubic symphysis, lying extraperitoneally deep to the fascia. Often, they are only recognized when they become

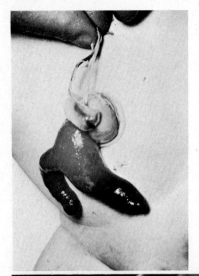

Fig. 19.4.
Intussusception of proximal and
distal ileum through persistent
omphalomesenteric duct
(see Fig. 19.1)

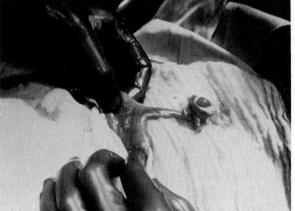

Fig. 19.5.   Findings at operation of persistent omphalomesenteric duct

infected (median abscess of the abdominal wall). If the entire urachus
remains open, urine discharges from the umbilicus (Fig. 19.6), which
increases when one applies pressure on the bladder. The urine may
produce inflammatory irritation of the umbilicus and the periumbilical area. Diagnosis is confirmed by injecting contrast material into
the urachal duct which then flows into the urinary bladder. Treat-

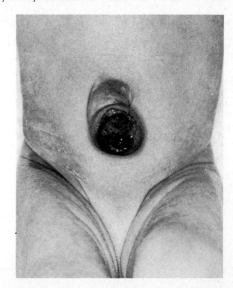

Fig 19.6.
Fistula of the urachus in
4-day-old infant. Urine is
discharging through the
fistula

ment consists of excising the entire sinus. Babies with a persistent urachal sinus often harbor additional urogenital malformations, especially obstructions of the lower urinary tract (see Chapter 18) which produce chronic or recurrent urinary infections. Therefore, intravenous pyelogram and a micturating cystouretherogram should always be carried out in children with a patent urachal fistula.

Congenital Defects of the Anterior Abdominal Wall

Congenital defects of the anterior abdominal wall usually cause severe malformations because of their early intrauterine occurrence (sixth to tenth fetal week). Fortunately, they are relatively rare. The four most important malformations are omphalocele (1 in 3000 to 6000 births), gastroschisis (1 in 30,000 births), exstrophy of the bladder (1 in 10,000 to 15,000 births) and vesicointestinal fissure (1 in 60,000 births). Exstrophy of the bladder is described in chapter 18. The other three malformations are discussed here.

Omphalocele (Exomphalos)

In this condition a thin-walled sac containing intestine protrudes through a congenital defect of varying size in the abdominal wall, situated in the umbilical area (Figs. 19.7, 19.8). The omphalocele

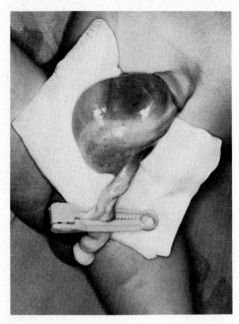

Fig. 19.7.
Small omphalocele of
one-day-old infant.
Primary repair is possible

differs from an umbilical hernia in that its sac is not covered with normal skin but consists of a translucent, avascular membrane representing peritoneum inside and amniotic membrane outside. In between these membranes lies Wharton's jelly.

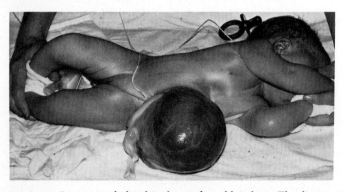

Fig. 19.8.   Large omphalocele of one-day-old infant. The liver and the intestine can be seen through the translucent membrane. Primary repair not possible

Embryology

Between the sixth and tenth weeks of gestation the coelom normally protrudes into the umbilical cord producing a physiological umbilical hernia. Between the tenth and twelfth weeks of gestation the midgut which had herniated into this umbilical pouch normally returns to the abdominal cavity. Omphalocele may be thought as simply failure of the midgut to return to the abdominal cavity. The etiology of this arrest of development is unknown.

Clinical Features

The size of omphaloceles is extremely variable (Figs. 19.7, 19.8); ranging from a few cm to a sac as big as a child's head. At birth the hernial sac is still intact. The umbilical cord is juxtaposed to the omphalocele, usually arising from its apex, and the umbilical vessels hug the wall of the sac. Visible through the extremely thin-walled sac are its herniated abdominal contents, generally consisting of intestinal loops and in large omphaloceles the stomach, liver, spleen, etc. The avascular sac desiccates within a few hours, becoming friable and opaque; infection and rupture then threaten. Rarely, the sac ruptures in utero or during passage through the birth canal; the baby is then born with extruded intestines. If the sac ruptures during delivery the intestines appear normal, but if rupture occurred earlier in utero, the intestinal loops are edematous, matted together, distended, brownish in color and covered with fibrin, the signs of an aseptic fetal peritonitis. The appearance of the intestine resembles closely that of gastroschisis (see below). About half of the children with omphalocele have additional malformations; gastrointestinal anomalies are most common (especially nonrotation of the midgut, see Chapter 5), cardiac malformations and malformations of the urogenital system.

Therapy

The omphalocele is a surgical emergency and requires immediate treatment.

Emergency Treatment by the Referring Physician

Babies with an omphalocele should be sent as quickly as possible to the nearest pediatric surgical center. Immediately after birth the omphalocele should be covered with gauze compresses moistened with warm normal saline or an antiseptic solution (e. g. betadine, mercurochrome). During transport the dressings must be kept moist; drying of the omphalocele sac increases the risk of peritonitis and rupture. A nasogastric tube should be passed and aspirated with a syringe every ten minutes. Stomach decompression obviates the threat of vomiting and aspiration, and also prevents the intestine from distending with gas; distended intestine rapidly enlarges the omphalocele sac and increases the likelihood of sac rupture.

Definitive Treatment in the Pediatric Surgical Center

Definitive management of omphalocele hinges on many factors: general condition of the baby, size of the hernial opening, consistency of the omphalocele sac and the existence of additional malformations. Tiny omphaloceles are adequately treated simply by twisting the umbilical sac around its axis and ligating its base. Omphaloceles with a fascial opening up to 5 cm in diameter (Fig. 19.7) are managed by resecting the sac and closing the abdominal wall in layers without undue tension.

In omphaloceles with a fascial defect larger than 5 cm in diameter (Fig. 19.8) it is usually dangerous to replace the contents of the omphalocele sac into the contracted abdominal cavity. Often primary closure under these conditions drastically elevates intra-abdominal pressure to produce two serious side-effects: 1) the diaphragm is elevated enough to cause serious respiratory embarrassment, and 2) the vena cava is compressed enough to reduce venous return and trigger heart failure. The following options are available to treat large omphaloceles:

Operation. Closure of the abdomen is performed in two stages. In the first stage only the umbilical cord is resected; the abdominal

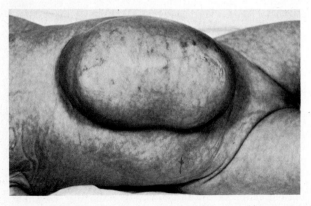

Fig. 19.9.   2-month-old infant who had a very large omphalocele which was covered by suturing the widely mobilized abdominal skin over it

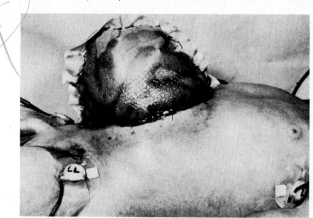

Fig. 19.10. Ruptured omphalocele. Treated by covering it with silicon rubber sheeting. Every one or two days the sac is made smaller until the abdominal wall can be closed within a period of 10 to 14 days

wall skin is mobilized sufficiently to close over the intact omphalocele sac (Fig. 19.9). Twelve to 24 months later the umbilical hernia thus formed must be repaired.

Recently, a silastic-dacron sheet has been developed which greatly expedites management of large omphaloceles. The umbilical cord and the omphalocele sac are resected and the eviscerated organs are surrounded by the silastic-dacron sheet. The sheet is sutured water-tight to the rim of the fascial defect and then closed over the top of the eviscerated bowel (see Fig. 19.10). During the subsequent days the prolapsed intestine gradually returns to the slowly enlarging abdominal cavity. Every one to two days the silastic sac is slightly reduced in size. After 10 to 14 days the remaining sheet can usually be removed and the abdomen is finally closed in layers. In cases of ruptured omphalocele and in gastroschisis (see below) this is the only possible treatment.

Conservative Treatment. This consists of painting the omphalocele sac with antiseptic solutions, e. g. a 2 % watery solution of mercuro-chrome. After one to two days a scar forms on the surface of the desiccated sac. The scar is slowly replaced by granulation tissue growing circumferentially over the sac. The size of the omphalocele decreases by scar contraction. After a few weeks it is completely covered by skin. After some months the resultant hernia is repaired. This procedure is especially valuable in children with very large omphaloceles who are in poor general condition or who also suffer from additional malformations. Its disadvantages are the long hospitalization, and the possibility of missing other malformations of the gastrointestinal tract.

Prognosis

In larger series the mortality of omphaloceles is still about 50 %. The causes for this high mortality are mainly additional malformations and prematurity. If the omphalocele sac ruptures in utero the mortality is even higher (from infection, sepsis, ileus).

Gastroschisis

In gastroschisis there is a defect in the anterior abdominal wall through which abdominal contents prolapse during several months of fetal life, mostly the stomach and small intestine (Fig. 19.11). The prolapsed intestinal loops show the typical changes of aseptic fetal peritonitis described earlier with in utero rupture of omphaloceles (see above).

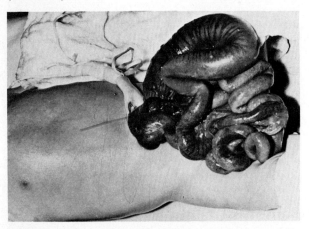

Fig. 19.11. Gastroschisis. The defect is situated beside the normally ending umbilical cord. The prolapsed intestine is stiff with edema. Treated by covering it with silicon rubber sheeting (see. Fig. 19.10)

Gastroschisis differs from omphalocele in that there is no vestige of a sac. The umbilical cord inserts in its normal place, generally to the left of the abdominal wall defect, sometimes separated from it by a narrow strip of skin. The abdominal wall defect in gastroschisis is usually only a few cm in diameter, but may extend from the xiphoid process to the symphysis. Additional malformations are rather rare, thus differing from omphalocele.

Therapy

In the maternity hospital the emergency treatment is the same as for a ruptured omphalocele. Before transfer of the baby to the pediatric surgical center a nasogastric tube is passed and the unprotected intestine is wrapped in warm, gauze dressings moistened with saline and antibiotics.

Since introduction of the silastic-dacron sheeting used as described above (Fig. 19.10), the prognosis of gastroschisis has improved measurably. While formerly only a few isolated survivors were reported, at present 30 % to 40 % of babies with gastroschisis can be saved.

Vesicointestinal Fissure (Exstrophy of the Cloaca)

This is the most serious, but fortunately the rarest congenital defect of the anterior abdominal wall (1 in 60,000 births). Fig. 19.12 schematically shows the anatomy of this most complex malformation.

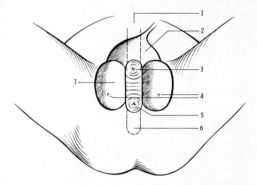

Fig. 19.12.
Schematic representation of vesicointestinal fissure:
1 Proximal intestine,
2 Omphalocele,
3 Proximal intestinal opening,
4 Left and right ureteral orifices,
5 Distal intestinal opening,
6 Distal intestine (usually ending blindly),
7 Right half of bladder exstrophy

To each side of the midline in the lower abdomen lie one half of an exstrophied bladder with its corresponding ureteral opening. A single exstrophic intestinal segment is situated between the bladder halves in the midline. It corresponds to the ileocecal region. The proximal intestinal opening lies cephalad to the distal one (Fig. 19.13). The bowel downstream from the exstrophied intestinal segment, i. e. the colon, is always atretic. Cephalad to the vesicointestinal fissure an omphalocele is frequently found. The pubic bones are always widely separated. The internal and external genitals show various malformations. Duplications of the genital tract are common.

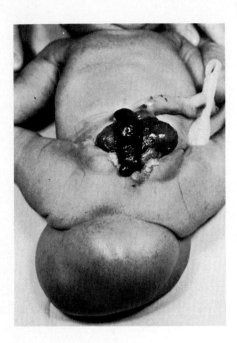

Fig. 19.13.
Vesicointestinal fissure. The prolapsed intestine can be seen between the two halves of the exstrophic bladder. The child also suffered from a large sacrococcygeal teratoma

Embryology

The malformation is caused by failure of mesoderm to ingrow between the layers of the infraumbilical membrane, which is part of the cloacal membrane. The endoderm and ectoderm are therefore in direct contact with each other, and disintegrate. If the urorectal septum has already formed, an exstrophy of the bladder results; if the disturbance appears earlier (during the cloacal stage) a vesicointestinal fissure presents. Fig. 19.14 shows schematically the probable development of this malformation.

Children with vesicointestinal fissure frequently have additional malformations, including myelomeningocele. They usually die during the first days or weeks after birth. Surgery should only be attempted in exceptional cases. Nevertheless, these children should still be sent to a specialized center immediately after birth.

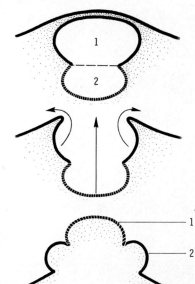

Fig. 19.14. Schematic representation of the formation of vesicointestinal fissure:

1 Bladder anlage,
2 Intestinal anlage (for description see text)

Congenital Hypoplasia of the Abdominal Wall Muscle (Prune Belly Syndrome)

In this condition there is faulty development of the muscles of the abdominal wall, caused by a disturbance during the early fetal period, All grades of hypoplasia occur, from a mild degree hardly noticeable clinically to the baby with apparently complete absence of abdominal muscles. Histological examination shows some hypoplastic muscle tissue even in the most serious cases. This malformation nearly always occurs in boys. There are usually serious additional malformations of the urogenital system, and occasionally gastrointestinal malformations.

Clinical Picture

In typical cases the children have a large, soft abdomen, which gravitates with position changes. The abdominal skin is wrinkled and adherent to the deep fascia (prune belly, Fig. 19.15). Isolated intestinal loops are visible through the thin abdominal wall and palpation of the abdominal organs is very easily accomplished. The rectus muscles above the umbilicus are frequently well formed; if so, the

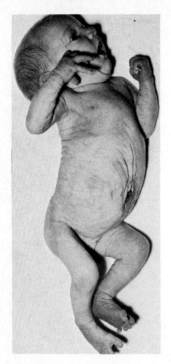

Fig. 19.15.   Prune belly syndrome. Typical wrinkled abdominal skin especially around the umbilicus

umbilicus appears to be pulled upwards. A greatly dilated urinary bladder is nearly always present; the bladder wall is markedly thickened by fibrous tissue, but there is often no bladder neck obstruction. Vesicoureteric reflux, hydroureters and hydronephroses are frequently found (see Chapter 18). Prognosis depends on the seriousness of the additional malformations of the urogenital system. Many of these children die of renal insufficiency when only a few years old. Treatment is directed to the underlying urological malformations. The weak abdomen is supported by a corset.

20 Surgical Diseases of the Skin and Adnexa

U. G. STAUFFER

Children harbor a very large number of congenital and acquired lesions of the skin. We shall limit our discussion to those conditions which may require surgical treatment. The most important among them are the different forms of pigmented nevi, portwine stains, hemangiomas, lymphangiomas and dermoid cysts. Hemangiomas and pigmented nevi are the two most common skin lesions of surgical importance; they can be very unsightly and cause grave psychological problems for the patient and his parents. In order to advise the parents correctly, the doctor must know something about their evolution and natural history. Hypertrophic scars and keloids are also of considerable practical importance, questions about their prevention and treatment being frequently voiced by parents, and they are therefore discussed here. Finally, a relatively rare congenital malformation, the so-called congenital amniotic band, is briefly described in this chapter.

Pigmented Nevi

Pigmented nevi are benign, tumor-like malformations of the skin which are either present at birth or develop during the first year of life. They belong to the group of hamartomas and occur very frequently. They are often found as multiple lesions; occasionally, a patient may harbor several hundred. Histologically they can be divided into the following types:

Epidermal or Marginal Nevus

These nevi present as flat, smooth, light brown spots and can occur anywhere on the body surface. They usually have a diameter of between 1 and 2 cm, but may be considerably larger. Histologically, one finds an increase of melanin in the cells. A nevus which is covered by hair is referred to as a hairy pigmented nevus. Epidermal nevi are frequently seen in connection with neurofibromatosis (von Recklinghausen's disease) and in this condition they are referred to as café au lait spots.

Several subdivisions of epidermal nevi can be made. Some nevi are only a few millimeters in diameter, dark brown and slightly raised above the skin surface (Fig. 20.1). Those on the face are frequently referred to as beauty spots. Histologically, they are characterized by an increase of melanin plus many light colored nevus cells, with an

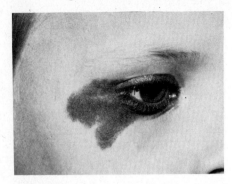

Fig. 20.1.
5-year-old boy. Pigmented nevus

increase of connective tissue in the neighboring skin. Excessive division of the nevus cells produces an elevated, tuberous skin tumor. The size usually varies in diameter from a few millimeters to several centimeters. Their color varies from light brown to black. The surface may be warty, or covered by hairs (Fig. 20.2). Occasionally, a hairy pigmented nevus may cover large areas of the body surface (Fig. 20.3). When melanoblasts penetrate the basement membrane into the dermis, they are referred to as compound nevi.

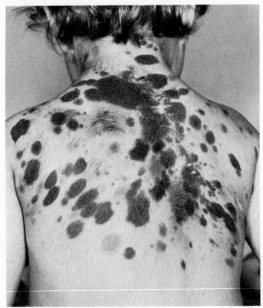

Fig. 20.2.
2-year-old girl.
Multiple pigmented hairy nevi treated by repeated partial excision

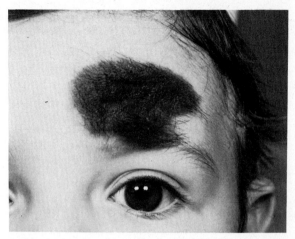

Fig. 20.3. 1-year-old girl. Large hairy nevus; should be treated by repeated partial excision

Blue Nevus

This usually presents as a bluish black, small spot. Histologically, it consists of interlacing fibroblasts with interspersed pigment cells. The best-known blue nevus is the so-called Mongolian spot, a more or less distinct blue discoloration over the sacral region which is occasionally seen in newborn infants.

Treatment

Malignant degeneration of a pigmented nevus hardly ever occurs in childhood. Indication for operation is therefore mainly cosmetic. Exceptions to this rule are nevi which are situated on especially exposed parts of the body, i. e. the palm, the sole and around the waist where they are subject to continuous irritation. These nevi should occasionally be excised in childhood because of the slight possibility that they may become malignant during adult life.

The small, flat and smooth nevi, the beauty spots and Mongolian spots hardly ever disturb the patient and are left alone. Large nevi, especially large hairy and warty ones, are often excised for cosmetic reasons. If they cover a very large surface they must be excised in multiple stages (Fig. 20.3). It is advisable to begin with these partial excisions during infancy because the nevus grows with the child and because the baby's skin is still very elastic and can be pulled together much more easily than in later life. Repeated partial excision usually eventuates in a much better cosmetic result than excision and grafting.

Telangiectatic Nevi

Telangiectatic nevi appear as bright red, well defined discolorations of the skin which are usually present at birth. Their bright red color may later change to bluish-red because of dilatation of the affected vessels. The skin discoloration disappears when the lesion is compressed with a glass slide. Histologically, these nevi consist of dilated capillaries without tumor-like proliferation of vessels which characterize the hemangiomas. Three types of telangiectatic nevi are distinguished:

Nevus Flammeus

These faintly red discolorations of skin are found in nearly half of all newborn babies (Fig. 20.4). They are usually situated in the mid-

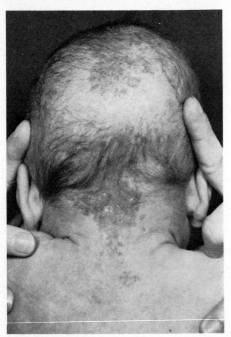

Fig. 20.4.
3-month-old girl. Nevus flammeus of the neck and back of head.

line, especially on the forehead, anterior aspect of the neck, root of the nose and eyelids. They usually fade within a few months; those on the face usually disappear after the second year of life.

Portwine Stain

Portwine stains are usually situated laterally to the midline and are bluish-red in color. They may be cosmetically very ugly. In many cases portwine stains are external signs of a more generalized vascular malformation. Those of the face may be associated with intracerebral vascular malformations (Sturge-Weber syndrome). If the portwine stain extends over large areas of the extremities, hyper-

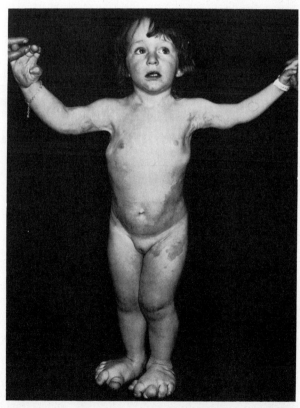

Fig. 20.5. 18-month-old girl. Klippel Trénaunay syndrome (lymphangiomatous gigantism especially of the feet with portwine stains)

trophy of the long bones of that limb plus lymphangiomatous swelling of the soft tissues with varicose veins may be seen. The hypertrophy is probably caused by chronic obstruction of lymphatic and venous return. The combination of portwine stains, gigantism and varicose veins is known as the Klippel-Trénaunay syndrome (Fig. 20.5).

Spider Nevi

These consist of a small dilated central venule from which a number of minute intracutaneous vessels radiate for a distance of several millimeters. They may be present at birth or develop later on. They frequently disappear during the course of years. They may also occur in association with cirrhosis of the liver.

Treatment

The nevus flammeus and the spider nevus hardly ever need treatment, usually disappearing spontaneously. A spider nevus is cured by coagulating its central vessel with the point of a diathermy needle. Treatment of portwine stains is difficult, especially when associated with widespread associated vascular deformities (Fig. 20.6). Being large in size, their excision leaves the patient with large, ugly scars. If at all possible surgical therapy is avoided, and the discolored skin

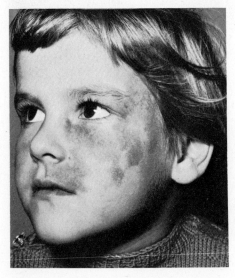

Fig. 20.6.
6-year-old girl. Portwine stain. The patient also suffers from jacksonian epilepsy and intracerebral vascular malformations

should be covered with masking cosmetics. Limb hypertrophy may require major cosmetic and even orthopedic operations. The results of these operations often leave much to be desired.

Hemangiomas

Hemangiomas are among the commonest malformations. They differ histologically from telangiectatic nevi by tumor-like proliferation of blood vessels. There may be large cavernous spaces filled with blood lined by markedly proliferating endothelial cells. Hemangiomas are not neoplasms in the strict sense since they never metastasize, and belong in the hamartoma family of abnormalities. While telangiectatic nevi are usually present at birth, hemangiomas generally appear during the first weeks or months of life. Hemangiomas occur nearly twice as commonly in girls than in boys, and can be found anywhere on the body surface. They grow for a number of months, usually at the same rate as the patient, but occasionally they grow considerably faster, especially those situated on the face. Coincident with growth, central necrosis of the hemangioma may occur, with ulceration and hemorrhage. If the ulcer heals, the hemangioma may disappear in the considerable scarring which occurs.

After the first year of life hemangiomas tend to regress, and by 4 to 5 years of age about 80 % of hemangiomas have spontaneously disappeared. There remains a scar which is often hardly noticeable and does not disturb the patient. Giant hemangiomas occasionally entrap platelets, leading to thrombocytopenic purpura (Kasabach-Merritt syndrome). Excision of the hemangioma will cure the thrombocytopenia.

Clinically, one often can distinguish superficial capillary hemangioma from the deeper-placed cavernous hemangioma, but the two forms may occur in conjunction with each other.

Capillary Hemangioma

They are mainly situated on the surface of the skin, but may extend into the subcuticular layers. They are distinct, well circumscribed, reddish, round or oval tumors which project slightly above the level of the skin (Figs. 20.7, 20.8). They vary in size from a few millimeters to several centimeters, with an average diameter of 2 to 3 centimeters (Fig. 20.7).

Cavernous Hemangioma

Here the skin is intact superficial to the hemangioma, which presents as a subcutaneous bluish mass. The tumor consists of numbers of

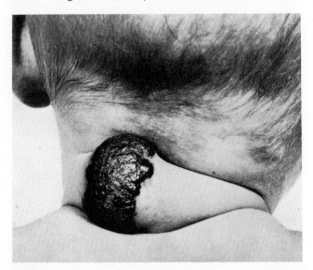

Fig. 20.7.   6-month-old infant. Capillary hemangioma of neck

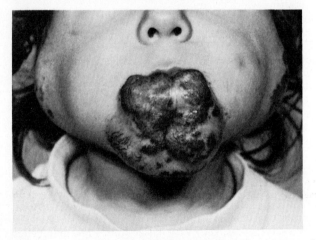

Fig. 20.8.   1-year-old girl with large capillary hemangioma lying superficial to a subcutaneous cavernous hemangioma of the chin

grape-like lobules filled with blood, surrounded by a connective tissue capsule. Cavernous hemangiomas often reach the skin surface, with a capillary hemangioma overlying a cavernous one (Fig. 20.9).

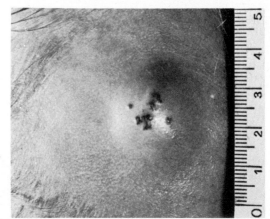

Fig. 20.9.
6-month-old infant.
Cavernous heman-
gioma of head with
additional small
intracutaneous
hemangiomas

Occasionally, deeply-situated cavernous hemangiomas may communicate with large feeding vessels.

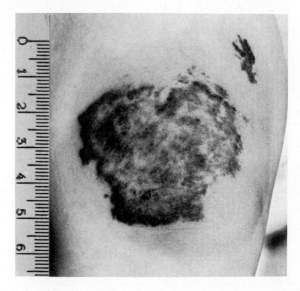

Fig. 20.10.   14-month-old girl. Capillary hemangioma showing central
healing without marked scar formation

Treatment

Since hemangiomas often heal spontaneously with a less-noticeable scar than those removed surgically, they are given every chance to heal spontaneously (Fig. 20.10). It is often difficult to persuade parents that nothing should be done. Surgical excision is indicated

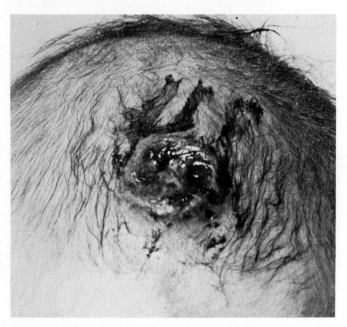

Fig. 20.11.   3-month-old infant. Ulcerated hemangioma

when complications like ulceration and hemorrhage develop, or when the hemangioma is situated where complications can be expected, i. e. on the scalp (hemorrhage when the hair is combed) or in the genital region (hemorrhage from maceration and friction) (Figs. 20.11, 20.12). A sclerosing solution (20 %/o saline) may be injected deep to the hemangioma, hoping to thrombose the feeding vessels. Although hemangiomas are very radio-sensitive, x-ray therapy should not be used because of the dangers of sequelae such as growth disturbances, necrosis of cartilage and bone, late neoplastic changes, etc.

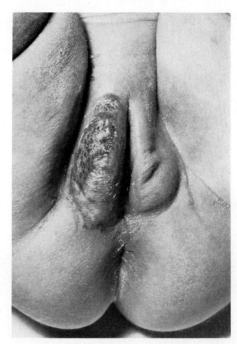

Fig. 20.12.
5-month-old infant.
Ulcerated hemangioma
of the labia

Lymphangioma

Lymphangiomas are considerably rarer than hemangiomas. They have a predilection for certain regions, such as the tongue, the neck, the axilla and more rarely the mediastinum. They may occur in any part of the body with lymphatic tissue. Lymphangiomas of the tongue give rise to a form of macroglossia. The tongue is swollen and thick, and on section is found to be permeated by innumerable small lymphatic cysts (Fig. 20.13). Neck lymphangiomas are referred to as cystic hygromas (see Chapter 11). Cystic hygromas more often involve the posterior triangle of the neck than the anterior triangle (Fig. 20.14), and frequently extend to the axilla, the thoracic wall, the upper arm and the mediastinum (Fig. 20.15).

Clinically, lymphangiomas are soft, fluctuant, non-tender tumors usually situated beneath the skin. The overlying skin may be normal in texture, or may be covered by small blister-like cysts. In contrast to hemangiomas, lymphangiomas are not sharply circumscribed, frequently extending into neighboring tissues and growing along vessels

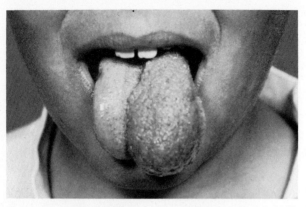

Fig. 20.13.   8-year-old boy. Lymphangioma of the left half of the tongue. The affected part is enlarged and covered with multiple small vesicles

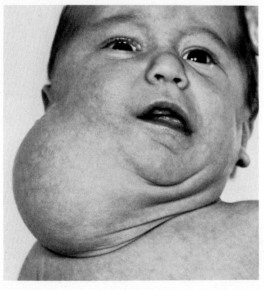

Fig. 20.14.
2-month-old infant.
Cystic lymphan-
gioma

and nerves to give the appearance of an infiltrating tumor. They brilliantly transilluminate.

Diffuse lymphangiomas occasionally involve the extremities, or in rare cases one-half of the body. These unfortunate patients harbor

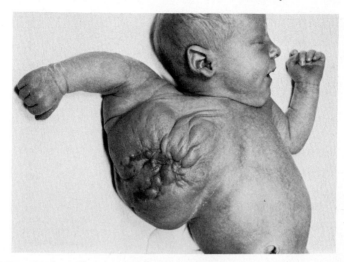

Fig. 20.15. 14-day-old infant. Giant lymphangioma in the right axilla extending to upper arm and lateral wall of thorax

thousands of small lymphangiomatous cysts in the subcutaneous tissues and muscles. As discussed previously (Klippel-Trénaunay syndrome) there may be associated gigantism, probably due to partial obstruction of lymphatic and venous return (Fig. 20.5).

Histologically, lymphangiomas consist of numerous small to enormously dilated cystic lymph vessels which are filled with a clear fluid. Like the hemangioma, lymphangiomas belong to the class of hamartomas and never become malignant.

Dermoid Cysts

The most frequent location for dermoid cysts is the head, especially lateral to the outer end of the eyebrow (Fig. 20.16). They also occur over the skull bones, especially superficial to the anterior fontanelle (Fig. 20.17) or at the root or bridge of the nose; a less common location is the median plane of the neck superficial to the thyroid cartilage or the suprasternal notch. They often arise during infancy. Histologically, dermoid cysts consist of elements derived from the skin and associated structures, surrounded by a connective tissue layer. They contain a white cheesy fluid consisting of sebaceous material, squamous epithelium and occasionally hair. Clinically, they

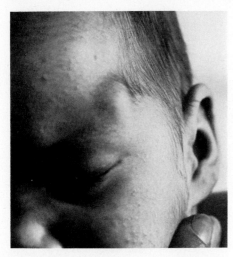

Fig. 20.16.
3-week-old infant. External
angular dermoid

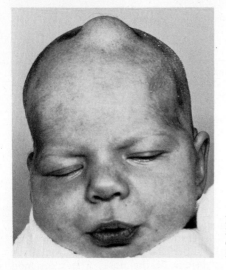

Fig. 20.17.
2-month-old infant. Dermoid
cyst overlying the anterior
fontanelle

appear as tense cysts which vary in size up to one centimeter,
enlarging slowly. They are not attached to the overlying skin, but
are firmly attached to the underlying structures. Dermoid cysts of
the skull are firmly connected to underlying periosteum, often lying
in a bony depression which can be clearly seen on radiography.

In the differential diagnosis of a dermoid cyst of the skull a meningo-cele must be considered (see Chapter 8). Dermoid cysts are usually much more tense than meningoceles. Furthermore, a meningocele enlarges and becomes more tense when the child cries or strains, which does not occur with a dermoid cyst. Treatment consists in excision of the dermoid cyst, which can usually be accomplished in toto without much difficulty.

Hypertrophic Scars, Keloids

Hypertrophic Scars

After certain types of trauma, lacerations, surgical operations, burns, etc., ugly, protruding and reddened scars result. However, these hypertrophied scars never grow beyond the site of the original trauma, differing them from keloids. In the usual course of events, hypertrophied scars regress over a period of years, becoming softer and paler, rendering surgical intervention unnecessary. The involution of scars may be accelerated by compression bandages: a layer of foam rubber is placed directly upon the scar and secured with elastic bandages enveloping the entire limb. This compression band-age must be kept in place day and night for many months, which may be impossible in small children. Furthermore, this treatment is impossible in the head and neck. Cortisone ointment applied topically for 4 to 8 weeks may cause some improvement. Hypertrophic scars which do not regress frequently cross flexion surfaces or skin lines at right angles, producing contractures which may be relieved by excision and skin grafting or by performing a Z-plasty to lengthen the scar. Surgical correction of a hypertrophied scar should not be carried out for at least one year after the original injury.

Keloids

True keloids are much rarer than hypertrophied scars. Some people seem to have a genetic predisposition for the overgrowth of fibrous scar tissue (especially Negrids). Keloids overgrow the limits of the original injury, in distinction to hypertrophied scars. A keloid starts as a small, firm lump which grows into a flat, fleshy band protruding beyond the surrounding skin, from which finger-like processes de-velop. The surface of a keloid is at first bright red and shiny, later turning pale; it may become covered with small telangiectases.

Even when keloids become paler in color, a very unsightly scar remains. Compression bandages are of limited value. Excision of the keloid scar is generally followed by formation of a new keloid, and is therefore discouraged. Sandpapering the scar often greatly improves its appearance. Steroids injected into the keloid may aid regression.

Amniotic Bands

Amniotic bands (Figs. 20.18, 20.19) are relatively rare, presenting in the newborn as a more or less annular scar around one of the extremities, especially the hands and feet. In the majority of cases these constrictions are confined to the skin, but occasionally may penetrate to the bone. In severe cases, the limb distal to the circular scar is amputated or is very deformed and hypoplastic; in less severe cases

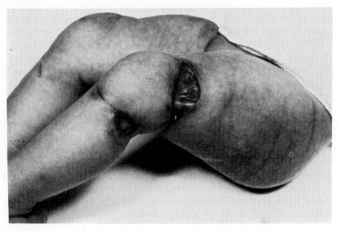

Fig. 20.18.   1-day-old infant. Congenital skin defects due to amniotic bands

the peripheral segment is merely swollen secondary to lymphatic stasis. An amniotic band on the head may cause either a circular scar or produce atrophic areas of skin.

Embryology

Amniotic bands are thought to be produced during the formation of the amniotic cavity. If formation of the amniotic cavity is incomplete, there remain columns of cells between the amnion and the ectoderm of the fetus. If these columns are invaded by mesenchyme they result in amniotic bands. When the bands traverse the amniotic cavity they may ensnare the fetal limbs.

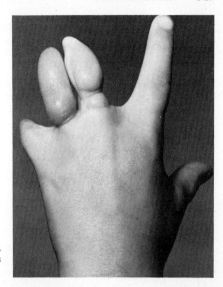

Fig. 20.19. 6-year-old boy. Scars due to amniotic bands around the fingers

Treatment

In simpler cases, excision and Z-plasty lengthening of the scar cures the condition. In very severe cases it may be necessary to amputate, the segment distal to the scar.

21 Malformation and Diseases of the Chest Wall

U. G. STAUFFER

In this chapter the different types of congenital and acquired lesions of the breast and chest wall are discussed. The acquired lesions are usually benign, but they often cause the parents a good deal of anxiety. Exact knowledge of the nature of these diseases is therefore of great practical importance to the doctor.

Abnormalities of the Breast

Neonatal Mastitis

The breasts of many newborn babies of both sexes undergo some enlargement between the third and seventh days after birth. The swelling is usually small (about 1 cm) but in exceptional cases may reach the size of a small lemon. The breasts are usually firm and are not painful. It may be possible to express some whitish secretion (witch's milk) from the nipples. These swellings usually subside within two to four weeks. The name neonatal mastitis is really misleading, because the condition is only a response of the breast tissue to estrogenic hormones which have crossed the placental barrier from the mother to the fetus. No treatment is required. Rarely a bacterial infection is superimposed, and an abscess may develop in the proliferating glandular tissue. If drainage of the abscess cannot be avoided, it is carried out through a small radial incision so that the fine glandular ducts are not injured.

Premature Breast Development

Occasionally, unilateral or bilateral development of the breasts occurs in females between the ages of two to five years (Fig. 21.1). There are no other signs of puberty. The breast enlargement is at first often unilateral, but a few months later the other breast often becomes affected. Palpation reveals a breast mass which is firm and 1 to 3 cm in size. In time the swelling may subside either completely or partially. The actual growth of the breast starts at about puberty, usually between eleven and twelve years of age.

Premature breast development is a benign condition with no associated endocrine disturbances. It is probably caused by a temporary increased susceptibility of the endorgans to circulating hormones. Awareness of this common physiological variation from normal

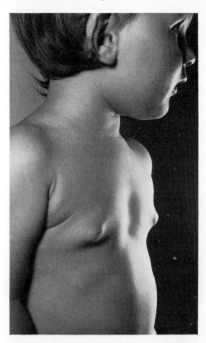

Fig. 21. 1.
3-year-old girl with premature
breast development

avoids unnecessary and dangerous investigations (such as biopsy)
which could injure the gland. Premature breast development must
be distinguished from the rare true precocious puberty. This is easy
as all the other signs of puberty are lacking and the height of the
children is normal. Radiography shows no signs of puberty (sesamoid
bones), and the bone age of the child is normal (for details see
textbook of pediatrics).

Gynecomastia

True gynecomastia is characterized by enlargement of glandular elements of one or both breasts in boys (Fig. 21.2). If the gynecomastia
is marked (prominence of the breast over a diameter of 5 cm) it
may be cosmetically unsightly and provoke serious psychological
disturbances in adolescent boys. In these cases the breast should be
excised. The best cosmetic results are obtained with a periareolar
incision. The curved submammary incision used in adults is not
recommended, as the scar accentuates the outline of the breast from
afar.

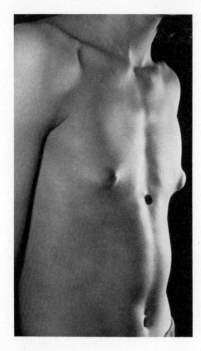

Fig. 21.2.
a) 13-year-old boy. True bilateral gynecomastia

Pseudogynecomastia

Marked accumulation of fat in the area of the breast simulates gynecomastia. The breast tissue itself is not enlarged. Additionally, patients develop striae around the hips and lateral thighs as part of their picture of general obesity. Frequently, the penis appears to be small as it disappears in the mass of suprapubic fat. The patients are usually tall and often have knock knees and flat feet.

There is no endocrine disturbance in these tall, fat patients with simple pseudogynecomastia. In contrast, patients with genuine endocrine disturbances associated with obesity almost without exception are shorter than normal (see textbooks of pediatrics). In pséudogynecomastia, mastectomy for cosmetic reasons is only rarely indicated. A reducing diet is the treatment of choice.

Prepubertal Mastitis

This painful breast enlargement occurs in many boys and girls before puberty. The complaints usually subside spontaneously. After

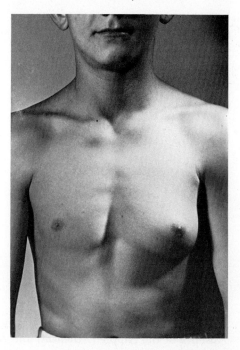

b) 13-year-old boy. Marked left gynecomastia

months or years the swelling often disappears partly or, completely. There is no endocrine disturbance.

Congenital Malformations of the Breast

Congenital malformations of the breast are rather rare, but may cause parents great anxiety.

Multiple Nipples (Polythelism)

There are occasionally supernumerary nipples situated on a curved line from the axilla to the region of the nipple and then down the trunk. They are usually located caudally of the normal nipple and are caused by a persistence of the primitive mammary line (Fig. 21.3). The accessory nipples are usually very small and contain no glandular tissue. The anomaly may be unilateral or bilateral. Treatment consists of excising the supernumerary nipples.

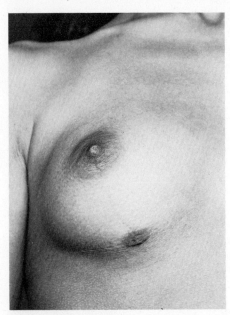

Fig. 21.3.
13-year-old girl. Accessory nipple. A faint pigmented strip runs towards the normal nipple

Absence of the Nipple (Athelism) and Absence of the Breast (Amastia)

This is a much rarer anomaly than multiple nipples. It is practically always unilateral. It is often only a symptom of a much wider dysplasia, with faulty development or absence of the pectoralis major muscle and dysplasia of the underlying ribs. The combination of dysplasia of the pectoralis muscle and underlying ribs may exist without athelia and amastia (Fig. 21.4). In girls at puberty surgical treatment consists in inserting a breast prothesis and creating an artificial nipple. This may be done by scraping off the corresponding skin area and replacing it with a free graft from the labia.

Malformations of the Chest Wall

Funnel Chest (Pectus Excavatum)

This consists of a more or less marked depression of the sternum and the adjacent cartilages. The cause of funnel chest is obscure. It sometimes occurs in several members of the same family, but there is no evidence of real hereditary factors.

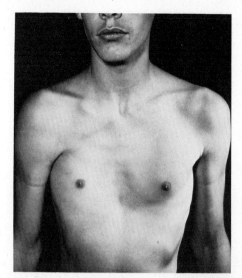

Fig. 21.4.
14-year-old boy with
aplasia of the right
pectoralis muscle. The
right nipple is slightly
higher than the left; slight
hypoplasia of the right
side of the thorax; slight
funnel chest

Clinical Features

Most children with a funnel chest are rather delicate and their muscles
are weak. They often have a typical postural kyphosis of the thoracic
spine, a lordosis of the lumbar spine, a hypotonic abdomen and
rounded shoulders (Fig. 21.5).

Funnel chest is often part and parcel of a general constitutional
weakness. Less commonly it is an isolated malformation in an otherwise normal or even athletic patient (Fig. 21.6). In some patients this
anomaly is present at birth, in others it only develops in the course
of the first year; it often becomes progressively worse until the child
is fully grown (Fig. 21.6). The depression usually begins at the 3rd
or 4th rib and is most marked at the junction of the sternum and
the xiphoid process. All degrees exist, from the mild, hardly noticeable deformity to the very marked, severe funnel chest in which the
posterior part of the lower sternum is situated only a few centimeters
in front of the spine. Occasionally, there is an asymmetrical form of
funnel chest with rotation around the axis of the sternum resulting
in unilateral depression of the ribs on one side and elevation of the
ribs on the opposite side.

Most children with funnel chest have no complaints. The parents
sometimes notice decreased exercise tolerance and the children may
complain of palpitation, precordial pain and dyspnea after prolonged
exercise. Spirometric examination usually is normal, even in the very
gravest types of funnel chest. Severely affected patients may have

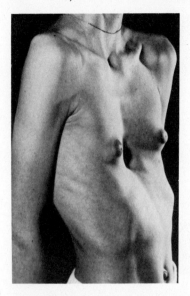

Fig. 21.5. 13-year-old girl. The funnel chest appears to be part and parcel of general muscular and postural weakness

an impediment in the filling of the right ventricle during diastole which may explain their slight diminution in work capacity.

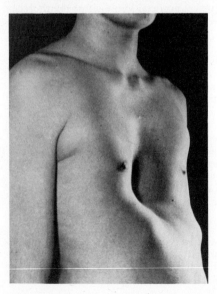

Fig. 21.6.
14-year-old boy. Athletic type. The funnel chest is an isolated malformation

Radiological and Laboratory Examinations

Radiography of the thorax usually shows a cardiac shift to the left. The right cardiac outline is hidden by the spinal shadow, as is the hilus (Fig. 21.7). Half of the cases develop systolic murmurs, probably caused by the cardiac shift. ECGs on severe cases show a slight rotation of the heart around its longitudinal axis. The severity of the funnel chest is best seen in a lateral radiography of the chest after the depression in the sternum has been marked by a barium sulfate strip. The shortest distance from the posterior part of the sternum to the anterior edge of the spine should be measured (Fig. 22.8 a, b). This is more accurate than measuring the distance between the xiphoid process and the spine with calipers.

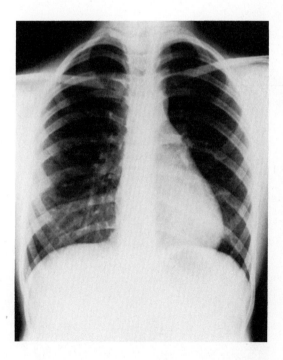

Fig. 21.7.
10-year-old girl
with funnel chest.
The heart is displaced towards the
left

Indications for Operation

As most children with funnel chests have no complaints, indication for operation is mainly on cosmetic grounds. Since the anomaly is very conspicuous and disturbing, the children may suffer from serious psychological disturbances. The child realizes that he is "different" and is frequently teased by his play- and schoolmates. The children become timid, dare not to undress, do not like to go swimming and withdraw. These symptoms have to be ascertained and considered when an operation is debated.

There is no general agreement concerning the optimal age for operative correction. We operate after the fifth year of age. The younger patient is unable to cooperate during pre- and postoperative breathing exercises and the subsequent important posture exercises. Also, the thoracic wall is often not sufficiently strong at younger ages.

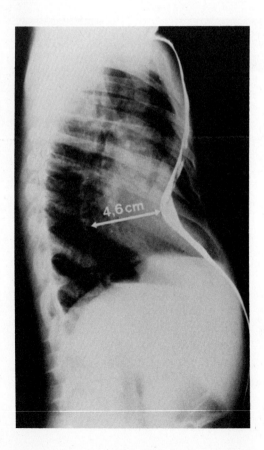

Fig. 21.8.
Boy with funnel chest. Lateral radiograph:
Fig. 21.8 a).
when 4 years old;

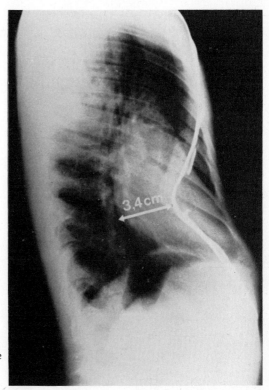

Fig. 21.8 b).
when 6 years old.
Definite increase of
the depression of the
sternum. Indication
for operation;

Surgical Correction

This consists of elevation of the funnel. The crack in the sternum itself is repaired by one or several osteotomies. Stability of the anterior chest wall is guaranteed by inserting a rib splint or by a metal pin which is pushed through the sternum. These pins are left in for at least 12 months (Fig. 21.8 c). Physiotherapy to improve the bad posture is indicated for one to two years.

Pigeon Breast

This condition occurs much more rarely than funnel chest. The sternum protrudes forward, the ribs are everted and the chest often appears relatively flat on its lateral surface. The sternum is frequently rotated round its longitudinal axis so that the anomaly is

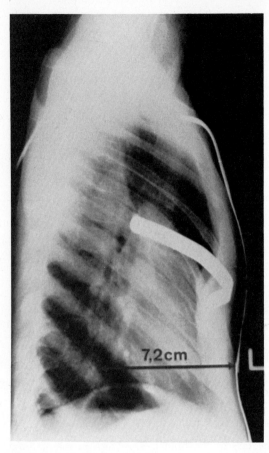

Fig. 21.8 c).
Situation after
operation and
fixation with metal
plate;

asymmetrical (Fig. 21.9). Similar to funnel chest, the pigeon breast
deformity has a tendency to become progressively worse until the
child is fully grown. Clinically, these patients have no complaints.
Serious cases are operated upon for cosmetic and psychological reasons. The operative technique is the same as for funnel chest, but
fixation of the sternum is not necessary. The cosmetic results are
generally good. The optimal time for operation is controversial. For
psychological reasons the operation should be performed before the
child starts school, but often is postponed until the eighth to tenth
year. Girls with mild deformities are not operated upon until puberty,
as the breast development may hide the cosmetic defect.

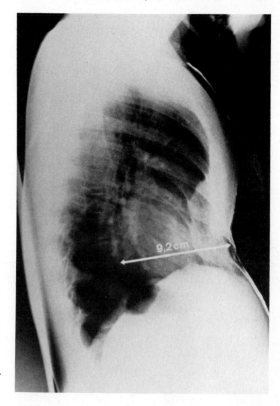

9,2 cm

Fig. 21.8 d).
Result 5 years after
operation

Cleft Sternum

The embryonic sternum is initially bifid, with longitudinal fusion of
both lateral parts occurring later. Analogous to disturbances of closure in the anterior abdominal wall, several characteristic malformations of different degrees of severity develop if fusion does not take
place. Fortunately, all these anomalies are rare. Different gradations
are found from the simple median, longitudinal hernia of the skin
over the manubrium (Fig. 21.10) to the complete sternal hernia. The
gravest form of hernia formation is associated with ectopia cordis.
The heart protrudes completely or partly into the gap. In this rare
malformation there is usually a simultaneous partial ventral defect
of the abdominal wall situated between the xiphisternum and the
umbilicus. There are frequently other malformations. Most of these
babies die during the first weeks of life.

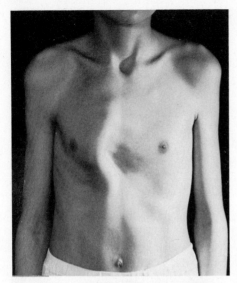

Fig. 21.9.
12-year-old boy.
Asymmetrical pigeon chest

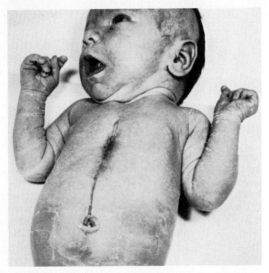

Fig. 21.10.   10-day-old newborn infant. Longitudinal median skin hernia

22 Accidents in Childhood

Introduction

U. G. Stauffer

One-third of pediatric surgical beds house children who have suffered trauma of one sort or another. Every fifth accident case involves a child under 16 years of age. Pediatric traumatology has therefore developed into one of the most important branches of pediatric surgery. It must also be remembered that accidents are the most frequent cause of death in children between one and 15 years of age.

About 20 % of all accidents in childhood occur at home, 30 % are traffic accidents and 50 % occur during sport and play activities. Certain types of accidents are typical for certain age groups. Children between two and five years of age typically incur accidents in the home such as scalds, falling from chairs and tables, pulling down heavy objects onto them, etc. In older children, traffic and sport accidents are most common. Not surprisingly, boys are affected two or three times more commonly than girls. The severity of the injuries extends from simple abrasions, contusions and fractures which can be treated in the outpatient department to severe brain injuries, rupture of organs and life-threatening hemorrhage.

The Child with Multiple Injuries

Multiple injuries endangering life comprise about 15 % of all trauma. We define multiple injuries as severe trauma to at least two organ systems, each of which endangers the child, i. e. a combination of brain injury and rupture of an intra-abdominal organ such as the spleen or liver. Ninety percent of these multiple injuries are incurred in traffic accidents. Multiple injuries occur most commonly at the age children begin school. Eighty percent of these injuries occur passively, i. e. the child is run over by a vehicle. In only 20 % is the child actively engaged while travelling in a car, while riding a bicycle, etc. The number of multiply injured children has paralleled the increase in road traffic. These injuries occur most frequently during the late afternoon or early evening and are especially common during the weekend. They are most frequent during summer and least common in winter.

The mortality of children with multiple injuries is high, from 15 % to 20 % in large series. An additional 20 % suffer more or less grave sequelae. The most common cause of death is brain injury, accounting for 80 % of all deaths; 20 % die of hemorrhagic shock, often before they have been admitted to hospital.

Life-saving initial management at the site of the accident, immediate transport to hospital and correct emergency treatment in hospital are vital to the survival and the quality of life of the injured child. Management of the various injured organ systems will be discussed separately below.

The Child with Multiple System Trauma

P. DANGEL

As in every life-endangering trauma situation adequate respiration must be the first priority. If the child is unconscious he is positioned prone to assure upper airway patency. In the absence of swallowing, gagging and cough reflexes, intubation should be carried out without delay. Even if the child makes respiratory efforts artificial respiration should be instituted. Causes of insufficient respiration are: head injuries with cerebral contusion, cerebral edema or hemorrhage, aspiration of stomach contents or blood, pneumothorax, hemothorax, pain secondary to fractures of the ribs, injuries of the upper abdomen, unstable thorax with multiple rib fractures, and laceration of the lung and bronchus. Children with perforating injuries of the thorax and hemorrhage into the tracheobronchial tree should be positioned on their side with the injured lung down to prevent aspiration into the healthy lung.

Secondly, the patient's circulation must be assessed. An intravenous infusion is started immediately to treat shock. The state of the circulation is monitored at short intervals. If necessary, central venous pressure is measured (see Chapter 3). External hemorrhage is controlled, if necessary by direct pressure. Shock without any external injuries always raises the suspicion of occult hemorrhage into the abdominal or thoracic cavities. Except in the newborn, head injuries per se never cause shock. On the other hand, unconsciousness is not caused by shock but by intracranial injury. Consciousness is lost only in the very terminal phases of shock.

Children with multiple trauma demand an organized evaluation based on priorities which roughly follow these guidelines:

1) Restore respiration.

2) Restore circulation.

3) Evaluate the central nervous system.

4) Evaluate the gastrointestinal system.

5) Evaluate the urological system.

6) Evaluate the muscles, skin and skeleton.

Every traumatized child must be examined for disturbances of the central nervous system. Coma is a late sign. Apathy, irritability, restlessness and excitement are signs of hypoxia secondary to deficient cerebral circulation. Unconscious patients are best transported lying on their side; one must consider the possibility of a spinal fracture, and move the patient with care. Cerebral injury is excluded only if the patient had no temporary unconsciousness, no disorientation, no retrograde amnesia and if the neurological examination shows no hemiparalysis, pupil difference, facial paralysis or pathological reflexes. When necessary, clinical examination is confirmed by echoencephalography and carotid angiography.

Respiration, circulation and consciousness are monitored repeatedly during the first few hours. Analgesics may mask disturbances of consciousness, and are often contraindicated until the extent of injury has been fully assessed.

Emergency treatment of a polytraumatized patient does not require many laboratory examinations. Hemoglobin and hematocrit should be determined at four-hour intervals. The younger the patient, the quicker he compensates for blood loss. A falling hemoglobin is therefore indicative of occult hemorrhage. The amount of urine excreted is measured every hour. Hematomas are looked for. Blood gases are obtained whenever even slight respiratory disturbances are found and in all children in shock. Crossmatching of blood is a wise precaution to take, although most cases of shock can initially be treated with Ringer's lactate or plasma (5 % albumin solution).

One should never forget the psychological management of the child with multiple injuries, not to speak of the psychological trauma to the distraught parents. Excitement of doctors and nurses triggered by the admission of a major trauma patient must be minimized.

Head Injuries

P. P. RICKHAM

Head injuries are very common in childhood. Over half the deaths due to trauma in childhood are due to head injuries; unfortunately, because of the increase in road traffic, this type of injury becomes more frequent every year. Only an outline of the more common types of injuries will be discussed here, special emphasis being given to findings which are typical for children.

Neonatal Head injuries

Intracranial hemorrhage from trauma secondary to a difficult or precipitous labor is common. Attacks of apnea, dyspnea, pallor, limpness or convulsions, profuse vomiting which may be bile-stained and a tense fontanelle often indicate the correct diagnosis, which may be confirmed by obtaining blood-stained cerebrospinal fluid by tap. Treatment centers around sedation and nursing the patient in an oxygen-enriched atmosphere. At times tracheal intubation and artificial respiration with a mechanical respirator may be required. The prognosis must be very guarded, as severe permanent neurological damage often results. It is wrong to keep a newborn with a severe intracranial hemorrhage alive by artificial respiration for prolonged periods, especially when the electroencephalogram shows cessation of all activities.

Subdural or Subarachnoid Hematoma

This condition also occurs in newborn infants. The signs are often non-specific: failure to thrive, occasional vomiting, a slightly elevated temperature and a bulging fontanelle. Diagnosis is confirmed by aspirating old blood or xanthochromic fluid through a needle inserted into the subarachnoid space at the lateral angle of the anterior fontanelle.

Treatment

Treatment consists of repeatedly aspirating the hematoma. Open operation is only resorted to if this simpler treatment fails.

Cephalhematoma

This is a subperiosteal hemorrhage producing a firm mass which is confined to one cranial bone (Fig. 22.1). It is often associated with a forceps delivery. It does not require any treatment as the blood will absorb in time.

Depressed Fracture

The bones may be indented without actually breaking (Fig. 22.2). Treatment consists of elevating the bone, but some of these fractures heal spontaneously.

Head Injuries in Older Infants and Children

Clinical picture

The symptoms of head injuries in children beyond infancy are not markedly different from that observed in adults (see adult textbook of surgery). The child's reactions tend to be more vigorous. Vomiting, high temperature, convulsions and shock are frequently observed

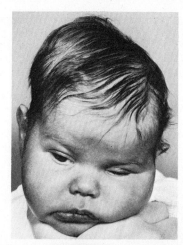

Fig. 22.1. Newborn infant with large, right-sided cephalhematoma

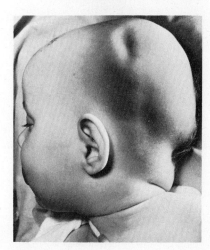

Fig. 22.2. Newborn infant with indentation of left parietal bone

even after relatively trivial intracranial trauma. Localizing signs are at times more difficult to elicit than in adults, and even a short lapse of consciousness may be associated with major intracranial damage. As in adults, one finds all degrees of consciousness from the deeply comatose flaccid child with stertorous breathing who does not react to external stimuli and who has fixed, dilated pupils to the apparently perfectly normal patient. Retrograde amnesia is uncommon in young children.

Diagnosis and Points of Management

The child's general condition must be assessed. Shock is treated (see above) although blood transfusions are given with caution as they may induce a fresh intracranial hemorrhage. Care is taken to exclude any serious trauma and hemorrhage elsewhere in the body (abdomen, thorax, limbs). Maintaining a patent airway is the most fundamental requirement of managing the unconscious patient, who is especially vulnerable to aspiration of vomitus or blood. The child should therefore be nursed flat lying on his side. Sometimes a plastic oral airway is required, and rarely an endotracheal tube must be passed. Hyperthermia and convulsions are treated by cooling and anticonvulsant medication respectively. A detailed neurological examination must of course be carried out. Fractures of the base of the skull may produce bleeding into the retro-orbital space (Fig. 22.3), pharynx, nose or from the ear.

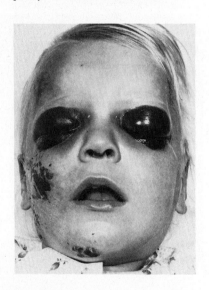

Fig. 22.3. Child with fracture of the base of the skull and bleeding into both retro-orbital spaces

Radiography

Roentgenograms

Roentgenograms should be taken in all suspected cases of skull fractures (Fig. 22.4), although the discovery of many of the minor fissure fractures of the vault is only of medico-legal importance.

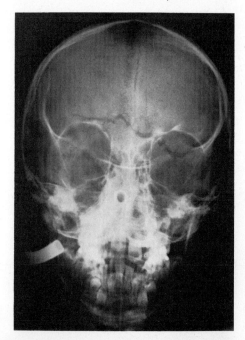

Fig. 22.4.
Roentgenogram of skull showing a widely fissured fracture.

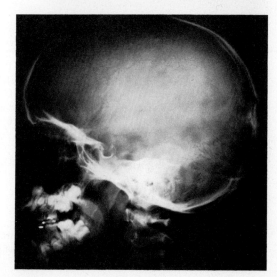

Fig. 22.5.
Tangential radiograph of skull showing depressed fracture in the region of the lambdoid suture

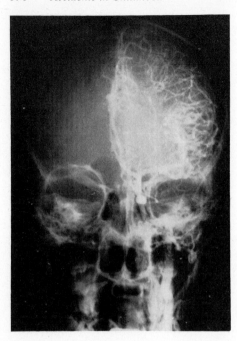

Fig. 22.6.
Cerebral angiogram
showing large subarach-
noid hemorrhage; the
vessels of the left parietal
cerebral cortex are dis-
placed inwards leaving a
space between the inner
table of the parietal bone
and the cortex

Further, small children may have severe intracranial damage without
any radiographic evidence of skull fracture, because the elastic skull
bones may indent on impact and snap back into place without
fracture, but still injure the underlying brain. Depressed fractures
are best outlined by tangential radiographs of the skull (Fig. 22.5).
Fractures of the base of the skull are often difficult to demonstrate
by radiography. In all cases of suspected intracranial hemorrhage a
cerebral angiogram should be performed (Fig. 22.6).

Conditions Necessitating Special Treatment

Depressed Fractures

Here the table of the skull is depressed below the surface, often
injuring the underlying dura mater and brain. In children early
operation, elevating the depressed bony fragments and repairing the
torn dura is always indicated. Untreated depressed fractures in children often produce focal epilepsy later on.

Extradural Hemorrhage

Intracranial hemorrhage from an extradural vessel is uncommon in childhood. There is a short period of unconsciousness after injury which in children may last only for a few seconds. This is followed by a "lucid interval" of full consciousness or improving consciousness succeeded by a rapid relapse. The classical signs of middle meningeal artery hemorrhage are a fixed dilated pupil on the side of the hemorrhage with muscular weakness and/or fits on the opposite side; regrettably, this is uncommonly seen in a pure form. It is a matter of utmost urgency to open the patient's skull, clear out the extradural blood clot and stop the bleeding. In children, extradural clots originate more commonly from diploic veins. As the pressure in these veins is low, the signs and symptoms of this type of extradural hemorrhage are sometimes vague and may take many hours to develop.

Subdural (Subarachnoid) Hemorrhage

Subdural bleeding occurs from tears in the large veins which overlie the convolutions of the brain or traverse the subdural space. A blood clot forms, but since the pressure in the veins is very low, bleeding will soon stop by itself without any immediate signs of increased intracranial pressure. The blood corpuscles in the center of the clot lyse, forming a highly concentrated osmotic solution surrounded by a semipermeable membrane. Water flows into the clot by osmotic pressure from the surrounding cerebrospinal fluid and the clot gradually expands. This expanding clot will slowly cause signs of increased intracranial pressure (headaches, vomiting, a slow pulse, etc.). In older infants and children these symptoms gradually develop after an initial period of concussion and a "lucid interval" of full consciousness which often lasts for many days or weeks. Treatment consists of evacuating the clot and in long-standing cases removing the semipermeable membrane as well (Fig. 22.7).

Compound Fractures of the Skull

Open fractures of the vault of the skull should be treated like any other open wound by débridement and removal of foreign material and dead tissue, including brain. The scalp is sutured, and the wound drained. This often leaves a bony defect which may have to be replaced by a plastic prothesis later on.

Open fractures of the base of the skull are often difficult to diagnose. In addition to the signs enumerated above, escape of cerebrospinal fluid from the nose, pharynx or middle ear should suggest diagnosis. Unfortunately, it is often impossible to distinguish pure blood

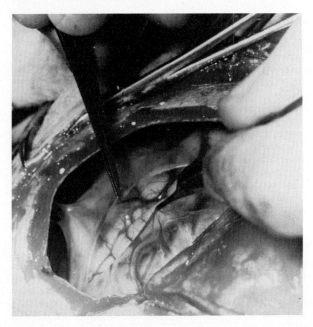

Fig. 22.7. Craniotomy for removal of membrane surrounding a chronic subarachnoidal hematoma. The translucent membrane has been incised and is held with forceps

from blood admixed with cerebrospinal fluid draining from the wound. Therefore, every basal skull fracture should be treated as an open fracture by rest in bed and antibiotics for at least three weeks. Only when the cerebrospinal fluid discharge persists is it necessary to surgically close the rent in the dura.

Cerebral Edema

This occurs either secondary to brain trauma or more commonly secondary to hypoxia following brain trauma. Signs of increased intracranial pressure often come on very rapidly. Intravenous administration of 30 % urea, mannitol or glucocorticoids has proved to be very effective in reducing cerebral edema. These solutions must be administered with great care as they produce marked shrinkage of the brain which may initiate a renewed hemorrhage. It is best to give these solutions during operation while the brain is under direct vision and possibly for the first 24—48 hours after operation.

General Treatment

The special points of treatment have been discussed above. The child with a head injury should be nursed in a quiet, semidarkened room until signs of cerebral irritation have disappeared. The unconscious child needs constant nursing care, special attention being devoted to maintaining an open airway to obviate inhalation of vomitus, mucus and blood (electric sucker at the bedside). Adequate nutrition must be provided (intravenous at first, later by gavage) bedsores prevented, feces and urine disposed of, etc.

Patients with closed head injuries require careful periodic neurological assessment to detect those who require surgical treatment. General worsening of the neurological status or the appearance of localizing signs favor operation, whereas gradual neurological improvement favors conservative treatment. Cerebral angiography and (as a last resort) drilling exploratory burr holes through the skull occasionally help to confirm the diagnosis of suspected intracranial hemorrhage.

All patients with open head injuries require antibiotics for at least two or three weeks.

Prognosis

On the whole, the prognosis for children with head injuries is better than for adults. Even children with lengthy unconsciousness and initially severe paralysis may recover virtually completely. The younger the child, the better the prognosis. Recovery may be prolonged and necessitates the help of physiotherapists, play therapists, teachers and parents, not to speak of the full cooperation of the patient. Fortunately, psychological disturbances following head injuries are uncommon in children; they tend to occur in children with considerable stress in the family environment.

Burns

M. Lehner

A burn is caused by thermal injury to body tissues, generally skin, which partly or completely destroys tissue. Severe burns produce temporary disturbances of circulation (shock), water and electrolyte equilibrium and metabolism, and may impair defense mechanisms against infection.

A burn produces basically the same injury in children as in adults, but in children differences in the response to trauma necessitate a different approach to treatment. In addition, the psychological make-up peculiar to the burned child must also be taken into account.

History of the Accident

Each age group has a rather typical setting in which burn injuries occur. Most burns in infants are caused by hot plates and hot water

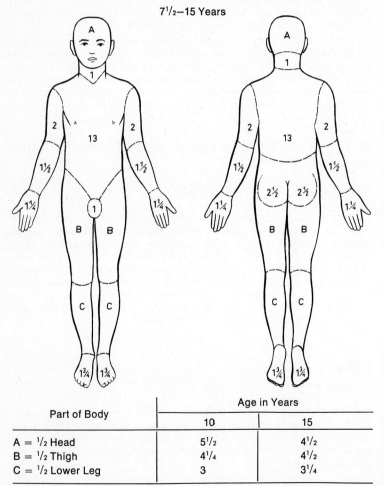

Part of Body	Age in Years	
	10	15
A = ½ Head	5½	4½
B = ½ Thigh	4¼	4½
C = ½ Lower Leg	3	3¼

Fig. 22.8 a).   Percentages of body surface in older children

bottles. Small children (toddlers) seem predisposed to scalds caused by upsetting or tripping over containers with hot water; also, electrical burns are incurred when they play with electric cords and plugs. Flame burns and explosions are more common in school age children.

Assessment of the Burn

The severity of a burn or scald is assessed according to both its area and depth.

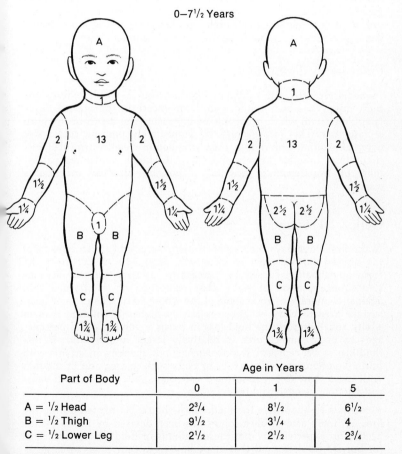

0–7½ Years

Part of Body	Age in Years		
	0	1	5
A = ½ Head	2¾	8½	6½
B = ½ Thigh	9½	3¼	4
C = ½ Lower Leg	2½	2½	2¾

Fig. 22.8 b). Percentages of body surface in infants and young children

The burn area is expressed in percentage of total body surface area. The usual "rule of nine" used for estimating body surface area in adults is useless in children, as proportions of the body alter with growth. Fig. 22.8 a, b diagramatically estimates body surface area in different childhood age groups.

The depth of a burn is described in degrees. A first degree burn produces vesicles and erythema and is the most minor thermal injury. A second degree burn results in partial necrosis, whereas the third degree burn induces complete dermal necrosis. A fourth degree burn destroys skin plus tissue which underlies the skin. Flame injury generally causes third degree burns. Scalds which in adults cause only first or second degree burns are likely to produce much deeper damage in infants, probably because of their thinner skin.

Emergency Treatment

Immediately after the offending thermal source which induces the burn injury has been withdrawn, temperature in the burned tissue is still elevated, which is capable of increasing the depth of the burn still further. This is prevented by immediately pouring cold water over the wound. The child is then wrapped in clean, warm blankets. If the burn involves more than 8 % of the body surface the patient must be transferred to hospital, if possible after an infusion is started.

General Treatment

In the first three days the loss of protein, water and electrolytes from the burned surface must be effectively dealt with. It occurs in the form of exudation caused by increase in capillary permeability, increased evaporation of water (less protection of the burned skin against evaporation) and edema of the whole body. The ratio of body surface area to body weight is relatively higher in children than in adults and therefore the fluid loss in burns involving equal percentages of body surface area is relatively larger in the child. If this fluid loss is not replaced, hypovolemic shock develops in infants with burns involving more than 8 % of body surface area and in children with more than 10 %. Associated with the shock is peripheral vasoconstriction, acidosis and renal failure.

A formula to quantitate the fluid which should be infused during the first 24 hours after a burn injury has been devised by Evans (Table 22.1). Our experience is that these amounts of fluid are not sufficient for burned children, and that amounts two to four times as large as those recommended by Evans are required. Table 22.2 documents the

Table 22.1.   **Evans' Rule**

Fluid Replacement in the First 24 Hours

2 ml/kg/%	of the burned surface
half	as electrolyte infusion
half	as colloid infusion (plasma)

Table 22.2.   **Minimal Fluid Replacement in the First 24 Hours in Children**

4 ml/kg/%	of the burned surface
$2/3$	as Ringer's lactate or Ringer's bicarbonate*
$1/3$	as Plasma

in addition to the normal fluid requirements of:

$$1800 \text{ ml/m}^2$$

$1/4$ per os	
The rest:	NaCl 0.9 % one part
	glucose 10 % four parts

* Composition of Ringer's bicarbonate solution:

Na^+	134 mEq/L
K^+	4 mEq/L
Cl^-	111 mEq/L
HCO_3^-	27 mEq/L

minimal amounts which have to be given to children during the first 24 hours after a major burn. The infused fluid rate is increased with tachycardia, fall of blood pressure or venous pressure, urine production less than 1 ml per kg per hour, elevation of urine specific gravity as well as with evidence of poor peripheral circulation. It must be stressed again that the fluid amounts shown in Table 22.2 are minimum quantities and must be increased whenever there are signs of circulatory failure.

Today it should be possible to avoid death from burn shock provided sufficient fluid is infused and the circulation is controlled. Pulmonary edema hardly ever occurs unless the lungs have been injured by smoke inhalation or previous disease. Maintenance of good peripheral circulation is the best precaution against cerebral edema. Renal failure has become extremely rare since adequate fluid replacement has been provided and if it occurs it is treated by dialysis.

Severe burns cause destruction of erythrocytes leading to anemia and edema which is treated by blood transfusions.

Burns of the face may produce edema of the larynx during the first few hours or days, and intubation may become necessary to assure adequate airway.

Inhalation of smoke damages bronchial mucosa and alveoli, resulting in pneumonia and pulmonary edema. Antibiotics are given for the pneumonia and positive pressure respiration improves the pulmonary edema.

Derangements in organic function and in metabolism are usually reversible. A negative nitrogen balance may develop from poor intake and loss of proteins from the burn which may deplete protein reserves. This is partly prevented by giving intravenous proteins and glucose or tube feeding a protein-rich diet.

Major loss of body heat from evaporation is minimized by nursing the patient in a warm and moist atmosphere.

There is danger of tetanus with every burn and tetanus prophylaxis must be administered.

A major burn may temporarily impair the victim's defence mechanism against infection. This factor, coupled with bacterial colonization of the burned surface may lead to septic complications. Frequent bacteriological culture of the burn surface and blood are therefore necessary. If septicemia occurs, appropriate parenteral antibiotics are given. Surface infection of the burn, however, should be treated only locally, as antibiotics are of little use in tissues with a poor circulation.

Local Treatment

The aim of local burn treatment is to combat infection and promote rapid epithelization.

Burned tissue is invaded by bacteria within 24 hours. The most dreaded organism is Pseudomonas. Infection by viruses and fungi is rare.

If the number of bacteria increases beyond 10^5 per gram of tissue there is danger that the burn may worsen because of destruction of still viable epithelial cells by leukocytes and bacteria. Thus, a second degree burn may be converted to a third degree burn because of infection. Quite apart from this, an infected burn may lead to septicemia and gravely endanger the patient's life.

The most important part of any treatment of a burn is the removal of necrotic material (burn eschar) as quickly as possible, because this material constitutes an ideal medium for bacterial growth. Immediately after the accident the blisters are removed under general anesthesia. Daily baths or showers remove further necrotic material. In patients with third degree burns the eschar is removed (debrided) under general anesthesia within the first two to three weeks. Necrosis from electric burns is best excised immediately as it extends deeply into the tissues and subsequent infection may worsen the injury.

The most important antiseptics for topical application to the burned surfaces are as follows:

0.5 % **silver nitrate solution** applied in moist dressings. It is a bacteriostatic solution. This has proved its value in children since the moist dressings can be removed without pain. There is, however, a danger of hyponatremia since the hypotonic solution removes ions from the body. Another disadvantage is that the healthy skin, walls, bedclothes, etc. are stained black. It is inadvisable to use silver nitrate in face burns of children as it may be swallowed, causing argyria.

Sulphamyloneacetate (Sulfamylon) in the form of an 11.2 % cream (acid salt of p-amino-methyl-benzol-sulphonamide) also acts as a bacteriostatic agent. It penetrates slightly more into tissues than silver nitrate. Open treatment with this cream is contraindicated since the child has to be constantly tied down. In addition, some patients suffer considerable pain when the cream is applied. Sulphamyloneacetate is absorbed, acting on the kidneys as a carbonic anhydrase inhibitor to produce acidosis.

Betadine (Providone-iodine cream) is a bacteriostatic agent useful in burn dressings. It is especially indicated for treating small burns in outpatients or treating burns of the face.

Unfortunately, silver nitrate and sulphamyloneacetate are ineffective against Pseudomonas. Gentamycin ointment is three times as effective in vitro against Pseudomonas than the other two drugs. 0.5 % of the drug is absorbed. Because there is a danger of resistance forming against Gentamycin, it is used only when Pseudomonas infection has been definitely proved.

Third degree burns are covered by split thickness skin grafts as soon as possible (0.25 to 0.35 mm in thickness). In children with extensive burns it may be life-saving to cover the burned surfaces temporarily with homografts (human skin from a donor) or heterografts (animal skin). Homografts or heterografts must be replaced every four to six days until the patient's own skin is available. This temporary coverage with homo- or heterografts diminishes protein loss from the burn and reduces its bacterial count dramatically.

In a patient with extensive burns, little of his skin may be available for grafting. In these cases the patient's split thickness skin grafts may be diced in a mesh by a special apparatus to then cover at least twice the area which simple split thickness skin grafts will cover. The spaces between the mesh then quickly epithelize.

Psychological Management

A burn is a severe psychological stress for the child. Pain is minimized with the help of short-acting anesthetics and drugs. Play therapy, personnel specialized in entertaining children and daily visits by the parents do much to help the child overcome the psychological trauma.

Later Complications

Hypertrophic scars are common and can be improved by compression bandages with foam rubber. Scar contractures form subsequent to burns of the axilla, neck and flexor surfaces of the joints. They must be treated by plastic operations with or without free skin grafts.

Thoracic and Abdominal Injuries

U. G. STAUFFER

Thoracic Injuries

Penetrating Injuries of the Thorax

Such lesions are rare in childhood. They are caused by gunshot or knife accidents, falls with impaling or penetrating injuries, etc. Each thoracic wound must be very carefully examined clinically and by radiographs. Pneumothorax or hemothorax must be drained if present.

Closed Injuries of the Thorax

Closed injuries are also much rarer in childhood than adulthood, usually occurring as one of multiple severe injuries following traffic accidents. Fractures of the ribs are uncommon because of the great elasticity of the child's rib cage. On the other hand, it is possible for children to suffer injuries to the lungs without rib fractures. Closed chest injuries are often overlooked because of the pre-eminence of other associated injuries, e. g. craniocerebral injuries, intra-abdominal hemorrhage, etc. In a patient with multiple trauma a chest radiograph should always be taken (Fig. 22.9).

Pulmonary Contusion (Traumatic Asphyxia)

This is caused by a sudden rise in intrathoracic pressure secondary to compression of the thorax while the glottis is reflexly closed. Areas of pulmonary hemorrhage occur, which are reflected radiographically by patchy areas of radio density comparable to the picture of bronchopneumonia. A large, isolated hemorrhage shows as a well-defined shadow. Tachypnea, dyspnea and in severe cases cyanosis highlight the clinical picture of acute pulmonary contusion. The condition usually disappears spontaneously within a few days and operation is not indicated. Analgesics are given for associated fractures of the ribs and antibiotics are begun in severe cases of pulmonary contusion because of the danger of a super-added infection. Oxygen is indicated for the severely afflicted child with cyanosis.

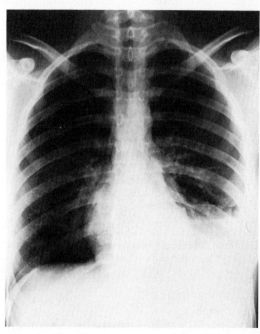

Fig. 22.9. Pneumohematothorax (left) in 10-year-old boy (traffic accident). Small apical pneumothorax (right). Fractures of 7th to 10th left ribs. Aspiration produced 500 ml of blood. Bilateral pleural drainage instituted

Laceration of the Lung

This occurs by lung injury incurred either directly by a sharp object such as the end of a broken rib, or secondary to sudden compression by the elastic thoracic cage.

The clinical picture depends on the severity and the type of injury and the complications which may arise (pulmonary hemorrhage, pneumothorax, hemothorax): shock, dyspnea, tachypnea and cyanosis. Hemoptysis and surgical emphysema are often observed. If there are associated rib fractures, breathing will be painful. The symptoms of other associated injuries frequently confuse the picture.

Treatment

Treatment consists in combating shock, tube drainage of pneumothorax or hemothorax, administering analgesics, antibiotics and at times oxygen. If these measures do not stabilize the patient, thoracotomy must be considered: small lacerations are oversewn, but larger lacerations require resecting the involved pulmonary segment or lobe. In most cases, however, conservative treatment suffices.

Traumatic Diaphragmatic Rupture

Although rare, knowledge of its possibility may be life-saving. It occurs only in patients with multiple injuries and is caused by a sudden severe change in the intrathoracic or intra-abdominal pressure. Because the liver cushions the right hemidiaphragm, traumatic rupture generally occurs on the left side.

Clinically, one finds a child with severe abdominal injuries who remains in shock with associated respiratory symptoms such as dyspnea, tachypnea and cyanosis. Pain in the tip of the shoulder (reflex pain transmitted via the phrenic nerve) is very characteristic. Chest radiographs reveal absence of the regular contour of the involved diaphragm; in addition, intestinal loops may be observed in the pleural cavity which often induce a contralateral shift of the mediastinal structures. At times the radiographic picture is less typical, and in the differential diagnosis eventration of the diaphragm and pulmonary atelectasis may be considered. Correct diagnosis and immediate laparotomy with repair of the tear may be life-saving.

Abdominal Injuries

Penetrating Wounds of the Abdomen

Wounds of this type are also rare in children, and occur from missiles or stab injuries (knives, arrows, branches, etc.). Every penetrating abdominal wound necessitates careful exploration of the wound under general anesthesia, and laparotomy if an internal injury cannot be excluded.

Closed Abdominal Injuries

Closed abdominal injuries occur in 2 %/0 to 5 %/0 of all childhood trauma. Statistically, they are most apt to occur between the 6th and the 8th years of life, or between the 14th and the 16th years. Boys are three times as commonly affected as girls. If the abdominal trauma is an isolated injury, it is usually (80 %/0) caused by a fall over a hard object, i. e. the bar of a bicycle, a stone, the edge of a table, etc. In only 20 %/0 is it caused by a traffic accident. However, in children with multiple injuries in addition to an abdominal injury, traffic accidents are by far the most common cause (60 %/0). Further, diagnosis may be very difficult, as the symptoms of the abdominal injury may be overshadowed by trauma to other major body systems. It is therefore most important that every child with multiple injuries has abdominal trauma specifically excluded. Timely diagnosis may be lifesaving.

Clinical Picture

An exact description of the accident (e. g. a fall onto a sharp edge or over the handlebar of a bicycle) as well as visible signs such as scratches, hematomas and contusions are important. Half the victims suffer only injury to the abdominal wall, but the other half harbor trauma to one or more intra-abdominal organs which require operation. Rupture or tearing of solid viscera (spleen, liver, kidney) represents the most common complication of severe abdominal injury producing hemorrhage which may either be intra- or extraperitoneal. Injuries to hollow viscera (colon, small intestine and urinary bladder) are less common, as are injuries of the pancreas. The question of injury to an intra-abdominal organ may be very difficult, occasionally necessitating exploratory laparotomy to answer.

Massive intra-abdominal hemorrhage is suggested by circulatory collapse which occurs in spite of intravenous therapy, localized abdominal tenderness and rigidity, pain in the left or the right shoulder tip, a falling hemoglobin concentration and an increase in abdominal circumference. Anteroposterior and lateral radiographs of the abdomen in the erect position may show fluid collections (hemorrhage) or free air beneath the diaphragm (rupture of GI tract). The urine must always be examined in patients with abdominal trauma, if necessary by catheterization; hematuria suggests urinary tract injury. Pelvis fractures also point toward injury to the lower urinary tract.

If the diagnosis is in doubt, the patient is examined repeatedly at short intervals by the same physician. Leukocytosis is of little diagnostic value, since it also occurs in cases with simple contusion of the abdominal wall as well as injuries to other parts of the body. Paracentesis may be very useful in the doubtful case. Aspiration of blood or intestinal contents demands immediate laparotomy. If the aspiration is negative, the peritoneal cavity is lavaged with 100 to 500 ml of warm, normal saline (depending on the age of the child); if the saline returns stained with blood or intestinal content, laparotomy is indicated. If the saline contains numerous leukocytes, a covered perforation should be suspected. Aspiration combined with peritoneal lavage will give the diagnosis in the majority of cases.

Contusion of the Abdominal Wall

The trauma is usually less severe than in cases with injuries to intra-abdominal organs, but at first there may be much tenderness and abdominal rigidity. The patient is frequently slightly shocked, but responds rapidly to intravenous therapy. The injury may cause a hematoma of the abdominal wall, a muscle or fascial tear, etc. Symptoms usually disappear within a few days.

Ruptured Spleen

This is the most common intra-abdominal organ to be injured by closed abdominal trauma. As the spleen contains a lot of blood and has only a thin capsule, rupture occurs relatively easily. The spleen is only partially protected by the lower left ribs which are very elastic in children. It is possible for the spleen to rupture in a large, heavy, newborn infant following a difficult labor.

Older children with splenic rupture usually harbor a hematoma or abrasion of the left upper abdominal quadrant, as well as tenderness and rigidity. Pain in the tip of the left shoulder is of special diagnostic value (seen in about 15 % of patients). There will be signs of shock secondary to hemorrhage. Occasionally a small tear may initially be tamponaded by a thrombus or omentum; these patients have hardly any complaints during the first few days, until they suddenly show all the signs of massive hemorrhage (delayed rupture of the spleen) when the tampon effect dissipates.

Treatment

In the case of ruptured spleen treatment consists of splenectomy. Children over five years of age have no disabilities following the operation, but below this age the spleen still plays a role in the immunological defense against infection. Therefore, in children below five years of age an attempt should be made to oversew the tear.

If the splenic rupture is an isolated injury, the prognosis is favorable with a postoperative mortality in the neighborhood of 1 %.

Rupture of the Liver

Because of its size and position the liver has little chance to escape from blunt injury to the right hypochondrium. The liver in children is relatively larger than in adults, and is less protected by the more elastic costal margin. Especially in newborns the liver takes up a disproportionately large amount of space within the peritoneal cavity; not surprisingly, rupture of the liver is the most common cause of intraperitoneal hemorrhage in the newborn. After a silent interval of between two and four days after birth there develops insidiously a progressively worsening state of shock, a drop in the hemoglobin concentration and increase in abdominal circumference. The mortality of neonatal hepatic rupture is high.

In older children the liver is the second most common intra-abdominal organ injured by closed trauma (the spleen is first). The right lobe of the liver is less well protected than the left, and is more commonly injured. All degrees of injury are seen, from small subcapsular hematomas to superficial tears to deep lacerations and avulsion of entire segments of the liver.

Shock, tenderness and rigidity in the right upper abdominal quadrant dominate the clinical scene, occasionally associated with gasping respiration and pain referred to the tip of the right shoulder.

Treatment

Hepatic lacerations are sutured, packed or drained, as appropriate; major avulsed segments are resected and drained. In contrast to adults with hepatic injury, postoperative complications like secondary hemorrhage, liver abscess, biliary fistula, etc., are relatively rare in children. Nevertheless, the mortality is high and relates directly to associated injuries, varying in large series from 10 % to 60 %.

Urinary Tract Injuries

Rupture of the Kidney

The kidneys in children are relatively larger and heavier than in adults, and are protected by less perirenal fat. Occasionally only relatively slight trauma ruptures a kidney in a child. The most characteristic sign of a ruptured kidney is hematuria; its absence practically excludes a severe injury to the kidney or lower urinary tract, with the exception of patients with total avulsion of the ureter. Abrasions, hematomas, tenderness and pain in the region of the costovertebral angle are common external signs of renal injury.

Every patient with either macroscopic or microscopic hematuria must have urologic investigation. Usually a plain radiograph of the abdomen and an intravenous pyelogram are all that are necessary. The abdominal radiograph may show an enlarged renal shadow or haziness of the psoas shadow (Fig. 22.10). The intravenous pyelogram often documents the extent of the injuries and is therefore very important when considering therapy. It also occasionally reveals a previously unknown malformation of the kidneys, i. e. a hydronephrosis, and ascertains function of the contralateral (uninjured) kidney.

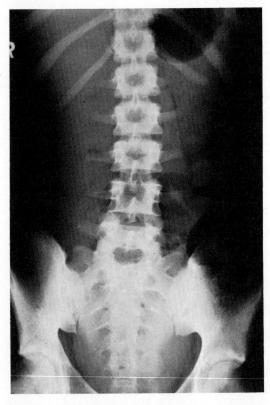

Fig. 22.10.
Right-sided rupture of kidney in 14-year-old girl (traffic accident). Plain abdominal radiograph shows protective scoliosis and absent psoas shadow

Treatment

A renal laceration which extends into the renal pelvis will extrude the contrast medium from the intravenous pyelogram into the perirenal tissues (Fig. 22.11). If the patient's general state is stable, immediate operation is indicated, where the surgeon concentrates on preserving renal tissue. Only non-vital sequestrated renal segments are removed. If the pyelogram shows only that the renal pelvis is displaced by

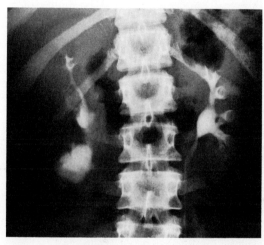

Fig. 22.11. Intravenous pyelogram in same patient as in Fig. 22.10. Only the upper calices can be seen on the right. There is extravasated contrast medium in the neighborhood of the lower renal pole. The ureter is not seen. At operation it was found that the lower pole of the right kidney and the ureter had been torn off. It was possible to save the upper pole and anastomose it to the ureter

a perirenal hematoma, non-surgical supportive treatment is indicated, including antibiotics to prevent a superadded infection. In doubtful cases, selective renal angiography may be helpful. During convalescence from a renal injury, serial pyelographs are obtained at intervals to detect complications such as strictures due to scar tissue and atrophic changes in the kidney.

Injuries to the Bladder and Urethra

Fortunately, injuries to the bladder and urethra of children are relatively rare, usually associated with fractures of the pelvis and multiple injuries following traffic accidents. Massive hematuria and pain on micturition, or anuria and a suprapubic swelling, are the presenting complaints.

Treatment

This depends on the severity of the injury. If necessary, a suprapubic catheter must be inserted. Urethral catheters splint the injured urethra. It is often difficult to reconstruct a urethra which has been completely avulsed.

Intestinal Injuries

Intestinal injuries are rarer than injuries of solid intra-abdominal organs, occurring only in about 5 % of all intra-abdominal injuries. They are caused by sudden, localized trauma applied to the abdominal wall. In children the muscles and supporting tissue of the abdominal wall are relatively thin and not enshrouded by much fat, offering relatively little protection to the underlying organs. As the distance between the abdominal wall and the spine is relatively short, compression injuries of intestine and pancreas can occur. Bowel fixed by natural (ligament of Treitz, mesosigmoid) or acquired adhesions is more vulnerable to injury.

Signs of peritonitis usually herald intestinal trauma with perforation, plain upright radiograph of the abdomen documenting the classical collection of air beneath the diaphragm. Perforation is

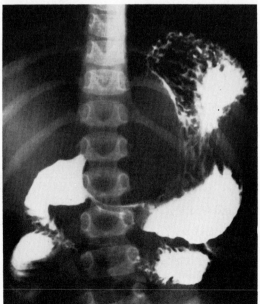

a

Fig. 22.12.
Traumatic pseudocyst of the pancreas in 7-year-old boy who had fallen over his tricycle.
Admitted to hospital 8 weeks after accident with increasing distention of abdomen, vomiting and loss of appetite. Barium meal;
a) A—P view. The lesser curvature is stretched over the pseudocyst and the stomach displaced laterally;
b) Lateral view. The stomach is pushed forward by the cyst

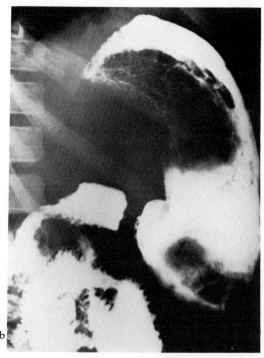

b

most common in the upper jejunum and in the retroperitoneal terminal portion of the duodenum because this part of the bowel is relatively fixed and therefore does not shift away from a directly applied force. The diagnosis of retroperitoneal intestinal rupture may be difficult. There are only localized signs of peritonitis and there is no air under the diaphragm on radiography. Occasionally an intramural hematoma of the duodenum causes intestinal obstruction.

Treatment

Intestinal injuries are treated by laparotomy, closure of the perforation and drainage of the peritoneal cavity.

Pancreatic Injuries

These are the rarest type of intra-abdominal injury, comprising 1 % to 2 % of the total. The history of trauma is usually quite typical: a fall over the handlebar of a bicycle or tricycle, or across a gym bar.

The clinical picture is rarely characteristic, but includes severe shock and indefinite abdominal symptoms. After a short symptom-free interval the child complains of pain around the waist radiating into both shoulders. Examination discloses tenderness and rigidity in the epigastric and hypogastric regions. The serum and urinary amylase are frequently, but not always, elevated.

Treatment

If the patient's general condition permits, laparotomy is indicated if there is marked suspicion of severe pancreatic injury. Incomplete rupture of the pancreas is treated by suture of the capsule and drainage; an avulsed segment requires terminal pancreatectomy. Milder pancreatic injury responds to non-surgical supportive care. A posttraumatic pancreatic pseudocyst may develop days, weeks or months after the original injury. The presenting complaint is usually increasing abdominal distention with a palpable epigastric mass. Pseudocysts of the pancreas may reach enormous proportions (Fig. 22.12 a, b). Treatment consists either of external drainage of the cyst (marsupialization) or preferably internal drainage into the stomach (cystogastrostomy) or jejunum (cystojejunostomy).

Fractures

U. G. STAUFFER

In addition to different locations, types and causes, fractures in children differ from those in adults in the following ways:

1) Fractures in children heal much quicker; the younger the child, the quicker the healing process.
2) Stiffness of joints, rightly feared as a complication of fractures in adults, hardly ever occurs in children even after prolonged immobilization.
3) Pseudoarthrosis and Sudeck's atrophy are extremely rare.
4) Axial, lateral and longitudinal malpositioning are largely compensated by increased growth; rotation malpositions, however, are permanent in children as in adults.

In general, treatment of fractures in children is conservative by closed reduction (manipulation) and immobilization with plaster of Paris casts. Because longitudinal growth in children is so rapid, precise end-to-end apposition of the fracture is unnecessary; in the femur it is even contraindicated. Increase of longitudinal growth after fractures in children up to 12 years of age amounts to 0.5 to

1 cm in the tibia and 1 to 1.5 cm in the femur. When considering this peculiarity of the growing skeleton in the child, a 1 cm shortening of the femur after a fracture can be tolerated easily (Fig. 22.13). Tibial shortening of up to 0.5 cm is tolerated, providing the axial repositioning is satisfactory. The reason for the increased longitudinal growth after fractures is not as yet clear, nor is the extent of the lengthening predictable. It does not depend on the type or site of fracture, nor on the degree of displacement.

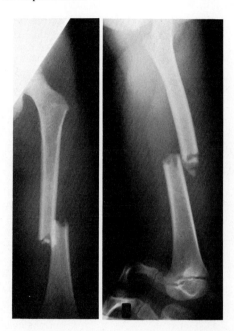

Fig. 22.13. Fracture of the femur of 8-year-old boy; good position with desired shortening of 1 cm

There are several important exceptions to the rule that fractures in children are treated conservatively (by closed reduction): fractures near joints and fractures of the shaft which cannot be reduced satisfactorily because of their location. Rotational malposition of fractures of the shaft must be corrected by operation. Once union occurs with a rotation malpositioning, premature degeneration and arthrosis of the neighboring joints may subsequently develop because of faulty weight bearing.

It is therefore important for the doctor who first treats the patient to know which fractures can be treated by simple conservative closed reduction and which must be operated upon. Table 22.3 summarizes

Table 22.3.   **Summary of Management of Fractures in Childhood**

A. Fractures of the Upper Extremities

1. Clavicle	Always conservative (closed). Figure-of-eight bandage 2 to 3 weeks.
2. Proximal humerus	Generally conservative (closed), bandaged to side of chest 1 to 2 weeks; rarely traction, occasionally operative reduction and fixation with Kirschner wires.
3. Shaft of humerus	Generally conservative (closed). Bandage to side of chest for 3 weeks, occasionally extension through olecranon. If radial nerve paralysis: operation.
4. Supracondylar fracture of humerus	
a) uncomplicated case	Reduction with Blount's method, plaster backsplint for 3 weeks, occasional longitudinal tension after Baumann. Operation only if position bad.
b) complicated cases, nerve and circulation damage	Operation.
5. Distal intraarticular fracture of humerus	Usually operation.
6. Radial condyle	Operation.
7. Epicondyle of ulna	Operation only if displacement more than 2 mm.
8. Head of radius	Usually conservative; operation only if angle of displacement more than 60°.
9. Olecranon	Operation only when displaced.
10. Forearm	Usually conservative (plaster backsplint extending to upper arm); rarely operation, fixation with Kirschner wires.
11. Finger	Conservative.

B. Trunk

1. Spine	Conservative (Plaster bed, later corset 4 to 10 weeks).
2. Pelvis	Mainly conservative (4 to 5 weeks bedrest).

C. Fractures of Lower Extremities

1. Neck of femur, Pertrochanteric fracture	Operation.
2. Subtrochanteric	Conservative if possible; operate if there is malposition, rotation (plate and screws).

3. Shaft of femur	Mainly conservative (traction with Kirschner wire 4 to 6 weeks). In older adolescents occasionally operative (plate and screws).
4. Distal femoral epiphysis (incl. separation of epiphysis)	Conservative.
5. Fracture of femoral condyle	Often operation (fixation with Kirschner wires).
6. Patella	
a) no displacement	Conservative immobilization in plaster 4 to 8 weeks.
b) fragments displaced	Operative wiring.
7. Intercondylar eminence	Operate if displaced (screws).
8. Tibial tuberosity	Mainly conservative.
9. Fractures of leg	Mainly conservative (plaster cast extending to thigh for 4 to 7 weeks) Occasionally traction with Kirschner wire for 3 weeks, then plaster cast for 3 to 4 weeks.
10. Fracture of malleolus	Operation if displaced (Aitken II and III).
11. Foot and toes	Conservative; plaster cast up to knee for 2 to 4 weeks.

the more important fractures in childhood and their treatment. Fractures close to joints, especially in the vicinity of the elbow, and the more common fractures of the shaft will be discussed in more detail below.

Postreduction Management of Fractures in Childhood

The postreduction management of children's fractures is basically different from that of adults. Treatment should be as simple as possible. Massage, passive excercises and other physiotherapy measures are usually unnecessary because of the short time of immobilization required and lack of joint stiffness. Forced mobilization of the joints under anesthesia should never be practiced in children. The best physiotherapy is active motion, which gives optimum functional results. Children who are still growing must be followed for lengthy periods, about two to four years; in special cases they must be followed until growth ceases in order to detect secondary deformities, increases of longitudinal growth, etc.

Fractures Near the Joints

We define fractures near joints as fractures which involve the epiphyseal line. If these fractures are not reduced anatomically correctly, premature fusion of the epiphyseal line leads to cessation of growth. If the fracture affects the joint itself and is not completely reduced, arthrosis will subsequently develop. If correct anatomical reduction is not possible with conservative therapy, open reduction and fixation of the fragments must be carried out. Roughly one in ten fractures in childhood affects the epiphyseal line. In the lower extremities these are mainly fractures of the malleolar region, more rarely fractures of the distal end of the femur; in the upper extremities they encompass fractures of the proximal end of the humerus or distal end of radius and ulna. Fractures round the elbow joint constitute a special problem.

The choice between conservative and operative management of fractures involving joints has been greatly facilitated by the classification devised by Aitken (Fig. 22.14). Simple separation of the epiphysis (Fig. 22.15) ("Aitken O") demands solely a reasonable reduction, and virtually never demands open operation; prognosis is good and

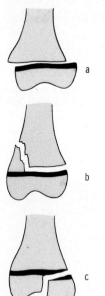

a) "Aitken 0". Separation of epiphysis;
b) "Aitken I". The epiphysial line is not involved;
c) "Aitken II". The fracture goes through the epiphyseal line into the joint;

Fig. 22.14.   Classification of joint fractures according to Aitken:

d) "Aitken III". The fracture runs from the metaphysis through the epiphyseal line and through
the epiphysis into the joint;
e) "Aitken IV". Longitudinal compression of the
epiphysis

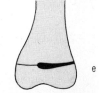

growth disturbances do not occur. The same holds true for an
Aitken I fracture (Fig. 22.16, 22.17).

In an Aitken II fracture, the epiphysis is involved and the fracture
line traverses the epiphyseal line. Absolutely correct anatomical
alignment is essential if growth of bony bridges across the epiphyseal

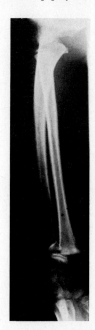

Fig. 22.15. Fracture of radius and ulna of 7-year-
old boy. Separation of distal epiphysis of radius
(Aitken 0) and distal fracture of ulna (Aitken I)

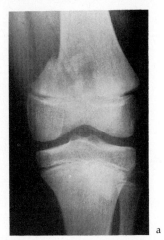
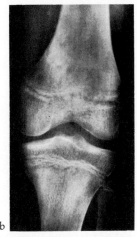

a   b

Fig. 22.16.   Aitken I fracture of distal femur of 10-year-old boy: a) On admission; b) After 6 weeks immobilization in plaster of Paris

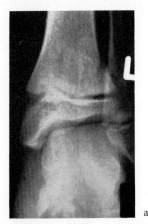
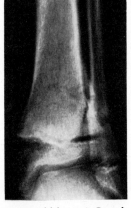

a   b

Fig. 22.17.   Aitken II fracture of distal tibia of 12-year-old boy. a) On admission; b) After 6 weeks immobilization in plaster of Paris

line and subsequent growth disturbances are to be avoided. If this is impossible by closed methods, operation is indicated (Fig. 22.18).

Aitken III fractures are usually treated by open operation unless there is no displacement of the fragments (Fig. 22.19). Kirschner wires and screws are used to fix the fragments; they hold well in the

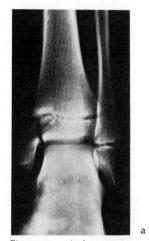 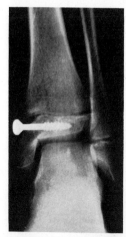

a   b

Fig. 22.18. Aitken II fracture of distal tibia of 11-year-old boy: a) On admission; b) Reduction and fixation by screw

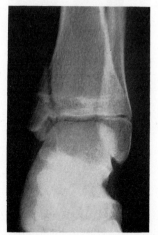 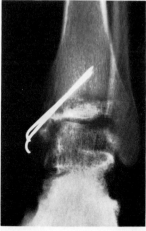

a   b

Fig. 22.19. Aitken III fracture of distal tibia of 13-year-old girl: a) On admission; b) After reduction and fixation with two Kirschner wires

child's hard spongiosa. If the epiphyseal line must be crossed, only Kirschner wires can be used (Fig. 22.19), as screws will damage the epiphyseal line and lead to premature ossification (Fig. 22.20).

The most difficult fracture is Aitken type IV, a compression fracture of the epiphyseal line. Diagnosis is not always easy, but is helped

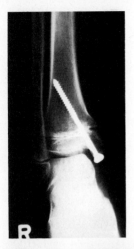

Fig. 22.20.   Aitken II fracture of distal tibia. Insufficient reduction and incorrect fixation with a screw running obliquely through the epiphyseal line which later may cause premature fusion of the epiphysis and possible arthrosis

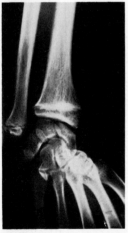

a   b

Fig. 22.21.   Aitken IV fracture of distal radius after 3 years a) Prematurely fused epiphysis with normal growth of ulna displacing the hand radially: b) Control picture of opposite side

by comparing the radiograph with that of the opposite side. Often the epiphyseal line is damaged to such a degree that severe growth disturbances result (Fig. 22.21). Long-term followup for months and years is therefore necessary. Later corrective operations may be necessary, such as a lengthening osteotomy.

Fractures of the Clavicle

Fractures of the clavicle are very common in childhood. Occasionally they are seen in the neonatal period as a result of birth trauma. The leading symptom is reluctance to move the affected arm (pseudo-paralysis). Clinical examination and radiography clinch diagnosis. Occasionally the fracture is discovered days or weeks afterwards when marked callus formation is already present. Placing the infant on his back is the only treatment necessary. Older children fracture the clavicle by falling on the outstretched hand. A "figure of eight" bandage for 3 weeks is the treatment of choice. Even with marked displacement of the fragments the fracture usually heals without complications.

Fractures in the Vicinity of the Elbow

Injuries in the vicinity of the elbow are more common in children than in adults. Correct management is vital.

Supracondylar Fracture of the Humerus

Supracondylar fracture of the humerus is the most common fracture in the vicinity of the elbow (60 % of all elbow fractures). It is a typical fracture of childhood, occurring only rarely in adults. Ninety-five per-

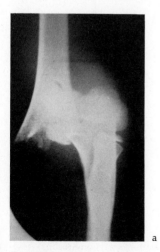
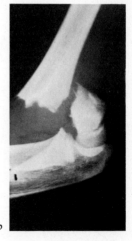

a   b

Fig. 22.22.   Supracondylar fracture of the humerus, extension type:
a) Anteroposterior view; b) Lateral view

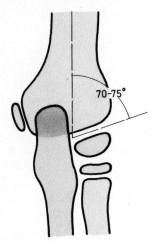

Fig. 22.23. Schematic representation of angle between epiphyseal line of the radial condyle and the longitudinal axis of the shaft of the humerus (see text)

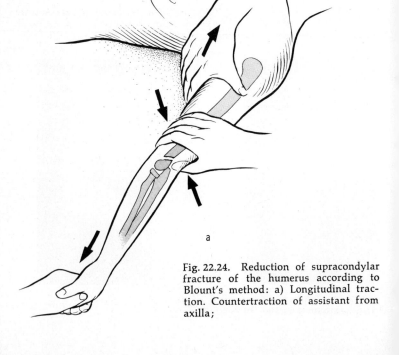

a

Fig. 22.24. Reduction of supracondylar fracture of the humerus according to Blount's method: a) Longitudinal traction. Countertraction of assistant from axilla;

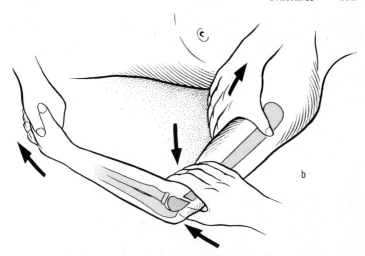

22.24 b). Correction of rotation and lateral displacement;

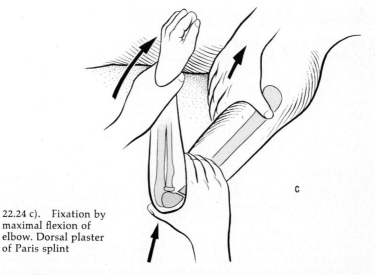

22.24 c). Fixation by maximal flexion of elbow. Dorsal plaster of Paris splint

cent of the time it is caused by a fall forward on the outstretched arm. The elbow is hyperextended and twisted (extension fracture); the distal fragment is displaced backwards, frequently with lateral rotation

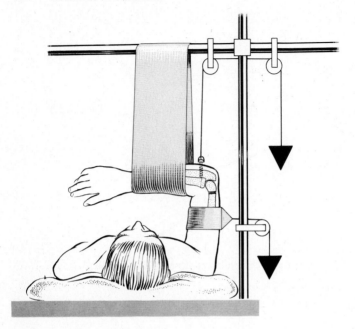

Fig. 22.25.   Supracondylar fracture of the humerus; ventral extension after the method of Baumann

and displacement (Fig. 22.22). The proximal fragment protrudes forward and may damage vessels and nerves of the antecubital fossa. Only about 5 % of supracondylar fractures occur by falling backwards on the benx elbow (flexion fracture); the distal segment is displaced forwards and nerve and vascular injuries do not occur.

Treatment

The aim of treatment is to maintain the angle between the epiphyseal line of the radial condyle and the long axis of the humerus, which normally is between 70° and 75° (Fig. 22.23). If the angle is smaller cubitus valgus results, if it is larger cubitus varus occurs. Most supracondylar fractures are treated conservatively after the method described by Blount (Fig. 22.24) or by extension (Fig. 22.25). If vascular or nerve damage exists open reduction must be performed; fixation by Kirschner wires generally suffices (Fig. 22.26). The elbow is then immobilized in a plaster of Paris backsplint for three weeks (Table 22.3). After the fracture has consolidated it may take

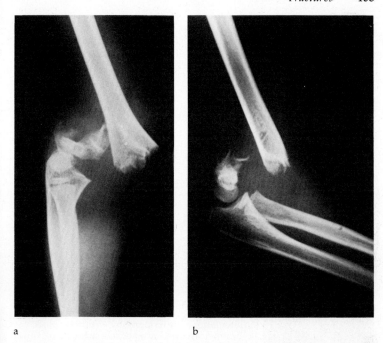

a   b

Fig. 22.26. Supracondylar fracture of the humerus, extension type: a) AP; b) lateral radiographs on admission; closed reduction produced a cold and pulseless arm;

weeks or months before full elbow joint function is restored; slight flexion and extension deficits commonly persist. Too vigorous physiotherapy (especially passive movements) should be avoided; they may tear the joint capsule, resulting in calcification and long-lasting or even permanent decrease in mobility.

Fracture of the Lateral Condyle of the Humerus

This fracture comprises about 20 % of all elbow fractures. It is caused by a fall on the outstretched arm with simultaneous medial rotation of the forearm. The fracture line runs from the lateral condyle obliquely medially and distally to the trochlea into the joint (Fig. 22.27). Traction of the extensors of the forearm usually cause rotation and dislocation of the bony fragment in a lateral and downward direction.

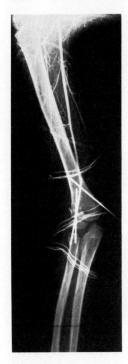

c) After open reduction and transfixion with Kirschner wires, there was no improvement in circulation; arteriography shows block in brachial artery. Thrombosed segment of vessel removed and ends reanastomosed;

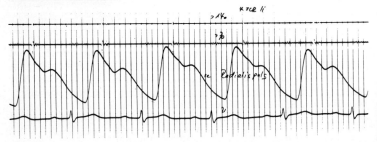

d) Pulse curve of radial artery 2 years after accident

Treatment

With associated elbow dislocation, open reduction must be carried out; the fragment is stabilized with one or two Kirschner wires (Fig. 22.27). The arm is then immobilized on a plaster of Paris back-

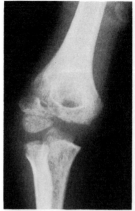 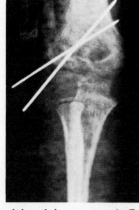

Fig. 22.27. Displaced fracture of lateral condyle of humerus: a) On admission; b) After open reduction and transfixion with two Kirschner wires

splint. The prognosis is usually good. If the epiphyseal line has been damaged an increasing cubitus valgus may subsequently develop, possibly requiring correction osteotomy. Therefore, followup examinations should be carried out for at least two years.

If a fracture of the lateral condyle has been overlooked or inadequately reduced, limitation of extension of the elbow results as well as painful pseudoarthrosis with damage to the ulnar nerve.

Fracture of the Medial Epicondyle of the Humerus

About 10 % of all elbow fractures are of this type, generally caused by forceful abduction of the extended forearm. Occasionally there is a coexisting dislocation of the elbow. In contrast to fractures of the medial condyle, the fracture line lies outside the elbow joint. With coexisting dislocation of the elbow the free bony fragment may be secondarily displaced into the joint. Radiographs usually show that the small epiphysis is torn off together with a thin, often hardly recognizable bony margin of the metaphysis, with lateral and downward displacement (Fig. 22.28).

Dislocations of more than 2 mm (in the anteroposterior radiograph) call for open reduction and fixation with a Kirschner wire. At the beginnning of the operation the ulnar nerve is exposed to prevent injury to the nerve. Following operation the elbow is immobilized in plaster for three weeks. If reduction is good, the prognosis is good;

Fracture of the Olecranon

This is rather rare, comprising only 1 % to 2 % of all elbow fractures of children. If there is no displacement treatment should be conservative, immobilizing the elbow in extension on a plaster backsplint for three to four weeks. With displacement, open reduction has to be performed. Suture with wires kept under tension as advised by Weber gives the best results; no postoperative immobilization is necessary (Fig. 22.30).

Monteggia Fracture

The so-called Monteggia fracture is a combination injury of the forearm; there is a transverse fracture of the ulna, usually at the junction of the proximal and the middle thirds of the shaft, plus dislocation of the head of the radius (Fig. 22.31). The Monteggia fracture is also a typical fracture of children. It is generally caused by a fall, the ulna hitting a hard corner; occasionally it results from a defense reaction against somebody trying to hit the patient. Monteggia fractures are usually treated by operation (Fig. 22.31). The annular ligament must be reconstructed.

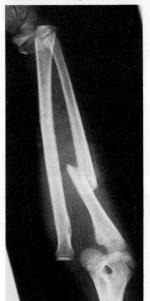 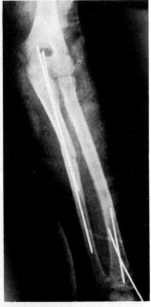

a   b

Fig. 22.31.   Classical Monteggia fracture, also Aitken I fracture of distal end of radius: a) On admission; b) Fixation with two Kirschner wires

Nursemaid's Elbow

This is a typical minor injury of childhood, with subluxation of the head of the radius beneath the annular ligament. It usually affects children under six years of age. At this age the head of the radius is not larger in diameter than the shaft, and subluxates beneath the annular ligament.

The injury typically occurs from a sudden longitudinal pull on the arm, as when someone pulls the child's hand to prevent him from tripping. The child complains immediately of severe elbow pain; the arm hangs limply down, the elbow is extended, the forearm pronated. Examination reveals tenderness over the head of the radius. The positioning of the arm and the accident are so typical that a radiograph need not be taken.

Treatment

This is very simple. Quick supination and simultaneous flexion of the elbow will reduce the subluxation. One often hears a click when the head of the radius slips into the correct position. A few minutes later the child moves the arm again perfectly normally.

Fractures of the Forearm

Most fractures of the forearm are treated conservatively (closed reduction) under anesthesia; the forearm is immobilized in a plaster of Paris backsplint for three weeks. In children greenstick fractures of radius and ulna are very typical and frequent. Here the bone is bent; the cortex is broken but the two fragments are held together by the periostium which is especially thick in children and prevents any lateral displacement (Fig. 22.32). These fractures are easy to reduce and usually heal without trouble.

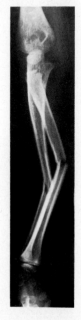

Fig. 22.32. Greenstick fracture of radius and ulna of 6-year-old boy

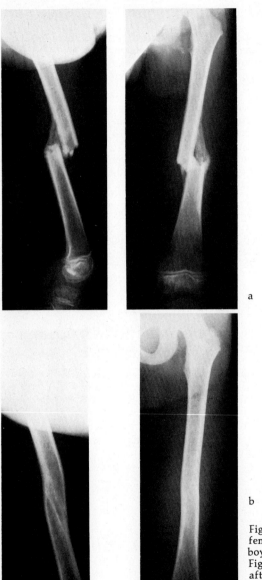

a

b

Fig. 22.33. Fracture of femur of 8-year-old boy. (Same patient as in Fig. 22.13). a) Healed after 6 week of traction; b) 4 years later; leg length equal

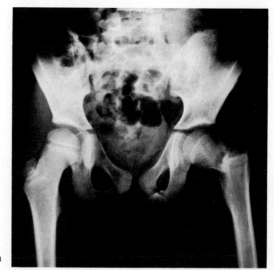

a

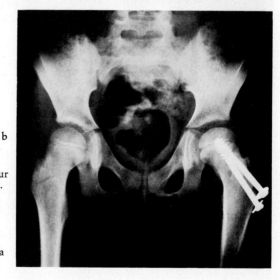

b

Fig. 22.34.
Lateral fracture of
the neck of the femur
of 11-year-old boy.
There is also a
fracture of the left
pubic bone:
a) On admission;
b) After fixation
with two spongiosa
screws

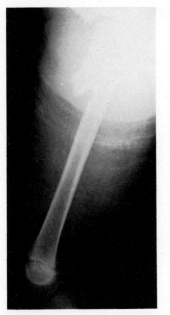 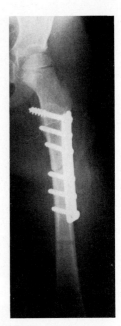

a   b

Fig. 22.35. Subtrochanteric fracture of femur of 5-year-old boy: a) Un-satisfactory position after traction; the proximal fragment is rotated forwards; b) After operative fixation with tension wiring according to the AO technique

Fractures of the Femur

All patients with fractures of the femur must be admitted to hospital. Most femoral fractures can be treated conservatively (closed), preferably by extension. An extension method should be applied allowing exact control of rotation. According to the age of the patient, these fractures heal within four to eight weeks. Transverse fractures need a little more time to heal than do oblique or longitudinal ones. Followup is extended to at least four years (Fig. 22.33).

Exceptions to the conservative management of femoral fractures are the relatively rare fractures of the neck of the femur (Fig. 22.34) and occasionally subtrochanteric fractures or supracondylar fractures. Subtrochanteric fractures require operative reduction when rotation displacements occur in spite of extension; fixation is achieved by a traction plate and screws according to the Swiss AO method (Fig. 22.35). After operation for femoral neck fracture the child must

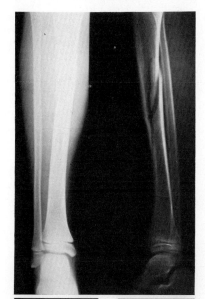

Fig. 22.36. Greenstick fracture in an 8-year-old boy:
a) On admission;

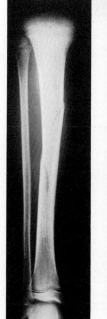

b) After 6 weeks; little callus has formed but the fracture is clinically firm

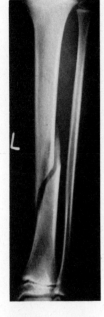

Fig. 22.37.   Torsion fracture of tibia with typical minimal varus displacement

wear an apparatus which prevents weight-bearing for weeks or months, such as a Thomas' calliper, to obviate aseptic necrosis of the femoral head.

Fractures of the Leg

These children are usually treated as outpatients with closed reduction under anesthesia and immobilization in a plaster of Paris cast extending to the thigh. Greenstick fractures (Fig. 22.36) may be treated by immobilization in plaster without anesthesia and without reduction. Immobilization should last for four to six weeks. Fractures of the tibia and fibula with marked displacement must be reduced under anesthesia. Followup is carried out in the outpatient department, radiographs being taken every two weeks to detect secondary displacements. A varus position up to 8 ° can be accepted since it usually is corrected by the increased growth. In small children one often finds slight varus displacement of the tibia, the fibula being intact (Fig. 22.37). Maximal recurvation of 5 ° to 6 ° is acceptable since it will correct itself spontaneously (Fig. 22.38). However, a valgus position must be avoided, since it does not spontaneously

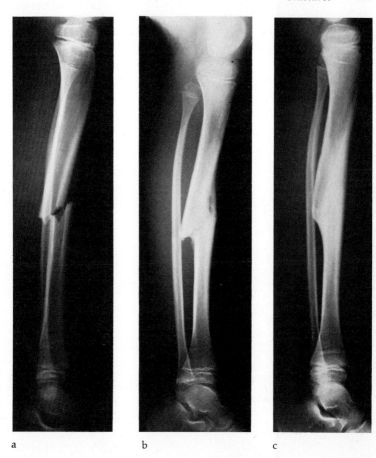

a   b   c

Fig. 22.38.   Transverse fracture of tibia with slight posterior angulation:
a) On admission; b) After 7 weeks; c) After 2 years

correct later on. More than 1 cm shortening, severe soft tissue injuries or displacement demand treatment by traction in hospital
(Fig. 22.39), but this is necessary in only one out of ten children.
On the average, traction is carried out for three weeks, after which
a plaster of Paris cast is applied for a further three weeks. Followup must approximate two years in order to judge final results.

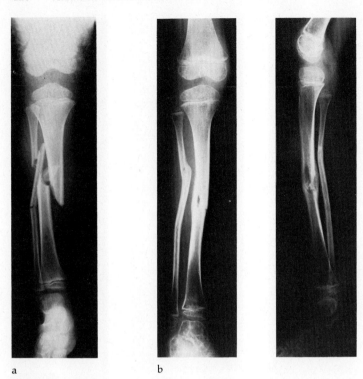

a   b

Fig. 22.39. Fracture of tibia and fibula with marked shortening treated with traction: a) On admission; b) 8 weeks later with 5 mm shortening;

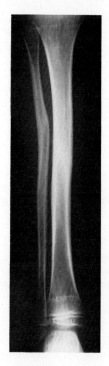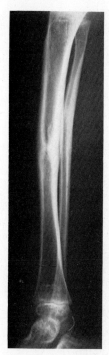

Fig. 22.39 c). 2 years later; both legs are same length

The Battered Child Syndrome

U. G. STAUFFER

This is a syndrome which is observed more and more frequently. It occurs in all social classes, but becomes more difficult to hide in the so-called lower income groups. The injuries are usually produced by the father, mother or both parents together. The parents are often young, immature and labile. On the one hand they are aggressive and impulsive, on the other they tend to be depressive and suffer from inferiority complexes. Psychoses are rare (under 5 %). Frequently the parents have had a hard, loveless childhood and they may have been maltreated by their parents. Because of their own childhood they are usually not able to establish a satisfactory parent-child relationship. Family tensions and at times financial worries are frequently found. Alcoholism often plays a part in the maltreatment of the child. Occasionally the condition is caused by overwork of the mother who has many children and is expecting another.

The battered child syndrome is frequently a distress sign of the whole family which cannot solve the problems which confront its various members. The factor which precipitates the maltreatment is usually trivial. Frequently the leading motive is a guilt complex of the parents who are frightened that the children do not respect them or love them sufficiently.

Clinical Picture

The children are frequently brought to the doctor by the parents themselves, although there is usually some delay. There is a vague and often contradictory history of an accident, or the possibility of trauma is denied by the parents. The objective findings and the history are contradictory and a suspicion of maltreatment will arise, which is hotly denied by the parents.

The battered child syndrome is most frequently found between the ages of 6 and 18 months; nearly all the children are under four years of age. Frequently one finds signs of neglect, malnutrition and backwardness apart from the signs of actual maltreatment. The children appear frightened, even apathic, but may be resentful or aggressive. They are often thirsting for some sign of love.

On examination characteristic lesions such as hematomas of the scalp, face or neck, small abrasions, wounds or scars on the trunk, and occasionally burns of the extremities are observed. In infants a subdural hematoma must always be looked for. Traumatic marks on the head, an increased skull circumference, gaping skull sutures, a tense fontanelle and retinal hemorrhages will confirm the diagnosis of subdural hematoma which occurs in 30 % of all battered children. Subdural hematomas are the cause of death in 70 % of the fatal cases. Severe visceral injuries are rare but because the diagnosis is usually delayed, 50 % of these injuries are fatal. Rupture of the stomach, duodenum, colon, spleen and liver, pancreatic injuries and even lacerations of lungs and heart have been described.

Laboratory Findings

If the child's general condition permits, all visible lesions have to be photographed for legal reasons. Tests for coagulation deficiency will exclude conditions which occasionally may simulate the battered child syndrome. Radiographs of all bones have to be taken. One may observe fractures in various stages of healing, separated epiphyses, etc. Subperiosteal hemorrhages are very typical, often surrounding the diaphysis. The bones tell a story which the child is too young or too frightened to tell.

Differential Diagnosis

It is often difficult for a doctor to believe the child could be maltreated and even rare differential diagnoses such as scurvy, vitamin D deficiency, etc. may be considered. The typical case is, however, easy to diagnose. Only children with the rare condition of congenital analgesia may present similar skin and bone lesions, but the clinical examination will exclude this condition.

Treatment

Severe cases such as subdural hematoma, visceral injuries, etc. must be treated as emergencies. Even children with relatively slight injuries should be admitted to hospital because only thus is one able to protect the child against further, more severe injuries. The doctor must not antagonize the parents or act as judge. Even in severe cases an attempt should be made to maintain a doctor-parent relationship. A carefully conducted talk may reveal the family problems. These parents are best managed by a specially trained team of doctors, social workers, etc. Individual care of the parents and close supervision after discharge from hospital are the best preventive treatment. If this is not done, 35 % to 80 % of the children are again maltreated. Between 5 % and 25 % of all battered children sustain permanent injuries, mainly secondary to brain damage. Psychological disturbances such as anxiety states, restlessness, insomnia, inferiority complexes, etc. are much more frequently observed. These children once grown up are likely again to maltreat their children. It is a vicious circle which can only be broken by a determined attack by the doctor and his helpers.

23 Benign and Malignant Bone Tumors

U. G. Stauffer

Bone tumors are more common in children than in adults; 80 % are benign and 20 % malignant. In large series, malignant bone tumors produce about 5 % of all cancer deaths in childhood.

Early recognition of benign bone tumors in childhood often saves the parents much worry and obviates unnecessarily major or ablative surgical procedures. In children with malignant bone tumors, early recognition may be life-saving. Unfortunately, diagnosis is often delayed for weeks and months because of the misapprehension that the child is suffering from "growing pains".

Only the more important bone tumors are discussed here.

Benign Bone Tumors

Four main types of benign bone tumors occur in childhood: osteochondromas or cartilaginous exostoses, juvenile bone cysts, the unossifying fibroma and the osteoid osteoma. Other benign tumors such as aneurysmal bone cysts and enchondromas are very rare.

The Osteochondroma (Exostosis)

Osteochondromas are the most common type of childhood bone tumors. Boys are more frequently affected than girls. These tumors frequently occur in families and are inherited as an autosomal dominant gene. Many sporadic cases are, however, observed. Osteochondromas occur either singly (Fig. 23.1) or multiple (Fig. 23.2). Multiple tumors may cause growth disturbances as well as severe deformities of the skeleton. Single tumors are mainly situated in the metaphysis of the long bones around the knee and the proximal metaphysis of the humerus. They assume variable shapes, from thin, bony spurs with a small base tilted towards the diaphysis or short, broad-based, knobby tumors (Fig. 23.2). Osteochondromas are composed of a loose spongiosum surrounded by a thin cortical layer of bone which in turn is covered by a layer of cartilage. The cartilagenous layer ossifies after cessation of growth. Radiographs show that the spongiosa of the metaphysis continues directly with the spongiosa of the exostosis (Fig. 23.1). Growth in the exostosis occurs as long as the parent bone grows, the exostosis slowly being displaced towards the diaphysis. Occasionally, the exostosis hinders the growth of the bone from which it arises, and multiple exostoses may cause distortion of the bone as well as diminution of growth.

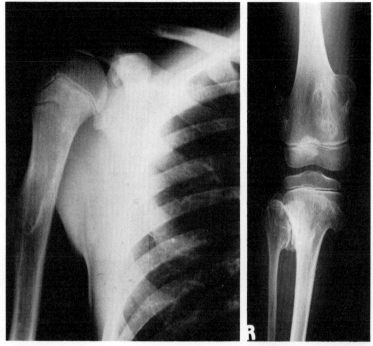

Fig. 23.1.   Fig. 23.2.

Fig. 23.1.   13-year-old boy. Solitary cartilagenous exostosis arising from the proximal metaphysis of the humerus

Fig. 23.2.   9-year-old boy. Multiple familial exostoses round the knee joint

Exostoses give rise to few complaints since they grow so slowly, and are usually discovered incidentally. Occasionally, pressure on tendons, muscles or nerves may cause discomfort which leads to their discovery.

Treatment

If an exostosis causes functional disturbances or symptoms, it should be removed early. Otherwise, operation is postponed if possible until the age of puberty, as experience has shown that exostoses frequently recur if removed before that age. After growth has ceased even asymptomatic solitary exostoses should be removed since 1 % become malignant later on. In patients with multiple exostoses one should only remove those which are symptomatic as malignant degeneration rarely occurs.

The Solitary Juvenile Bone Cyst

This is a typical disease of the skeleton in childhood. The etiology is not clearly understood. Bone cysts are mainly located in the proximal metaphysis of the long bones, especially the humerus, femur and tibia. Radiographs show a sharply-delineated round area of radiolucency with a thin cortical layer (Fig. 23.3). No periosteal reaction is seen, and the cyst does not traverse the epiphyseal line. As the cyst grows it slowly travels toward the diaphysis. It usually contains clear, slightly yellow fluid and is lined with a thin, velvety membrane of reticular connective tissue.

Bone cysts hardly ever cause complaints spontaneously. The majority are discovered only when a pathological fracture develops (Fig. 23.3). Occasionally they are incidentally seen on a radiograph taken for other purposes.

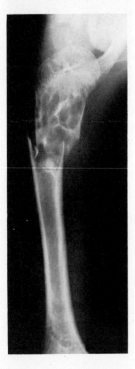

Fig. 23.3.   7-year-old boy. Solitary juvenile bone cyst in the proximal metaphysis of the humerus. Pathological fracture

Treatment

If a spontaneous fracture occurs, one can usually wait for normal healing to occur. Rarely, healing of the fracture may promote healing of the cyst, but usually the cyst must be dealt with surgically later on. At operation the lining membrane is carefully removed and the cavity is filled with bone chips usually taken from the iliac crest.

If a bone cyst is discovered incidentally, one should operate immediately only if there seems to be imminent danger of spontaneous fracture. In most cases it is better to wait until a small zone of normal bone develops between the margin of the cyst and the epiphyseal line, as operation on the cyst may otherwise interfere with bone growth. In children under 10 years of age, the cyst occasionally recurs after operation.

The Non-Ossifying Fibroma of Bone

Bone fibromas are relatively common, being mainly situated in the area of the distal metaphysis of the femur and in the proximal and distal metaphysis of the tibia. They hardly ever cause complaints and are usually discovered only incidentally. Only rarely does an especially large fibroma lead to a spontaneous fracture.

Radiological findings are quite typical (Fig. 23.4). The fibroma is always located near the periphery of the bone as a single or multiple grape-like circular area of radiolucency. They vary in size; the overlying cortical bone is always intact; only rarely is it somewhat thinned. Fibromas differ from bone cysts in that they do not protrude over the normal bone contour. There is no periosteal reaction and the fibroma is usually separated from the spongiosa by a thin sclerotic margin. Histologically one finds cellular fibrous tissue arranged in strands and whorls.

The fibroma is frequently small and limited to the cortical bone (so-called fibrous defect of the bony cortex) (Fig. 23.5). These small defects are found in upwards of 40 % of children, and disappear during later growth of the patient. They never become malignant.

Treatment

The smaller fibromas, especially those situated in the bony cortex, cause no disability and no treatment is necessary. Large defects should be curetted and the resulting cavity filled by cancellous bone chips. Recurrence is very rare.

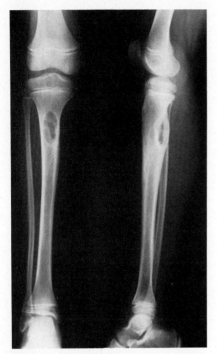 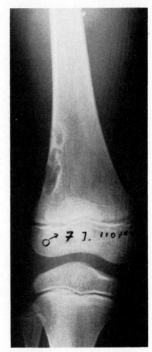

Fig. 23.4.   Fig. 23.5.

Fig. 23.4.   8-year-old girl. Large, non-ossifying fibroma in the proximal metaphysis of the tibia, producing slight pain in the knee. Slight secondary reaction of the periosteum following minimal trauma. Condition cured by curettage and filling the resulting cavity with bone chips

Fig. 23.5.   7-year-old boy. Fibrous defect of the cortex. Accidental finding. No treatment necessary

Osteoid Osteoma

This is a rather rare tumor; boys are more often affected than girls. The tumor may occur anywhere in the skeleton except the skull, but is most common in the femur and tibia. It rarely becomes larger than 1 cm in diameter. The radiographic findings are characteristic: a central radiolucent area in the afflicted bone with a sclerosed layer of bone around it. The bony cortex shows a fusiform thickness (Fig. 23.6).

Clinically, patients characteristically complain of persistent, localized pain which occurs mainly at night; there is tenderness and thickening

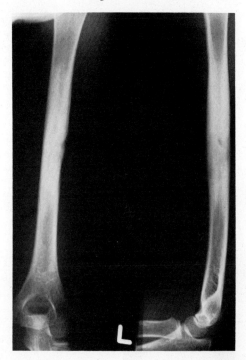

Fig. 23.6.
8-year-old boy. Osteoid osteoma in the shaft of the humerus. There is a central lucent area with sclerosing bone around it and a thickening of the cortex

of the bone on palpation. It is possible to mistake an osteoid osteoma for a localized chronic osteomyelitis (Brodie's abscess). Histologically, the tumor consists of osteoid tissue; there are no signs of infection. It should be curretted.

Malignant Bone Tumors

The most important malignant bone tumors of childhood are the osteogenic sarcoma, Ewing's tumor and reticulum cell sarcoma. These tumors occur relatively more commonly in childhood than in adults. Fibrosarcomas and chondrosarcomas, on the other hand, usually occur in patients beyond 20 years of age and will therefore not be discussed here. Although there are histological differences between Ewing's tumor and reticulum cell sarcoma, these two tumors are clinically so similar that they will be discussed together. Osteogenic sarcoma and Ewing's tumor number among the most malignant growths in childhood. Even by using all modern treatment methods (surgery, radiotherapy and chemotherapy) only about 20 % of victims will be cured. The doctor therefore has a grave responsibility in dealing with the parents, the frequently bad outcome triggering great problems in the doctor-parent relationship. It is of prime importance that the parents trust the doctor, as otherwise the parents in their despair may consult quacks who only increase their child's misery. Treatment must be continued even in hopeless cases.

Osteogenic Sarcoma

This tumor occurs most frequently near puberty when maximal osteogenic activity (growth) occurs; during this period of life these tumors arise from osteoblasts in the medullary cavity, haversian canals and beneath the periosteum, and grow rapidly to considerable size (Fig. 23.7). Histologically, they are composed of very polymorphous tissue including spindle cells and giant cells with islands of hyaline tissue, cartilage and bone.

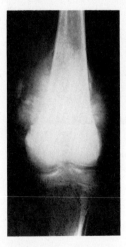

Fig. 23.7. 13-year-old boy. Large, rapidly growing tumor of the distal femur. Mainly osteoplastic, osteogenic sarcoma shows typical spicules of new bone formation

More than two-thirds of osteogenic sarcomas arise round the knee, in the distal femoral or the proximal tibial metaphysis. The proximal metaphysis of the humerus is the next most common site. The main clinical symptoms of osteogenic sarcoma are localized pain and a rapidly growing, tender and warm swelling. Radiographs typically show a soft tissue swelling and extensive osteolytic foci (Fig. 23.8) with marked new formation of bone under the elevated periosteum (Fig. 23.7). The bony spicules run perpendicular to the shaft of the bone, but are by no means always present (Fig. 23.8). The tumor metastasizes early to the lungs.

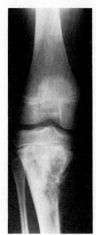 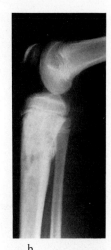

Fig. 23.8.
11-year-old girl. Mainly osteoplastic, osteogenic sarcoma of the proximal metaphysis of the tibia. The bony structure is blurred and the cortex eroded. There is only little new formation of bone arising from the periosteum

a   b

Treatment and Prognosis

The best type of treatment is still debated. We recommend open surgical biopsy when the patient is receiving chemotherapeutic drugs. When the diagnosis is certain, early amputation is carried out. Following this, patients are treated with cytostatic drugs (at present adriamycin) for at least one year. Radiotherapy appears to be of little value. Solitary lung metastases can be removed surgically later under cytostatic cover.

In large series the cure rate of osteogenic sarcoma is only 10 % to 15 %. Most patients die of pulmonary metastases during the first two years after diagnosis. This bad prognosis justifies the radical treatment. If the parents are wisely counseled they will accept an amputation, which is usually tolerated well. The patient is able to walk two days after amputation on a primary prosthesis, and usually leaves the hospital within three to four weeks.

Ewing's Tumor

Ewing's tumor (reticulum cell sarcoma) is the most common malignant bone tumor in children under 10 years of age. It has occurred as early as during the first two years of life. About one-half of these tumors are situated in the large bones (femur, tibia, humerus, etc.), the remainder arise in the flat bones (scapula, the skull bones) and vertebrae. Ewing's sarcoma does not arise from the bone proper, but

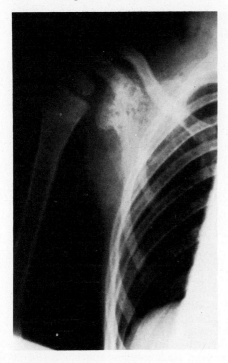

Fig. 23.9.
3-year-old boy. Ewing's sarcoma of the left scapula. Blurring of the bony cortex and multiple areas of radiolucency

from the bone marrow. Histologically, it consists of closely packed small round cells which may be arranged in rosettes like a neuroblastoma. Radiographs often reveal that the entire diaphysis is affected; the spongiosa contains areas of radiolucency and the cortex is blurred (Fig. 23.9). Early subperiosteal new bone formation is common which in typical cases form an onion-skin-like appearance. The bone is fusiformly enlarged. The radiographs are not always typical.

The main clinical features of Ewing's tumor are intermittent pain in an extremity which bears a hard, warm swelling in a child with an elevated temperature. Early Ewing's tumor is easily mistaken for subacute or chronic osteomyelitis.

Treatment

The diagnosis is confirmed by open biopsy carried out while the child is receiving chemotherapy. Once the diagnosis is confirmed the tumor should be irradiated (3000 to 6000 r), following which the child is given cytostatic drugs for at least a year (mainly cyclo-phosphamide and vincristine). The mass characteristically melts away with radiotherapy. However, the ultimate prognosis of Ewing's tumor is unfavorable, early metastases occurring to other parts of the skeleton or the lungs. Solitary pulmonary metastases can be excised. Although the prognosis of Ewing's tumor is today somewhat better than for osteogenic sarcoma, permanent cures occur only in about 20 % to 25 % of cases.

References

Readers who wish to obtain more detailed information on any specific point are referred to the following books:

Gans, S. L.: Surgical Pediatrics. Grune & Stratton Inc., New York 1973

Johnston, J. H., R. J. Scholtmeijer: Problems in Paediatric Urology. Excerpta Medica Foundation, Amsterdam 1972

Matson, D. D.: Neurosurgery of Infancy and Childhood. Thomas, Springfield, Ill. 1969

Mustardé, J. C.: Plastic Surgery in Infancy and Childhood. Livingstone, Edinburgh 1971

Mustard, W. T., M. M. Ravitch, W. H. Snyder, K. J. Welch, C. D. Benson: Pediatric Surgery. Year Book Medical Publishers Inc., Chicago 1969

Rickham, P. P., Johnston, J. H.: Neonatal Surgery. Butterworth, London, 1969

Sharrard, W. J. W.: Paediatric Orthopaedics and Fractures. Blackwell, Oxford 1971

Subject Index